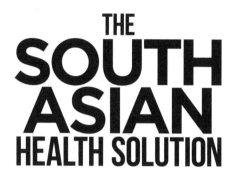

THE
SOUTH
ASIAN
HEALTH SOLUTION

RONESH SINHA, MD

Library of Congress Control Number: 2013915701
Library of Congress Cataloging-in-Publication Data is on file with the publisher
Sinha, Ronesh 1971-
The South Asian Health Solution/Ronesh Sinha

ISBN: 978-1-939563-05-7
1. Health 2. Weight Loss 3. Diet 4. Physical Fitness

Editor: Amy Lucas
Design and Layout: Caroline De Vita
Illustrations: Caroline De Vita
Cover Design: Janée Meadows
Index: Sara Beatty
Consultants: Shally Sinha, MD; Mark Sisson

Publisher: Primal Blueprint Publishing.
23805 Stuart Ranch Rd. Suite 145 Malibu, CA 90265
For information on quantity discounts, please call 888-774-6259,
email: info@primalblueprint.com, or visit PrimalBlueprintPublishing.com.

For my late father, Dr. Ramananda Sinha,
a physician who inspired me to write, teach,
and question everything.

TABLE OF CONTENTS

ACKNOWLEDGMENTS

To my wife Shally, who has officially joined the circle of author's neglected spouses. Thank you for supporting me, believing in me, and acting as a single parent so often during this process. (And thank you for helping me write the children's chapter!) Thank you to my sons Rohan and Avi, who teach me to connect with my inner child every single day. To my mom, for her unconditional love and ingenuity with the recipes. To my brother Robin, who kept checking in on me no matter how much I drowned myself in this book and my work.

Special thanks to my publisher Mark Sisson who allowed me to take a decade long dream and turn it into a book that exceeded my expectations. You are living proof that you don't need an MD to save lives and help people achieve optimal health. Huge thanks to Brad Kearns from the Primal Blueprint Publishing team. You are an unbelievable coach who kept me motivated, kept me laughing, and always found a way to extract great content out of me. Thanks to my editor, Amy Lucas, for patiently helping me uncover my inner author, amidst a pile of complex scientific jargon. Thank you Caroline De Vita for designing a beautiful interior layout for the book that reflects the richness of South Asian culture. To the very talented Janée Meadows for crafting a brilliant book cover.

A special thanks to Janet Lederer, VP of Health Education from the Palo Alto Medical Foundation (PAMF), who has been an inspiration and huge supporter of all of my South Asian and culturally tailored health initiatives. I want to thank all of the wonderful people from PAMF's marketing department (Sarah Chan, Erin Macartney, Sapna Parekh, Cynthia Greaves, and Ed Bierman to name a few), who help me take my message to the diverse communities and workforces in Northern California and beyond.

And finally, I want to thank all the dedicated HR team members—from companies across Silicon Valley—who have allowed me to deliver culturally tailored health education programs to such diverse workforces. Your employees inspired so much of the material in this book, and I am committed to helping them find innovative solutions to lead healthier lives.

CHAPTER 1

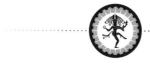

INFLAMMATION AND INSULIN: THE REAL CULPRITS

WHY ARE SOUTH ASIANS AT SUCH a high risk for diabetes and heart disease? This is the most common question I face in my clinic, during lectures…even at cocktail parties where I'm often surrounded by South Asians puzzled by this epidemic. Regardless of my response, many South Asians are convinced they know the answer. Do any of the following sound familiar?

- "My husband puts too much ghee on his rice, or too much sugar and cream in his tea."

- "My wife can't stop worrying about everything so I'm sure stress is the reason her blood sugar is so high."

- "I can't find the time to exercise, but I'm sure once I do, I'll lose the weight and improve my heart health."

Each of these reasons carries a certain degree of truth (except the ghee—keep reading and you'll find out how ghee can actually be good for health), but pay close attention to the verifiable and scientifically validated answer:

Excess insulin, resulting from a condition called insulin resistance, is by far the most common cause for pandemic heart disease and its associated risks in South Asians.

Excess insulin is the underlying thread that weaves together virtually every chronic ailment currently afflicting South Asians. There is no controversy here. Talk to any primary care doctor or specialist who has stayed on top of the research and they will agree that insulin disorders are the root cause of the health crisis plaguing South Asians.

Instead of debating whether to eat a low-carb vs. low-fat meal, or vegetarian vs. non-vegetarian diet, your goal is to implement a low-insulin lifestyle—and this book arms you with all the tools you need to make this radical shift in your health.

Along with insulin resistance, chronic inflammation has emerged as a powerful threat to health and longevity. Chronic inflammation occurs when an overactive and defective immune system does more harm than good. Aberrant and untethered inflammation—a direct consequence of poor lifestyle decisions coupled with potentially high-risk genes—is the root cause of almost every imaginable chronic disease… from heart attacks and strokes to Alzheimer's disease. Inflammation is also responsible for accelerated aging, a phenomenon I frequently observe in South Asians and which we'll discuss in detail in Chapter 11.

WHEN INSULIN AND INFLAMMATION STRIKE

You can fortify and protect your heart's health by shifting your focus to controlling insulin and inflammation, which, when properly regulated, will help to prevent most life-threatening and disabling conditions that reduce longevity and impair quality of life. Let's start off with the story of a former patient of mine to see just how insulin and inflammation led to his tragic death.

Case Study: Ravi

Ravi, a 41-year-old accountant and father of two sons, came to me after sustaining his first heart attack at age 39. He had a significant family history of early heart disease. (His father passed away at 47 from a fatal heart attack.)

Prior to his first heart attack, Ravi was a non-smoking vegetarian with a body mass index of 25, abdominal obesity, and gout (a painful arthritis condition usually localized to pain in the big toe). After his first heart attack, surgeons inserted stents to open up his clogged arteries. He underwent an intense post-heart attack cardiac rehabilitation program and lost 15 pounds. He was put on the standard post-heart attack regimen of cholesterol-lowering medications and blood thinners.

He saw me for a South Asian consultation two years later, accompanied by his wife.

When I asked Ravi about stress, he told me he was dealing with the usual stress of work and raising young, active boys, but felt he had his overall stress levels under control. His wife disagreed and vented that Ravi was back to being a workaholic. He kept up with visits to the gym three to four times a week and stuck to his prescribed low-fat diet, but unfortunately he had regained 10 pounds. His arms and legs looked fairly muscular, but he had the typical protuberant South Asian belly.

One of the main components I recall from that consultation was the sense of tension in the exam room between Ravi and his wife. It was obvious that even though Ravi was trying to portray a relaxed attitude, he was, like so many of my other South Asian clients (especially men), internalizing a great deal of stress. The other notable factor was that he was consuming a tremendous amount of carbohydrates in his diet, albeit in the form of whole grains. His lab work showed normal blood pressure, medication-lowered LDL (bad) cholesterol levels at 60 mg/dL, elevated triglycerides at 185 mg/dL, and low HDL (healthy cholesterol) at 32 mg/dL. His blood sugar was in the prediabetes range. The only other abnormal lab was an elevated hs-CRP (highly sensitive C-reactive protein), a marker for inflammation.

Together we outlined a detailed lifestyle plan that included a complete overhaul of his diet with a focus on reduced carbohydrates. We also incorporated yoga and mindfulness practices to help manage his stress. One month later I received a message from Ravi's wife that he had died from a massive heart attack on a Sunday morning. He leaves behind his wife, and six- and four-year old sons.

I promise not all my case summaries end so dismally, but I'm haunted by stories such as Ravi's all too often. Fortunately, most are lucky enough to get a second chance, but others leave behind devastated families that struggle to move forward, constantly reflecting on what might have been done differently to prevent such a tragedy. Ravi made the right changes, but these changes came too late. Let's discuss Ravi's case by illustrating how insulin and inflammation caused his untimely demise. I have simplified these complex processes as much as possible to help you understand how to make the right lifestyle changes and prevent a tragedy like Ravi's.

Inflammation: A Case of a Sprained Artery

Inflammation is your body's protective response to injury. Let's say you are playing a game of badminton and are running to make a forehand return. Unfortunately, your foot slips and your ankle turns inward, causing you to fall to the ground. Your body instantly senses the injury and activates the inflammation process. Blood vessels open up around the injured ligaments to allow an army of different cells, such as white blood cells, red blood cells, and platelets, to flood the injured ankle and start making repairs. During this healing response you notice the hallmark symptoms of inflammation: swelling (from fluid accumulation), redness and heat (from a rush of blood into the area), and pain (from the chemical irritation of your nerves). The swelling actually keeps the ankle stable, much like an internal ankle brace, and the pain prevents you from moving your ankle in directions that would worsen the injury. As you can see, the inflammatory process safeguards the ankle and helps with the repair process.

What's the connection between a sprained ankle and Ravi's fatal heart attack? A sprained, or injured, artery activates the inflammatory response in a similar manner. Arteries are the blood vessels that carry blood from your heart to your vital organs, muscles, tendons, ligaments, and joints, thereby nourishing every part of your body with oxygen and nutrients. Arteries that extend from the heart are large, but as they travel farther from the heart and closer to their destination (body part, vital organ, etc.), they gradually taper into a mesh of tiny arteries called capillaries. Capillaries wrap around their target, be it a sprained ankle or an injured artery, delivering oxygen-rich blood, nutrients, and immune system cells that activate healing.

Think of these tiny arteries as narrow straws. If you were to suck mango juice through one of these straws (or arteries), the juice would come into contact with the inner surface of the straw, or the blood vessel layer known as the ECL (endothelial cell layer). The difference between a healthy ECL and a damaged one can mean the difference between life and death, or optimal health and chronic disease. A healthy ECL is a relatively tight barrier, just like your straw, that prevents juice from leaking.

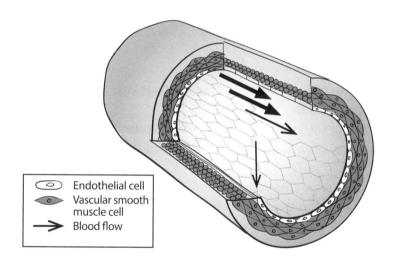

Endothelial cell
Vascular smooth muscle cell
Blood flow

Aside from acting as a barrier, the ECL keeps tabs on every aspect of your health because it is constantly in contact with your blood. Are you sneaking in bites of Indian sweets hidden in the back of the fridge thinking no one will find out? Your ECL knows your secret because it immediately senses the increase in blood sugar! If you are embroiled in an ongoing conflict with a family member or friend, your ECL feels the rush of cortisol and other stress hormones coursing through your blood. Your ECL knows your deepest, darkest secrets, and when it becomes injured or feels threatened it reacts by signaling the inflammation alarm, just as your body would if you were to sprain your ankle. All those white blood cells, platelets, and numerous inflammatory substances immediately arrive at the ECL to assess and repair any damage to the artery. Before we move on, let's summarize:

> Your ECL is in constant contact with your blood and can detect even the subtlest chemical disturbances arising from poor nutrition or negative emotions; it responds to any damage or perceived threats by sounding the inflammation alarm.

In a healthy body, the inflammation crew is remarkably effective at making repairs and keeping the ECL in great condition. However, in an unhealthy body, this emergency response system, which is called upon far too often and in desperate need of some time off, often does more damage than good.

Ravi's Death: A Case of Immune System Corruption and Overactivation

In order to better understand how Ravi's immune system backfired, let's discuss two other key characters involved in inflammation:

Macrophages: Your immune system commands these mini-vacuum cleaner cells to suck up dust and debris from the ECL. Macrophages are key players in triggering atherosclerosis, the process that forms artery-clogging plaques.

Platelets: These sticky cells in your blood repair damage to the ECL and prevent bleeding. However, they can also escort macrophages across the damaged ECL where these cleaner cells start building and destabilizing dangerous plaque.

Ravi's ECL clearly sensed multiple threats. Tremendous emotional stress and elevated blood sugar from excess carbohydrates in his diet were most likely factors. Other threats to the ECL include excess free radicals from a diet full of processed foods and lacking in healthy antioxidant sources such as fresh vegetables and fruit. Conditions such as high blood pressure, which we'll discuss in Chapter 3, can also injure the blood vessel wall.

Inflammatory cells arrive with honest intentions to heal and repair but often become corrupted by various factors. Macrophages that come to vacuum up the dust may detect some tasty oxidized LDL cholesterol under the ECL surface. They then penetrate the ECL, gobbling up the LDL cholesterol, which is subsequently transformed into foam cells. These foam cells not only lay the foundation for plaque, but also release chemicals called cytokines, which recruit even more white blood cells into the area, thereby increasing inflammatory damage.

Let's break down the three major steps contributing to Ravi's heart attack:

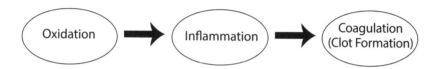

1. **Oxidation:** Oxidation occurs when substances called free radicals damage your body's cells. Free radicals are the harmful byproducts of an unhealthy lifestyle. Free radicals steal electrons (negatively charged particles) from healthy cells. When a cell loses an electron, it becomes unstable, degenerates, and eventually dies. Free radicals are the culprits behind an endless number of maladies from heart disease and cancer, to Alzheimer's disease and accelerated aging. Free radical oxidation damages your sensitive ECL, and in doing so, triggers inflammation.

    South Asians lead a highly oxidative lifestyle with a severe lack of protective natural antioxidants. One or two servings of overcooked vegetable curry dishes hardly provide sufficient antioxidant protection against the gross amount of free radicals most South Asians consume. Ravi most likely suffered from oxidation fueled by a diet low in antioxidants and high in free radical generating foods such as crispy snacks full of excess carbs. Coupled with high stress levels, oxidation was a persistent process in Ravi's life.

2. **Inflammation:** A major trigger for the inflammation that sparked Ravi's heart attack is the presence of oxidized LDL cholesterol particles, also known as ox-LDL. LDL cholesterol, despite being labeled "bad cholesterol," is primarily harmful in the presence of free radicals capable of transforming it into ox-LDL. Macrophages that penetrate the ECL have an appetite for ox-LDL, which they digest and convert into foam cells. Foam cells lay the foundation for new plaques from an early age, which is why the entire family, including kids, needs to lead a healthy lifestyle. Foam cells also trigger rampant inflammation, which in Ravi's case made existing plaque unstable. The other major source of inflammation for Ravi and so many other South Asians is excess belly fat. Belly fat is a storehouse of inflammatory chemicals!

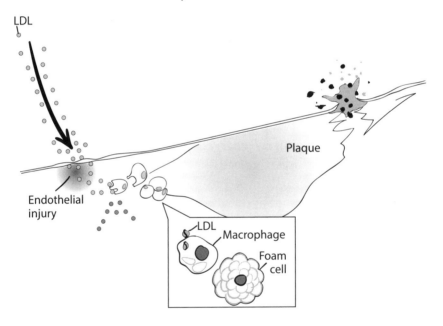

3. **Coagulation:** A plaque is like a dormant volcano, and its lava is a blood clot created by a process called coagulation. When the plaque is inactive, there is no harm done. However, Ravi's risky lifestyle choices caused the plaque to start rumbling. His

plaque eventually erupted through the ECL, spewing a blood clot that blocked off his artery and caused his heart attack. The goal is not to develop a plaque in the first place, but if you already have one, the trick is to make sure it stays stable.

Insulin Resistance at the Train Station

Now that we understand the role inflammation played in Ravi's heart attack, let's delve deeper into insulin resistance, a core concept throughout this book. We'll focus on your muscle cells, where insulin resistance usually begins. To make the process more accessible, let's use a train station analogy, since nearly every South Asian has experienced a crowded train station at some point in his/her life.

Take a look at our train station symbols:

- Muscle cells are the train cars

- Glucose (sugar) molecules are the passengers

- Train tickets represent the hormone insulin

- The railway platform where passengers wait to board stands in for your bloodstream

- The conductors are the insulin receptors on your fat and muscle cells

After a meal, and under normal circumstances, insulin carries most of your glucose to your muscle cells to use as energy. Insulin is able to usher sugar into your cells by latching onto the cell's insulin receptors. In other words, passengers (glucose) board the train (muscle cells) by presenting their ticket (insulin) to the conductor (insulin receptor). When your body regulates insulin correctly, blood sugar levels stay balanced; an appropriate number of passengers board the train without crowds of passengers waiting on the railway platform (your bloodstream). However, when you become insulin resistant, chaos breaks out at the train station. First of all, you have a stubborn or resistant conductor who refuses to allow anyone aboard the train (your muscle cells preventing glucose from entering). The result is a crowd of angry passengers rioting on the platform…or glucose molecules accumulating in your bloodstream and causing your blood sugar to rise. In the early stages of insulin resistance there is one train that does remain open…your fat cells. The glucose passengers rejected from the muscle train load onto your fat cells where they are stored as triglycerides. When fat cells swell with triglycerides, you experience an increase in body fat.

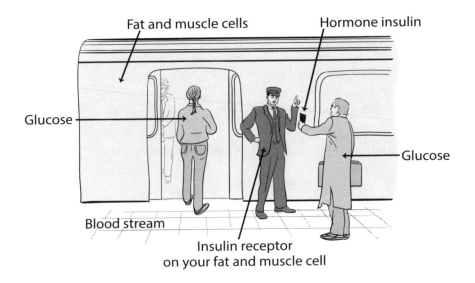

Eventually other trains (fat, liver, etc.) will also become resistant to the effects of insulin. As a result, blood sugar levels will continue to climb high enough to instigate prediabetes and diabetes. The blood sugar level cutoffs are below.

Prediabetes is diagnosed when your fasting blood sugar (glucose blood test done after an 8-12 hour fast) is 100 mg/dl or above, or your A1C test (aka glycohemoglobin) is between 5.7 and 6.4 percent. The A1C is an estimate of your average blood sugar over the past 2-3 months.

Diabetes is diagnosed when your fasting blood sugar is 126 mg/dl or above, or your A1C test is 6.5 percent or higher.

Elevated blood sugar isn't the only expression of insulin resistance. An insulin resistant liver converts glucose into triglycerides, which are then dumped into the bloodstream as cholesterol packages called lipoproteins. Looks like excess carbohydrates in an insulin resistant individual lead to high blood sugars and elevated triglyceride levels!

Even though the more common type 2 diabetes is deemed "non-insulin dependent," if you do not make significant lifestyle changes, your pancreas will eventually tire out and will no longer be able to pump out insulin to help control your blood sugar. Once you become insulin deficient, you will likely need to take injectable insulin to regulate your blood sugar. We can think of the whole process as a spectrum:

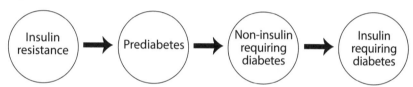

The earlier you intervene, the better your chance of preventing this life-threatening progression. Making changes early means recognizing clues for insulin resistance—such as excess abdominal fat and high triglycerides—before your blood sugar becomes irreversibly abnormal. In fact, your cholesterol panel can provide early clues to insulin resistance and can indicate a future risk of prediabetes, diabetes, and heart disease 5 to 10 years <u>before</u> your blood sugar rises into the abnormal range. If you wait for your blood sugar to become abnormal, then you may have already missed the boat...or shall we say the train! We'll discuss how to interpret your cholesterol panel accurately in Chapter 2.

How Insulin Resistance Fuels Inflammation

High blood sugar, or hyperglycemia, causes microvascular complications that affect the smaller blood vessels. These conditions, including neuropathy (nerve disease), nephropathy (kidney disease), and retinopathy (eye disease), are commonly linked to diabetes. Even prediabetic patients can develop complications like neuropathy before becoming diabetic.

Macrovascular diseases involve larger blood vessel complications, including heart attacks and strokes. Those resistant cells that aren't letting glucose inside send a signal to your pancreas to keep pumping out more insulin in a desperate effort to normalize the excess sugar in your blood. More insulin leads to more issues. In fact, excess insulin causes most of the heart disease (major macrovascular complication) seen in South Asians. You don't have to be diabetic to develop these macrovascular complications. You can have perfectly normal blood sugar levels and still drop dead from a heart attack or become paralyzed by a stroke due to the more subtle signs of insulin resistance (excess belly fat, high triglycerides, etc.).

Some of the conditions potentially caused by insulin resistance, as well as an explanation of their link to inflammation, are below.

> *You can have perfectly normal blood sugar levels and still drop dead from a heart attack or become paralyzed by a stroke due to the more subtle signs of insulin resistance.*

High blood pressure: Increased insulin makes blood vessels stiffer and causes them to retain more salt and water, thereby elevating blood pressure. Elevated blood pressure damages the ECL, which then promotes inflammation.

Abnormal cholesterol: Insulin resistance increases triglycerides, lowers HDL (good cholesterol), and increases harmful type B LDL cholesterol. Type B LDL in particular triggers inflammation when it is gobbled up by hungry macrophage immune cells underneath the ECL surface. Triglycerides promote inflammation through the creation of more type B LDL particles. HDL has several anti-inflammatory effects, such as blocking macrophages from attaching to the ECL, thereby reducing oxidation of LDL. The combination of high triglycerides and low anti-inflammatory HDL leads to excess inflammation.

Obesity: Insulin promotes the selective storage of abdominal fat, which is a major storehouse of inflammatory chemicals. Difficulty losing weight can be a sign of underlying insulin resistance, because high insulin levels make it notoriously difficult to lose fat. Chapter 4 discusses the dangers of belly fat in detail, while Chapter 6 explores how to burn that stubborn fat.

Hopefully it's becoming clear just how insulin resistance and chronic inflammation shape the dangerous pathways that lead straight to heart disease, diabetes, and a growing list of other chronic conditions.

Signs of Insulin Resistance and the Metabolic 6-pack

Insulin resistance is so common in South Asians that I now assume all South Asians are to some degree insulin resistant until proven otherwise. Just take a look around you. When was the last time you saw a South Asian without excess belly fat? Most of the South Asians who appear slim are likely "skinny-fat." Their fat lurks under the surface, blanketing their liver and other internal organs. Even if you are not technically insulin resistant, eating excess carbs, as most South Asians do, will eventually lead to high insulin levels in your body.

In the enlightening book, *Syndrome X: Overcoming The Silent Killer That Can Give You A Heart Attack,* Dr. Gerald Reaven, a Stanford endocrinologist and world renown expert in diabetes research, coined the term "metabolic syndrome" (aka "Syndrome X") to describe individuals who have a high degree of insulin resistance that significantly increases their risk of developing diabetes and heart disease.

His criteria include abdominal obesity (aka belly fat), high triglycerides, low HDL, high blood pressure, and elevated blood sugar. The International Diabetes Federation (IDF) has further modified these key measures of insulin resistance, including ethnic-adjusted waist circumference measurements. I've included IDF criteria and the waist measurement table in the appendix.

I've modified and turned the metabolic syndrome criteria into a set of goals called the Metabolic 6-pack:

- Trim your waist circumference to less than 90 cm (35 inches) in males and 80 cm (31 inches) in females

- Drop your triglyceride level to less than 100 mg/dL (1.13 mmol/L)

- Raise your HDL cholesterol above 40 mg/dL (1.03 mmol/L) if you're male and above 50 mg/dL (1.29 mmol/L) if you're female

- Reduce systolic BP (top number) at or below 120 and diastolic BP (bottom number) at or below 80 mm Hg

- Decrease fasting blood glucose below 100mg/dL (5.6 mmol/L) and HbA1c less than 5.7%

- Get hs-CRP level below 1.0 mg/dL

The basic modifications to the standard criteria are lower triglyceride and blood pressure goals and the addition of the HbA1c and hs-CRP tests. The HbA1C (glycohemoglobin) test, which represents your average blood sugar over the last three months, gives a more detailed snapshot of your blood glucose status than a single reading does. The hs-CRP is a good test to measure heart inflammation, which is elevated in many of my insulin resistant South Asian patients. According to the American Heart Association and Centers for Disease Control, 1.0-3.0 is low risk, >3.0-10.0 is high risk, and >10.0 may represent inflammation from somewhere outside the heart, such as an inflammatory joint condition.

Keep your Metabolic 6-pack numbers in check, and you will have likely successfully attacked insulin and inflammation!

I would rather you prioritize moving your Metabolic 6-pack numbers into their goal range than obsess over having a six-pack of abdominal muscles or chasing an unrealistic goal weight on your scale. Another quick quantitative measure that can help you assess heart attack risk is the triglyceride-to-HDL ratio, which is your triglyceride level divided by your HDL level. A value less than 3.0 is associated with a low risk of insulin resistance. When you keep these numbers in check, you will have likely successfully attacked insulin and inflammation…even if your weight is above your body mass index target!

Notice that one particular number has been omitted from the metabolic syndrome criteria, and that's the LDL cholesterol measurement that doctors and drug companies put so much emphasis on. Insulin resistant individuals usually have normal to low LDL levels, which often give both physicians and patients a false sense of security despite the fact that these patients are extremely high risk. I have also seen numerous fit, healthy non-insulin resistant individuals with elevated LDL levels needlessly put on statin medications despite leading extremely healthy, anti-inflammatory lifestyles that put them at a very low risk for heart disease.

Apart from the metabolic syndrome criteria, additional clues to insulin resistance include:

- A family history of diabetes or early heart disease

- A history of gout (painful inflammatory arthritis usually involving the big toe)

- A history of polycystic ovarian syndrome (PCOS)

- A history of gestational diabetes (diabetes during pregnancy)

- A history of exceptional difficulty losing weight

- A skin condition called acanthosis nigricans (dark, hyperpigmented, velvety rash over skin folds—neck, armpits, groin, etc.)

HOW DID WE GET INTO THIS MESS?

Obesity is a global health issue, but South Asians continue to lead the race to the top…or shall we say the bottom of the health curve. I run wellness programs for high tech firms with diverse demographics. There are a few consistent factors: every employee sits in front of a computer all day, is under high stress, and eats similar foods from the company cafeteria and the micro-kitchen stocked with junk snacks. What is so disturbing is that the risk profiles consistently show more insulin resistance in South Asians, even those at a lower body weight than employees of other ethnicities. Are South Asians just dealt a bad deck of genes, or do cultural and lifestyle components put them at an even higher risk? The answer is both.

Genes and Evolution

Excess abdominal fat is a hallmark of the South Asian body and one of the core features of insulin resistance. Why did South Asians develop this high-risk disposition? There are several theories that go beyond the scope of this book, but let's highlight three in particular, which, when analyzed together, may explain the evolutionary adaptations of our South Asian ancestors to life on the Indian subcontinent.

1. **Famine:** The thrifty gene theory argues that certain ethnic groups, such as South Asians, who used to live in a year-round feast-famine cycle, inherited a gene that predisposed them to store body fat during times of famine.[1] Famine has been an intrinsic part of South Asian life for thousands of years, particularly during agricultural times when the unpredictable

monsoon patterns often resulted in droughts, killing millions of South Asians on a regular basis. The extra body fat was intended to provide energy when food was scarce. Researchers think the intensity and duration of these periods of famine may have made South Asians more susceptible to the gene.[2]

2. **Tropical climate:** Mitochondria are the power-generating units inside your body's cells. They either produce ATP, which is chemical energy that helps propel your body, or they generate heat. For primitive South Asians living in warmer climates, mitochondria prioritized ATP (energy) production over heat production to produce enough fuel to do the hard physical work characteristic of that era. However, when South Asians are inactive and consume a high-calorie diet, this adaptation becomes a "metabolic inefficiency" that promotes excess fat accumulation and insulin resistance.[3]

3. **Infection:** The Wells hypothesis states that reserving fat energy helped support immune system function during times when infections were rampant.[4] Recall how abdominal fat in particular is a major source of inflammation and immune activation, thereby contributing to chronic disease when calories are abundant. However, in times when food is scarce, this type of immune activation may have protected against life-threatening infections. Studies show that a higher body mass index up to a certain point reduces infection risk, especially in seniors.[5]

Evolutionary theories such as these are gradually being validated by solid molecular and genetic evidence. For example, ENPP1 is a protein associated with insulin resistance; South Asians, compared to other ethnic groups, have an even more aggressive version of this insulin resistant protein called the K121Q mutation.

The protective fat storage tendencies of our ancestors are producing an epidemic of obesity, diabetes, and heart disease in our modern world.

Let's fast-forward to modern times, when we live in a year-round feast-feast cycle, are exposed to indoor climate control, and no longer have to deal with frequent infections thanks to vaccines and modern medications. The tradeoff is that sedentary behavior has become the norm. The protective fat storage tendencies of our ancestors are producing an epidemic of obesity, diabetes, and heart disease in our modern world.

High Risk Moms Produce High Risk Babies

The nutritional status of a pregnant woman can influence whether her child develops insulin resistance and its associated complications later in life. There is a growing body of evidence that suggests low-birth-weight South Asian babies are at an increased risk of developing diabetes and heart disease, particularly when they are overfed early in life.[6] It is common practice for anxious South Asian parents and family members to overfeed thin South Asian infants in order to achieve catch-up growth. This can backfire and put babies at risk for developing adult diabetes and heart disease later in life. I detail the implementation and disastrous consequences of this deleterious cultural practice in Chapter 10.

Pregnant South Asian women are experiencing an epidemic of gestational diabetes (diabetes during pregnancy). In fact 30 to 60 percent of mothers with gestational diabetes will go on to develop adult onset diabetes after delivering their babies. There are many cultural myths that promote excessive caloric intake and limited activity levels during pregnancy. These outmoded ways of thinking result in out of shape mothers who gain excessive body fat beyond what is required to support a healthy pregnancy. The end result is a diabetic mother who may pass on her insulin resistance to her baby, thereby increasing the child's odds of developing diabetes later in life.

Are South Asians Less Active Than Other Ethnic Groups?

All ethnic groups are shifting towards increasingly sedentary life-styles, but the question is whether South Asians rank highest among the inactive. Some of the most detailed studies on South Asian risk factors have been conducted in the UK and Canada; both countries have a nationalized health program and a large South Asian popula-tion. The British and Canadian governments are feeling the financial pinch of funding health care for this high-risk population, and as a result have dedicated extensive resources to evaluating risk factors in South Asians. A Canadian study compared physical activity levels in all major ethnic groups, including South Asian, Caucasian, Latin American, East Asian, Black, West Asian/Arab, NA Aboriginal, and those classified as other. South Asians came in last place out of all the groups![7] A similar study carried out in the UK confirmed lower physical activity rates in South Asians compared to all other ethnic groups.[8]

The sedentary epidemic is not just confined to adults, but has hit South Asian children, who often model their behavior after inactive parents. The British Heart Foundation conducted a study made up of 208 children of whom 96 were white European, 65 were South Asian, and 47 were from other ethnic backgrounds. The children kept dia-ries and wore activity and heart rate monitors for eight days. The South Asian children were found to be the least active; most of this difference was seen during afterschool hours, when children spent more time performing sedentary activities such as doing homework, playing video games, or visiting a religious place of worship.

Vitamin D Deficiency and Insulin Resistance

As we spend more time sedentary indoors and out of the vitamin-D producing sun we grow more susceptible to vitamin D deficiency. Dr. Michael Holick, author of *The Vitamin D Solution* and one of the world's leading experts on the subject, reports that some 75 percent of the US population is vitamin D-deficient due to indoor-dominant lifestyles and irrational fears of skin cancer from sun exposure. Vir-tually every South Asian patient I see has some degree of vitamin D deficiency, and the average levels tend to run much lower than those of most other ethnic groups. This is due to a combination of darker skin pigment and a predominantly indoor lifestyle. (Chapter 11 features a special section on vitamin D with recommendations for screening and treatment.)

Vitamin D deficiency is associated with a growing list of disorders, including insulin resistance. In fact, a study made up of women with an insulin resistant condition called PCOS (polycystic ovarian syndrome), showed that low vitamin D levels were the best predictor of insulin resistance.[9] Vitamin D has also been shown to exhibit potent anti-inflammatory effects by reducing the production of inflammatory cytokines such as IL-2, TNF-alpha, and Interferon-gamma.[10]

Now, don't think that taking vitamin D supplements is going to cure all your insulin issues. Vitamin D deficiency is a potential contributor that still pales in comparison to the effects of an unhealthy diet and inactivity, both of which result in excess body fat. Keep in mind that studies show a correlation between vitamin D deficiency and insulin resistance, but this link does not necessarily indicate that vitamin D causes insulin resistance and that taking a supplement will make a difference. There was, however, one randomized control trial done in New Zealand that found that insulin resistant South Asian women supplementing with vitamin D exhibited reduced insulin resistance. The greatest improvements occurred when vitamin D levels were increased above 80 nmol/L, much higher than the standard cutoff of 30 nmol/L currently used.[11] Further studies need to be conducted to see if vitamin D supplementation does indeed play a therapeutic role.

The South Asian Diet: A Major Health Risk

A characteristic feature of the South Asian diet is the abundance of carbohydrates, especially in the vegetarian diet. The core of most South Asian diets is a combination of flat breads, rice, and lentils. These foods alone are enough to promote excess fat deposition and insulin resistance in inactive South Asians. Top that off with the typical South Asian crispy snacks fried in dangerous trans fats… and the sweets, sodas, and influx of Western fast food chains and processed foods…and you end up with a dangerous combination of high-risk genes and an even higher risk diet. In my consult practice, I actually do an intake of how many grams of carbs patients consume on a daily basis. The average South Asian patient easily takes in 150-200 grams more of carbohydrates than do patients of other ethnic groups. The good news is that even my patients who appear to have the strongest genetic predisposition towards insulin resistance (as measured by virtually every family member being diabetic) are often able to overcome most, if not all, risk factors once they make the recommended lifestyle changes. Don't let your genes get you down!

The Immigrant Effect

South Asian immigrants to Western countries have a three to four times higher prevalence of diabetes than their native counterparts.[12] I see this time and time again in the clinic when I examine patients who have just emigrated from India. Within the first year they often gain an average of 15 pounds (what I refer to as the "immigrant 15"). Most of this weight gain can be attributed to the toxic nutritional environment of countries like the United States, where portion sizes are much larger and processed foods with high fructose corn syrup and other insulin-releasing ingredients much more abundant. Physical activity levels also go down considerably. I had one patient take his pedometer to India where he was stationed for three months on a work assignment. Lack of easy car accessibility—which we enjoy in the US—increased his baseline activity, and he routinely walked 5,000 more steps daily when in India. Unfortunately, Western foods and an increasingly sedentary lifestyle have spread to India and all over the world, so the immigrant effect is now a global phenomenon.

ACHIEVING YOUR METABOLIC 6-PACK

Now you understand how Ravi had his heart attack, how inflammation is related to chronic disease, and how insulin resistance is a major fuel source for inflammation. You also know how to recognize signs of insulin resistance so that you can initiate the immediate lifestyle interventions outlined in the following chapters. However, before you do anything, I strongly suggest that you outline your personal goals. Many of my South Asian patients are strongly driven by numbers, but unfortunately they are chasing the wrong ones. Here are the most common mistakes I see:

- Trying to lower LDL cholesterol when triglycerides are the real problem

- Trying to reduce total body weight, rather than focusing on waist size and adding muscle

- Lowering the grams of fat consumed, which by the way can be anti-inflammatory, rather than lowering the grams of carbs

Target a weight that helps you achieve your Metabolic 6-pack. Any additional pounds you want to lose beyond the Metabolic 6-pack may be related to improving your fitness, increasing your energy, or fitting into your pre-pregnancy dress size. Fat burning is a process that occurs from the inside out. Fat cells deep within your belly will need to be emptied of years of stored triglycerides before you start to notice significant external changes. Be patient. Once you start chipping away at these goals, you should start to see some physical changes as your body sheds fat and energy increases.

Other Useful Markers for Inflammation and Heart Health

Liver inflammation: Non-alcoholic fatty liver inflammation is very common in South Asians and is another repercussion of insulin resistance. You can screen for liver inflammation with a simple test called the ALT (alanine aminotransferase or SGPT).

Heart rate measures: A useful measure of blood vessel health and inflammation is your pulse (heart rate). More specifically, heart rate recovery time (HRR) is an excellent indicator of fitness and heart health. HRR is discussed in Chapter 7. Heart rate variability (HRV) is another type of heart rate measure that can be used to gauge emotional stress, which, as we discussed, is also correlated with inflammation. HRV is discussed in Chapter 8.

Controlling the Flames of Inflammation

Inflammation, fueled by insulin resistance and excess insulin, is a force we all need to control if we want to improve our health. Think of inflammation as a fire with three major categories of flammable factors:

1. **Food:** High fructose corn syrup, trans fats and interesterified fats, excess sugar and carbohydrates, and other artificial chemicals from processed foods can fuel oxidation and inflammation, especially if there is a lack of antioxidant rich foods in the diet.

2. **Fat:** Not *dietary fat*, but *body fat*—which is primarily triggered by inactivity and the foods listed above—promotes fat storage and impairs lipolysis (fat burning). Belly fat in particular is a major source of inflammation.

3. **Feelings:** Stress, depression, anger, hostility, internalized negative emotions, etc. These can be considered "inflammatory emotions," which we'll discuss in more detail in Chapter 8.

Any or all of the above can stoke the fires of inflammation. Since inflammation, especially at a low-level, cannot be reliably measured by any test (hs-CRP may not always be elevated), you have to rely on your body's signals. If inflammation is a fire, there are two types of smoke signals that can alert you to its presence:

External smoke signals: These are symptoms you can feel, like rapid breathing, heart palpitations, a sore neck or back from muscle tension, sweaty palms, fatigue from chronic stress or sleep deprivation, or any of the aforementioned inflammatory emotions.

Measurable smoke signals: These are the biometric values (blood pressure, cholesterol, etc.) that make up your Metabolic 6-pack.

Your goal is to be so in-tune with your body, that you can detect the external smoke signals before they cause deeper level inflammation. Ravi had a lifelong problem with stress and internalized negative emotions, which likely prompted oxidative damage and inflammation to flicker on and off for years. Additional factors, such as the accumulation of belly fat and insulin resistance, further magnified this inflammation, leading to atherosclerosis and ultimately the plaque rupture that caused his fatal heart attack. This type of tragedy may have been preventable… if only Ravi had detected and reversed these early warning signs sooner! The following chapters will teach you how to sense and monitor your body's cautionary signals and intervene with effective lifestyle modifications that will prevent the occasional flickering flames of inflammation from turning into full-blown forest fires.

Being fitter and healthier has given my patients and me a sense of inner peace, clarity, creativity, and energy that has helped us realize our full potential in all areas of life.

Beating Insulin Resistance, Taking Responsibility and Maximizing Your Genetic Potential

In order to fight the epidemic of insulin resistance, you must apply the same level of discipline and dedication to your lifestyle as you do to your academic and professional pursuits. What if your grades or your paycheck depended on how healthy and fit you were? Would that get you motivated? If so, then why doesn't the thought of having a heart attack, a stroke, a diagnosis of diabetes, premature aging, and arthritis…or the possibility of turning your kids into orphans, your spouse into a widow, and handing your loved ones the burden of having to take care of you… motivate you to take control of your health? What about the fact that your behaviors and eating habits are having an adverse effect on your children, who look to you as a role model? Imagine having to qualify your child's success: "Yes, my son graduated first in his class and runs his own company, but unfortunately he takes insulin injections for his diabetes and is probably going to have a heart attack at any moment."

In Silicon Valley I take care of quite a few South Asian CEOs who graduated top of their class but are now victims of chronic health issues due to unhealthy lifestyle habits. Why aren't health factors worth more than money or an A+ grade? There is no rule saying you have to choose one or the other. Being fitter and healthier has given my patients and me a sense of inner peace, clarity, creativity, and energy that has helped us realize our full potential in all areas of life.

Despite the role of genes and evolution, you will be amazed by the resiliency and potential of the South Asian body to overcome years of abuse and transform into a leaner, more energetic, insulin sensitive, fat-burning machine within just a few months. You will thank your body for being so forgiving, and I guarantee you will never want to turn back to the life you had before. All those foods you thought you couldn't live without will be a distant memory and an occasional indulgence rather than an addiction. So keep reading to uncover your true genetic potential and to live the long and healthy life you were meant to.

Summary

- Insulin resistance is the predominant cause of heart disease and related conditions in South Asians.

- Metabolic syndrome is a cluster of insulin resistant conditions that can clue you in to early heart disease risk.

- Many standard risk factors and tools measured by physicians often overlook insulin resistance in South Asians.

- Attack insulin resistance early at the root, rather than medicating its branches.

For Professionals

- Emphasize the role of inflammation and its relation to heart attacks and chronic disease.

- Rather than prescribing the usual "eat more vegetables and fruits," emphasize how consuming more natural antioxidants reduces blood vessel inflammation.

- Motivate patients to manage stress and negative emotions as an anti-inflammatory strategy so they understand how their thoughts and feelings directly impact their health.

- Physicians, nutritionists, and employers who run health screens should focus on the Metabolic 6-pack measurements to pick up on important risk factors in all patients, particularly South Asians.

- Recognize that South Asians who have eliminated "junk food" from their diet may still be at risk for major sources of inflammation, including an antioxidant-poor, carb-heavy diet, excessive sedentary behavior, high stress, and abdominal obesity.

CHAPTER 2

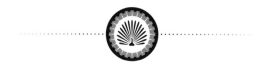

CHOLESTEROL AND HEART DISEASE

IT'S CRITICAL TO UNDERSTAND THE ROLE that cholesterol plays in heart disease, because we have been egregiously misled in this area by conventional wisdom. Physicians and patients generally have a severely distorted view of the true mechanisms and risk factors for heart disease. We harbor the oversimplified beliefs that LDL causes heart disease (so you shouldn't eat cholesterol-containing foods) and that if your LDL cholesterol is too high you should take statin medications to lower it. Nothing could be further from the truth! This chapter will present a complete and easily understandable picture of cholesterol's role in the body and the true risk factors for heart disease.

Case Study: Vinod

Vinod is a 34-year-old software engineer who came to see me for a physical exam. He couldn't remember the last time he had a physical and admitted that his wife "forced him to make the appointment." He denied having any active medical issues other than high job stress, and reported feeling in good health overall. He rarely exercised, did not smoke, and ate a vegetarian diet. His family history revealed that his father had diabetes and his mother had high cholesterol.

Unfortunately, Vinod did not follow up with me as recommended and did not adhere to lifestyle suggestions. Approximately nine months after his physical, I received a call from his cardiologist informing me that Vinod had been admitted to Stanford University Medical Center due to a heart attack.

Vinod's fasting cholesterol panel at the time of his physical showed the following numbers:

Total Cholesterol:	190
LDL:	108
HDL:	32
Triglycerides:	250

This is a very common cholesterol panel among South Asians. At first glance, you would not expect these numbers to cause a heart attack in a thirty-something. The total cholesterol level is less than 200 and the LDL (bad cholesterol) level is considered normal by most doctors. However, these results reveal some danger signs. Before we discuss Vinod's results in greater detail, let's garner a little background information about cholesterol since most patients and physicians are misinformed about this important topic.

CHOLESTEROL CONFUSION

A cholesterol panel is the most overhyped, misinterpreted, misunderstood, and misleading lab test I deal with in my clinic. As a result of the cholesterol fixation, we now have a population that is grossly overtreated with statin medications and undertreated with proper lifestyle changes. Statins are so incredibly effective at treating high cholesterol numbers within a few weeks, that many patients, feeling falsely protected by these drugs, continue their downward trend of unhealthy habits.

How protected are you when you take a medication to control your cholesterol without making healthy lifestyle changes? Not very! A UCLA study found that 75 percent of patients hospitalized for a heart attack had an LDL within the acceptable range of less than 130 mg/dl, and half had levels of less than 100 mg/dl, which is considered ideal.[1] These results seem to indicate that we've gotten very good at treating numbers without treating the underlying causes discussed in Chapter 1—insulin resistance and inflammation!

As a result of the cholesterol fixation, we now have a population that is grossly over-treated with statin medications and under-treated with proper lifestyle changes.

Fortunately, the new 2013 cholesterol guidelines, drafted by the ACC/AHA (American College of Cardiology and American Heart Association) discourage treating with statins to achieve specific LDL target numbers. This faulty approach has led to millions of statin users taking higher than normal statin doses or multiple cholesterol medications in an attempt to achieve goal LDL numbers. Medications like Zetia have helped patients reach goal LDL numbers, but they have never been proven to reduce the incidence of heart disease, the real goal. The new guidelines finally acknowledge the safety concerns of statin use, but unfortunately recommend the use of an inaccurate risk calculator tool to assess the need for statins. Dr. Nancy Cook and Dr. Paul M. Ridker of Harvard Medical School conducted a rigorous analysis of more than 100,000 healthy patients and found that this risk calculator tool overestimated heart attack and stroke risk by 75 to 150 percent. They stated in a commentary published in the prestigious journal *The Lancet*:

> "It is possible that as many as 40 to 50 percent of the 33 million middle-aged Americans targeted by the new guidelines for statin therapy do not actually have risk thresholds exceeding the 7.5 percent level suggested for treatment."

In addition to overestimating risk, this calculator also underestimates risk in South Asians by ignoring key markers such as high triglycerides, prediabetic blood sugar levels, and abdominal obesity. I've personally used this tool in South Asian patients who have had a heart attack and it frequently predicts a very low risk! If doctors use this tool, they will be telling many insulin resistant patients they have nothing to worry about, when in fact they are actually ticking time bombs.

Unfortunately, the calculator is based on outdated studies featuring predominantly Caucasian patients. Rather than relying on this imprecise tool, you can accurately interpret your numbers using the six cholesterol rules in this chapter, as well as the Metabolic 6-pack outlined in Chapter 1.

Statin use shows no indication of declining. Even more outrageous is the fact that drug companies are lobbying to use statins to treat children with high cholesterol, despite the lack of safety data. Adult side effects such as musculoskeletal pain and liver inflammation may be more pronounced in a growing child. Putting children on statins, means exposing patients to several decades of potential toxicity.

To make matters worse, dietary misconceptions about cholesterol have created flawed nutrition guidelines and further confusion. Most of this misinformation stems from the "diet-heart hypothesis," which erroneously states that cholesterol and saturated fat in the diet increase heart disease risk. This is based on the belief that dietary cholesterol and saturated fat raise blood cholesterol, which then leads to atherosclerosis, the process that forms heart attack-causing plaques. Cholesterol does play a critical role in triggering atherosclerosis, but not the type of cholesterol or saturated fat obtained from the diet. This is good news for you egg lovers out there! If you're still having doubts, I've provided a brief summary below of just some of the evidence disproving the diet-heart disease hypothesis.

DIET-HEART DISEASE HYPOTHESIS HOOPLA

→ In 1997, the father of the diet-heart disease hypothesis, Ancel Keys, conceded the following: "There's no connection whatsoever between cholesterol in food and cholesterol in the blood. And we've known that all along..."

→ A meta-analysis of 21 studies that collectively followed 350,000 people for up to 23 years concluded the following: "There is insufficient evidence from prospective epidemiologic studies to conclude that dietary saturated fat is associated with an increased risk of CHD, stroke, or cardiovascular disease (CVD)."[2]

→ Three large trials involving health professionals—the Women's Health Initiative,[3] the Nurse's Health Study[4] and the Health Professional's Study[5]—found no link between saturated fat intake and heart disease, obesity, and chronic diseases like cancer.

If you are still skeptical, I recommend reading further to learn how to accurately interpret your current cholesterol levels. Don't stop there: follow the lifestyle principles outlined in this book, and then recheck your numbers in six to eight weeks. No study is more convincing than the one you perform on yourself.

Heart Disease: The Real Role of Cholesterol

If you skipped Chapter 1 and anxiously started here because of concerns about your cholesterol results, I strongly recommend you go back and read the first chapter, since it explains how artery-clogging plaques are formed—a process known as atherosclerosis. I summarized the three main steps (oxidation, inflammation, coagulation) that caused Ravi's fatal heart attack.

I'd like to take the time now to expand on cholesterol's role in atherosclerosis in order to reinforce the principle that high cholesterol alone does not normally cause heart attacks. Heart attack risk is more heavily influenced by the type of cholesterol you have and the type of blood vessel environment your cholesterol is exposed to. These two factors are dependent on your lifestyle choices. If you lead a low oxidative, anti-inflammatory lifestyle with none of the other criteria in the Metabolic 6-pack (such as increased belly fat, high triglycerides, and low HDL cholesterol), an isolated abnormal cholesterol measurement is unlikely to cause heart disease. On the other hand, even if your cholesterol levels are normal (with or without medications) and you have one or more criteria from the Metabolic 6-pack, then you remain at higher risk for heart disease. You must focus on reversing these risks, regardless of what your cholesterol results show.

LDL Cholesterol: A Tale of Two Boats

We talked about trains when we discussed insulin resistance, but now I'd like to use another mode of transportation when describing cholesterol metabolism—boats.

Lipoproteins are the carriers or "boats" that transport cholesterol and another type of fat called triglycerides throughout the body via the blood. So, when I mention "boat" I'm talking about lipoproteins, and the primary passengers on this boat are triglycerides and cholesterol.

How do these cholesterol boats trigger atherosclerosis, the process that forms dangerous plaques? LDL, or low-density lipoprotein, is the most commonly known lipoprotein that can cause plaques to form. You'll see this lipoprotein on your cholesterol results. (LDL cholesterol is also the target of the blockbuster class of cholesterol drugs known as statins.) However, there are two forms of LDL. Large, fluffy LDL, known as type A; and small, dense LDL, known as type B. Think of type "B" as standing for "B"ad.

So, we have two types of boats, the small "B"ad boats and the larger, relatively harmless, A boats. Both type A and B LDL can contribute to atherosclerosis, especially if someone with type A LDL has other risk factors (abdominal obesity, high CRP levels, strong family history, smoking, etc.), but type B LDL typically carries the higher risk.

THE IMPACT OF FAMILY HISTORY

A "strong" or "significant" family history is defined for males as having a first-degree male relative (father, brother, or son) with a history of heart disease, stroke, or some other form of atherosclerosis at an age less than 55, and for females as having a first-degree female relative (mother, sister, or daughter) with a similar condition at an age less than 65. A grandfather who had a heart attack at age 45 would technically not be considered a "strong" or "significant" family history, but should still be a consideration that motivates you to minimize your personal risk factors. If your mother and father lived to be 85 with no history of heart disease, you aren't necessarily protected. Older generations were often more physically active, ate more natural foods, and had normal vitamin D levels due to sufficient sun exposure. I have seen several instances of today's generation being the first to present with diabetes or heart disease due to significantly unhealthier modern lifestyles. On the other hand, I've had patients with a very strong family history of heart disease and diabetes escape this fate because they implemented healthier lifestyle plans. Bottom line is that family history provides a rough estimate of genetic risk, which can be influenced by a nutritious diet and sufficient physical activity.

Why are the smaller, type B boats more dangerous? Instead of floating innocently down your blood vessels, these boats are constantly looking for trouble. Type B LDL anchor to the inside of the blood vessel wall (the ECL from Chapter 1), penetrating snugly under the surface. (By the way, my runner-up for what "B" should stand for is "bullet" since these particles embed themselves into the blood vessel wall and trigger the gunfire we refer to as inflammation.) The larger, fluffy type A LDL particles are more likely to bounce innocently by like beach balls, not hanging out long enough to do any damage to the blood vessel.

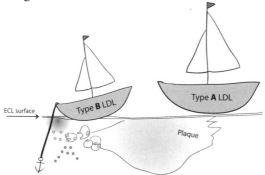

Notice how the smaller type B boat has docked itself on the ECL surface, waiting to be oxidized and ingested by macrophages, while the type A boat floats by without causing any waves.

There's one other transformation that type B LDL is more likely to undergo before it inflicts damage, and that is oxidation. Oxidized LDL (ox-LDL) specifically attracts the hungry immune system macrophages that gobble them up and turn them into plaque-forming foam cells. Foam cells are basically macrophages that have devoured cholesterol in the form of ox-LDL, giving them a "foamy" appearance. Foam cells also produce large amounts of a chemical called myeloperoxidase, which further oxidizes LDL particles.

Not only could you have the wrong type of boats (type B), but you could also have too many boats! Each LDL boat is what we call an LDL particle, and your LDL particle number (LDL-P) represents the number of cholesterol boats bobbing down your bloodstream. When elevated, you're contending with major boat traffic on the high seas. When excess LDL particles hang out for too long in one place, they are more likely to dock onto the ECL and start the hazardous process of building plaque. In general, the more type B LDL you have, the more likely you are to have a greater number of LDL particles. Because type B boats are smaller, you'd need a lot more of them than larger type A boats to haul the same amount of cholesterol cargo. In fact, studies are repeatedly showing that your LDL particle number (measured on advanced lipid tests) may be one of the best cholesterol indicators of heart disease risk.

Surprisingly, the LDL result on your cholesterol panel, a number that doctors and drug companies cling to, provides very limited information. It just tells you how much cholesterol cargo your LDL boats are carrying. In other words, it tells you the LDL-C, which is the concentration of cholesterol inside each LDL particle. It tells you nothing about LDL size (big versus small boats), whether the LDL is oxidized, or the number of LDL particles in your bloodstream.

Both the type and number of cholesterol boats increase the probability that your LDL may undergo oxidation. But there are many other factors, such as major lifestyle considerations that cause LDL oxidation and trigger inflammation. For example, trans or hydrogenated fats are a dangerous form of fat, which, unlike saturated fats or dietary cholesterol, can cause abnormal cholesterol levels and excess inflammation, and lead to increased heart disease risk. Abundant polyunsaturated fats, which come mostly in the form of vegetable oils, can also lead to increased inflammation, especially when they outnumber healthier omega-3 fats found in fish and plant-based sources. Below are some other factors that may raise the risk of LDL oxidation and overall inflammation.

- Diet low in antioxidants (found in vegetables, fruits, nuts, and seeds)

- Lack of adequate sleep (promotes systemic inflammation and compromised immune function)

- Stress and related emotional disorders (anxiety, depression, etc.)

- Other unhealthy lifestyle practices (smoking, inactivity, environmental pollution, and even excessive cardiovascular exercise, aka "chronic cardio" as fitness expert Mark Sisson calls it)

Many of the foods we limit due to high cholesterol content, such as shrimp, eggs, and meat, typically have no adverse impact on cholesterol profiles and are far less harmful than the excessive carbohydrate sources prevalent in the South Asian diet.

Many of the foods we limit due to high cholesterol content, such as shrimp, eggs, and meat, typically have no adverse impact on cholesterol profiles and are far less harmful than the excessive carbohydrate sources prevalent in the South Asian diet. For example, I've had far more patients lower their triglycerides by switching their breakfasts from oatmeal or cereals, like Honey Bunches of Oats (a South Asian favorite!), to eggs.

<u>Low</u> Cholesterol Causes More Heart Disease in South Asians than <u>High</u> Cholesterol Does!

Hopefully that headline caught your attention. Whenever I ask people what they define as an abnormal cholesterol level, they answer, "a total cholesterol level above 200 mg/dL." I think we should stop talking about this misleading number altogether. In order to do so, I'd like to propose something radical—completely eliminating the total cholesterol level from lipid panels! Clinging to this obsolete definition of abnormal cholesterol may keep you mired in the high-risk health category without you even knowing it. The truth is that most of my South Asian patients with a high risk of heart disease have <u>low</u> cholesterol levels with a total cholesterol number less than 200 mg/dL. If you can get past the total cholesterol and instead follow the six simple rules for reading cholesterol, then you will know more about interpreting your results than most doctors do!

Most high-risk, insulin resistant South Asians have cholesterol levels lower than 200 because while a standard cholesterol test directly measures the amount of triglycerides and HDL in your blood, it does not measure the LDL cholesterol. The Friedewald equation uses the measured triglycerides and HDL to provide an estimate for the LDL. If we manipulate the equation a bit, your total cholesterol turns out to be the following, assuming you are using mg/dL as your lab unit of measure:

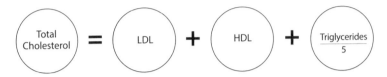

Recall from Chapter 1 that a typical South Asian lipid panel indicates an insulin resistant profile where HDL (good cholesterol) is low and triglycerides are high. If HDL is low, your total cholesterol number will be lower. But low HDL puts you at higher risk! If your triglyceride levels are high, they will have minimal impact on the total cholesterol, since triglycerides are divided by 5. Finally, the LDL number in insulin resistant South Asians is often lower because these individuals are plagued by the smaller, more dangerous type B LDL. Since LDL measures how much cholesterol cargo each boat carries, a smaller boat carries less cholesterol, which means LDL levels will be lower. It's easy to see how a low total cholesterol number can be dangerously deceptive when it comes to measuring your cardiovascular risk. To summarize:

> Total cholesterol levels tend to be lower in South Asians due to a combination of low HDL, a triglyceride level that is divided by 5, and more dangerous small, dense LDL particles that result in a lower LDL value since they hold less cholesterol.

Vinod is a perfect example of a patient who suffers from this all-too-common scenario. His total cholesterol is below 200 because he has low HDL levels and most likely has type B LDL based on his high triglycerides. Why are high triglycerides a sign of dangerous type B LDL cholesterol? High triglycerides latch onto HDL and LDL lipoproteins, turning them into oily, greasy, appetizing particles voraciously consumed by hungry enzymes called lipases (hepatic and endothelial lipases to be exact). Once lipases devour these LDL and HDL particles, they shrink in size, producing the smaller and dangerous type B

LDL. Smaller HDL particles aren't harmful, but they are easily metabolized and excreted in the urine, causing a drop in HDL levels.

You can see how high triglycerides are the initial culprit, but did you know that high carbohydrates are the major instigator of high triglycerides? Dietary cholesterol and saturated fat, on the other hand, are neutral bystanders that for years have been falsely implicated as the primary offenders in the diet-heart hypothesis. Turns out carbohydrates have been guilty all along.

SIX CHOLESTEROL RULES

Many physicians are misled by the seemingly normal LDL measurement on Vinod's cholesterol panel and overlook the fact that there are actually dangerous type B particles present. A total cholesterol level less than 200 doesn't merit congratulations, but requires an in-depth analysis using the cholesterol rules that follow.

Rule 1: Get Checked Early and Often

Abnormal cholesterol results appear in South Asians from an early age, often 10 years earlier than they do in other ethnic groups. Many experts recommend starting cholesterol screening at age 35 for the general population. Amazingly, this can be too late for many South Asians! By age 35, many have already succumbed to the onset of heart disease.

Abnormal cholesterol levels typically don't manifest symptoms until you suffer a complication (heart attack, stroke, etc.), so it is important to get monitored regularly. In general, most South Asians should have their first cholesterol panel by age 18. If your results are abnormal based on the criteria that follows, you should have your cholesterol checked a minimum of once a year. If risk factors occur early in life—such as diabetes, obesity, or a significant family history—then preliminary screening in childhood may be necessary. Discuss cholesterol screening with your child's pediatrician. Sadly, legitimate heart disease risk factors are showing up in South Asian children as a result of the childhood obesity epidemic, which I discuss in greater detail in Chapter 10.

Rule 2: Ignore Your Total Cholesterol Level

The total cholesterol alone is misleading and fails to give you the big picture on heart disease risk. It's critical to assess the individual components of the cholesterol panel and how they relate to one another.

Rule 3: When It Comes to LDL, Size Matters

On a standard lipid panel, the LDL result only reflects the concentration of cholesterol, which is not useful. If your triglycerides are over 200 mg/dL, and for many even over 150 mg/dL, you likely have the smaller, higher risk type B LDL regardless of what your LDL level is. Vinod's LDL before his heart attack looked deceptively normal at 108 and wasn't flagged as abnormal on his lab report. However, since his triglycerides were high at 250, he almost certainly had type B LDL. There are more advanced lipid tests that show you the type A/B breakdown, but for now high triglycerides can serve as a rough guide.

Rule 4: Focus on Triglycerides, an Early Measure of Risk and Lifestyle

High triglycerides have become so common in South Asians that I once had a physician colleague tell me that he doesn't worry unless the triglyceride level in his Indian patients peaks at over 300! I call this high triglyceride desensitization! Just because high triglycerides are common doesn't mean such numbers are safe. In fact most labs to date are using 150 mg/dL as the cutoff for abnormal triglycerides. Some even use 200 mg/dL as their cutoff, which, without a doubt, places you in the danger zone. Remember: high triglycerides are the inciting event that leads to the transformation of good boats into bad ones and triggers the loss of valuable HDL. This process leads to the cholesterol hallmark of insulin resistance and metabolic syndrome: high triglycerides, low HDL, and type B LDL cholesterol.

Let's bullet the top three traits of dangerous triglycerides:

- **Early marker of insulin resistance:** High triglycerides are an early warning sign of future diabetes and heart disease risk.

When your body becomes insulin resistant, triglycerides often increase long before blood sugar goes up. I refer to high triglycerides as a marker of "pre-pre-diabetes." Remember, the earlier you detect warning signs of insulin resistance and intervene, the better your chances of avoiding diabetes altogether.

> *High triglycerides are an early warning sign of future diabetes and heart disease risk.*

- **Early marker of unhealthy dietary choices, especially carb intake:** Triglyceride levels typically correlate with carbohydrate intake and can drop by a few hundred points within a month after making the carb reductions discussed in Chapter 6. I tell patients that triglycerides are their "carbohydrate truth test" because if levels haven't dropped after I've made my recommendations, they are probably sneaking in a few more crispy snacks, sweets, servings of rice, Indian breads, or other carbohydrate-rich foods.

- **Early marker of heart disease:** The lower the triglycerides, the lower your risk of heart disease. A triglyceride level of less than 150 mg/dL is considered normal by most labs and standard guidelines, but studies now show that less than 100 is the preferred measurement. In fact, many experts such as Dr. William Castelli, former director of the Framingham Heart Study, advocate a triglyceride level less than 60.[6] Not only does this range minimize heart disease risk, but it also indicates that most patients have shifted into the fat-burning zone discussed in Chapter 5.

Rule 5: Know Your Ratios

According to Rule 2 you are to ignore your total cholesterol level. Instead, I'd like you to focus on the following two ratios:

Total cholesterol-to-HDL ratio: This is your total cholesterol divided by your HDL and is a much better risk indicator than your total cholesterol measurement. Follow this ratio when comparing prior results and aim for a ratio of less than 4.0. (Less than 3.5 would be ideal.) Vinod had a total cholesterol of 190 and an HDL of 32, so his ratio was close to 6.0, putting him significantly above the cutoff. Sometimes your total cholesterol will go up because your HDL goes up, but your progress will be marked by a drop in your ratio.

Triglyceride-to-HDL ratio: This represents your triglyceride divided by your HDL, an excellent early marker of insulin resistance and future diabetes risk, along with associated complications such as kidney disease. This ratio becomes abnormal long before your blood sugar does. Experts agree that your ratio should be 3.0 or less. The lower the better, with 1:1 an excellent ultimate goal. Just triple your HDL level and see if your triglycerides fall below that number. Vinod's HDL was 32, so for his ratio to fall below 3.0, his triglycerides would have to be less than 96 (32 x 3). His was 250, far above this goal. My superstar patients have been so vigilant with controlling this ratio through lifestyle changes that often their HDL cholesterol ends up equaling or even exceeding their triglyceride level...now that is what I call an impressive reduction in risk!

Rule 6: Raise that HDL, but Be Patient

Rule 4 touched on how triglyceride levels respond quickly to lifestyle changes. HDL levels may take longer to respond. Lowering carbohydrate intake is one of the most effective ways to not only lower your triglycerides, but to also improve your HDL levels over the long run. Recall how high triglycerides lower your HDL levels, so it makes sense that if you lower triglycerides, HDL levels should increase.

Unfortunately, genetics can keep HDL low regardless of how much you improve your lifestyle. Don't lose hope. Keep working on your other numbers (triglycerides, weight, etc.).

Men should aim for an HDL over 40 and women should aim for an HDL over 50. Again, rather than focusing on individual numbers follow the ratios in Rule 5. Also keep in mind that regular exercise (aerobic and strength training) can help improve HDL levels.

Vinod's Results

Using our newfound knowledge, let's take a look at Vinod's cholesterol panel and see what his numbers truly represent.

Total Cholesterol:	190
LDL:	108
HDL:	32
Triglycerides:	250

For most physicians, Vinod's cholesterol profile may not set off any major alarms. He has low total cholesterol and a reasonable LDL level, correct? Not so fast…you now know that his deceptively normal looking LDL is anything but. Since his triglycerides are above 200 mg/dl, his LDLs are most likely the dangerous type B cholesterol.

What about Vinod's ratios? His total cholesterol/HDL ratio is nearly 6.0, which is far above the target ratio of less than 4.0. His triglyceride/HDL ratio is 7.8, which is at the level of significant insulin resistance and heart disease risk. Without even seeing Vinod in person, you can visualize excess belly fat contributing to his insulin resistant profile. Without knowing what he eats, you can already surmise from his labs that his diet is made up of excessive carbohydrates, which have led to the dangerous cholesterol triad of high triglycerides, high type B LDL, and low HDL. A cholesterol panel, when viewed through the right lens, can actually provide an insightful snapshot into the underlying risks and lifestyle of an individual. Unfortunately, most healthcare providers are using the wrong cholesterol lens and focusing too much on total cholesterol and LDL cholesterol values.

ADVANCED TESTING

Advanced lipid testing and additional blood tests can provide valuable information to help manage health conditions and risk factors. Physicians often use these tests for patients considered "intermediate risk." These are patients whose risk factors put them in the gray zone, making it difficult to determine whether more aggressive interventions or medications are necessary.

hs-CRP (highly sensitive C-reactive protein): Physicians order this test to measure the level of blood vessel inflammation. CRP molecules are not just passive markers of inflammation, but contribute directly to atherosclerosis. They allow dangerous macrophages to bind to the ECL surface and inflict damage to the blood vessels. In South Asians, elevated hs-CRP can be attributed to many different lifestyle and body composition factors, of which excess belly fat is one of the most significant. The minute I see inches coming off the waist, the hs-CRP usually starts dropping back down to normal.

Lipoprotein(a): I recommend this test if you have a direct family member (sibling or parent) who has experienced a heart attack, stroke, or vascular disease, especially before age 70. Lipoprotein(a), or Lp(a) as it appears on blood tests, is a lipoprotein boat similar to LDL. However, Lp(a) also activates coagulation (blood clotting). Recall the three steps in heart disease: oxidation, inflammation, and coagulation. Compared to other ethnic groups, South Asians have one of the highest levels of Lp(a), a marker that is strongly associated with early and aggressive forms of heart disease.[7] Although there is no proven drug treatment to significantly reduce elevated Lp(a) (niacin and estrogen may modestly lower it), a high value should motivate immediate and more aggressive lifestyle changes, and may indicate the need for further testing.

Advanced lipid profiling: These tests examine more detailed information such as the different cholesterol subclasses, separate values for your type A LDL and type B LDL, and your LDL particle number (LDL-P). I often order these tests for patients who have an isolated elevation in LDL with no other risk factors. This is also a useful test if you have very high triglyceride levels, which interfere with the estimated LDL on a standard lipid test. As noted, LDL is not directly measured on a standard lipid panel, but instead calculated from the measured triglycerides and HDL. If your triglycerides are high, the calculation can be inaccurate. The advanced tests, on the other hand, directly measure LDL, so the results are accurate regardless of triglyceride level.

There are additional risk markers included in these profiles that may be of some use if you are in the care of a physician familiar with advanced lipid profiling. Examples of advanced lipid tests include the Berkeley Heart Lab, the VAP (vertical assisted profile), and the NMR lipoprofile test, which is currently the only FDA-approved method for measuring LDL particle numbers. Health Diagnostic Laboratory (HDL) also runs a detailed cholesterol panel.

There are many other numbers on these advanced lipid profiles—which look like detailed report cards, often color coded—that can be difficult to interpret. I would not obsess over these tests and don't recommend getting them done repeatedly. They don't add much more value than a standard lipid profile, and the lifestyle changes you need to make are usually the same. Advanced testing may be useful if you have borderline to abnormal cholesterol despite leading a healthy lifestyle with no other risk factors. Remember, your heart disease risk goes far beyond your cholesterol numbers regardless of how much cutting-edge data these panels provide. In that respect, the Metabolic 6-pack discussed in Chapter 1 gives you far more useful data about the health of your heart and blood vessels.

WORKING WITH YOUR DOCTOR

To date, most doctors rely on the traditional reading of cholesterol panels and miss the critical nuances of an insulin resistant lipid profile. Current clinical and nutrition guidelines for medication and dietary management of abnormal cholesterol are outdated. These seeds are planted early in medical training and reinforced repeatedly by continuing medical education (conferences, lectures, most medical journals, textbooks, etc.). I practiced this outmoded approach for a long time and only made these discoveries through my personal experience with cholesterol issues and the pandemic challenges faced by my patients. I had metabolic syndrome with a triglyceride level over 300, type B LDL, and an HDL that had dropped into the 20s despite the fact that I followed a strict, low-fat diet! I couldn't continue on such a health-compromising path, so I delved deeper into the research and discovered that if I fixed my triglycerides by lowering my carbohydrate intake, the other numbers would improve. Sure enough, I watched my triglycerides drop into the 70s, my HDL rise above 40, my LDL shift to type A, and my body fat drop into the single digit range. After applying these same principles to my patients and noticing similar results, I was convinced! Fortunately, I've found most doctors open to and inspired by this updated approach to cholesterol management, especially once they've witnessed remarkable improvements in patients who have implemented the recommended lifestyle changes. Choose a physician who is flexible and open to letting you try this health-saving approach. If you've failed the standard three-month low-fat diet trial, ask for another two- to three-month trial period in which to implement the dietary guidance outlined in Chapter 6. Don't let your physician prescribe medications (unless you are a true high-risk candidate who needs prescriptions) without first applying lifestyle modifications to turn your cholesterol numbers around. Be sure to have your numbers checked before and after, and discuss with your doctor the ratios outlined in the six cholesterol rules. If you feel your numbers are still not being accurately interpreted and your doctor prescribes lifelong medication therapy, seek a second opinion or a referral to a lipid specialist. You may need advanced lipid testing and want to make sure your doctor knows how to interpret these results.

The days of handing complete management of your medical condition to your doctor are over. It's important to take responsibility and conduct your own research. It's your body that's being potentially committed to decades of cholesterol medication, so make sure it's the right decision!

Coronary calcium testing: This non-invasive CT scan imaging test of your coronary arteries (your heart's blood vessels) measures calcium build-up using a standard scoring system called the Agatson score (named after Dr. Arthur Agatson, author of the *South Beach Diet*). Calcium build-up in your coronary arteries is a surrogate marker for atherosclerosis. The higher your Agatson score, the greater your risk. A score above 400 indicates an increased risk for a heart procedure (bypass surgery, stent, etc.) or cardiovascular event (heart attack, stroke) within two to five years. A score over 1000 indicates a 20 percent chance of suffering a heart attack or death due to a heart event within one year! A negative score is a fairly accurate predictor that you will not have a heart event in the next two to five years. Often the score report gives you an annual "cardiac mortality risk," which is a percent value, such as a 0.2% risk of heart disease death annually. It's important to understand that these reports do not account for your individual risk factors and often underestimate risk in South Asians. Any amount of plaque, especially when combined with one or more of the Metabolic 6-pack factors, needs to be taken seriously. Even a tiny plaque formation can instantly rupture and block off a blood vessel.

IMPROVING YOUR CHOLESTEROL LEVELS

Lifestyle changes can significantly and rapidly improve cholesterol levels. In some cases, making the right changes can completely eliminate the need for cholesterol medications. The following information will give you some guiding principles for improving your cholesterol and lowering overall heart disease risk.

Remember...don't obsess over the cholesterol numbers. I have patients who have incorporated exercise, shed pounds, decreased stress levels, added fresh vegetables and other antioxidant-rich foods to their diets, but only noted modest improvements in their total cholesterol, HDL cholesterol, and LDL cholesterol levels. What they don't immediately appreciate is that these changes, independent of their effects on cholesterol levels, have lowered the risk of heart attack by at least half. They have significantly reduced the toxic environment of inflammation and oxidation—which are prerequisites for atherosclerosis to occur—not to mention decreased the risk of multiple other chronic medical conditions ranging from cancer to Alzheimer's disease. You can't always measure these effects with a simple blood test, but countless studies have shown that these changes substantially improve longevity and quality of life.

A Big Picture View of Your Basic Cholesterol Panel

Instead of obsessing over individual numbers, take a broader view of your cholesterol panel. Treat it as one small component in the grand battle against heart disease and chronic disease. Remember the UCLA study that found that 75 percent of patients hospitalized for a heart attack had normal LDL levels? Such findings are an indication that lab results were overemphasized while key risk factors like stress, sedentary behavior, excess carbohydrate intake, and subsequent elevated insulin were underemphasized. Rather than succumb to the tempting idea that a particular set of numbers on your blood test makes you heart attack proof, it's imperative that you take in the big picture of the assorted risk factors of heart disease, particularly the fertile (or rather, "infertile") ground required for oxidation and inflammation of cholesterol particles. Rather than focusing only on your cholesterol results, think more about how to attack insulin resistance and inflammation by paying closer attention to your Metabolic 6-pack.

When looking at your cholesterol panel, see if it provides early clues to insulin resistance, especially one or more signs of the deadly lipid triad of high triglycerides, low HDL, and small, dense LDL. Remember that this dangerous combination is triggered by high triglycerides. If you do have an insulin resistant lipid profile, consider the chain of events that led to these results, often initiated by high triglycerides. Let's summarize:

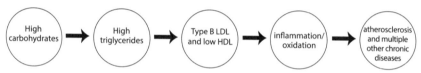

Lower your carbohydrate intake sufficiently and you potentially reverse most, if not all, of these adverse conditions. Sure, cutting out a large amount of carbs might be a big lifestyle challenge, but the improvement in your test results and the decrease in your heart disease risk can occur quickly and dramatically, making the change swift and quite literally painless.

Rather than focusing only on your cholesterol results, think more about how to attack insulin resistance and inflammation by paying closer attention to your Metabolic 6-pack. As you proceed with lifestyle modifications, your LDL can and often does elevate initially.

However, this frequently reflects a good consequence of shifting your LDL from bad type B to better type A. Bigger type A LDL boats can hold more cholesterol cargo, which is why LDL levels tend to drift up. Triglyceride-lowering medications like fibrates and fish oil can cause a similar increase in LDL levels, so don't panic if your numbers rise, especially if your ratios simultaneously improve, and don't let your doctor automatically prescribe a statin for what is actually a healthy LDL makeover.

Reducing Inflammation and Insulin Resistance

Even if you have reversed that deadly lipid triad, you still have the inflammation/oxidation problem to deal with. Having plenty of lower risk type A LDL boats won't protect you from a heart attack if you lead a highly inflammatory lifestyle. Many atherosclerotic experts believe that tackling inflammation should be the primary goal of our lifestyle and pharmaceutical efforts. I completely agree. So how do we do this?

Reduce carbohydrates: Carbohydrate reduction is the backbone of your lifestyle plan. Excess carbohydrate intake raises glucose levels, which triggers a host of inflammatory responses. How does this happen?

Glucose binds to protein in the blood to form what are called advanced glycation end products, or AGEs. (How's that for a fitting acronym? AGEs cause you to age...literally!) In atherosclerosis, AGEs bind to receptors on immune cells called receptors for advanced glycation end-products, or RAGEs. RAGEs stimulate a chemical called NF-kB. When activated, NF-kB triggers the production of a whole family of inflammatory chemicals that invoke the nasty blood vessel changes that cause atherosclerosis.

This chain of events is incentivized by excess glucose in the blood, which sparks the production of more AGEs. This AGE-->RAGE reaction has been linked to a growing list of chronic conditions, including Alzheimer's disease, cancer, and accelerated aging. When consumed to excess, carbohydrates are one of the most inflammatory substances you can put in your body. The worse the carb (i.e., high fructose corn syrup, sugar, etc.), the greater the inflammatory response.

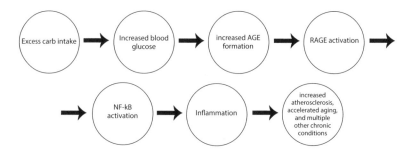

Exercise: We've focused primarily on dietary changes to slow down atherosclerosis, but we can't overlook the potent anti-inflammatory effects of a sensible exercise program. Notice the qualifier "sensible," because extreme exercise—such as marathon running or ironman triathlon training—can often be pro-inflammatory and actually elevate cardiac risk factors. A sensible workout pattern and an increased effort to move more each day improves your metabolizing (breaking down) of lipids and glucose. Being more active helps lower your triglycerides, the inciting factor leading to the insulin resistant cholesterol triad.

By improving your ability to break down sugar, exercise reduces the formation of those nasty AGE-RAGE complexes that promote inflammation. Exercise works on multiple other levels to reduce inflammation, including controlling the damaging effects of stress. One study showed that increased physical activity reduced heart disease and overall death rates in patients who had elevated hs-CRP levels, suggesting that physical activity has an anti-inflammatory effect.[8] We'll discuss exercise in more detail in Chapter 7.

Stress reduction: Never underestimate the role of stress in chronic disease. It's not coincidental that a stressful situation often triggered a devastating health event in my patients who already had existing risk factors. High stress levels are often the tipping factor that leads to plaque rupture. Not to mention, stress promotes high-risk behaviors like unhealthy eating, smoking, and reduced activity levels due to feelings of overwhelm.

Fortunately, there are mind-body healing modalities—such as yoga and meditation—that can help you significantly reduce and consistently monitor your stress levels. A UCLA study led by Steven W. Cole showed a reduction in NF-kB expression (a gene that triggers increased inflammation) after an eight-week program of a meditation technique called mindfulness based stress reduction (mbsr).[9] Stress reduction is discussed in further detail in Chapter 8.

Antioxidant-rich diet: Adding antioxidant-rich foods to your diet helps to moderate inflammation. For example, increased vegetable and fruit intake has been shown to lower hs-CRP levels.[10] We'll discuss foods with high concentrations of antioxidants in more detail in Chapter 6, but here's a quick list to get you started:

- Vegetables and fruits

- Fish

- Nuts and seeds

- Healthy fats

- Dark chocolate (in moderation)

- Red wine (in moderation)

Reduced abdominal fat: Belly fat is one of the most inflammatory regions of your body. If you were to look at belly fat cells under a microscope versus fat cells elsewhere (arms, legs, etc.), you would see an inflammatory factory at work. Belly fat actually produces a wide range of inflammatory chemicals, such as IL-6, an inflammatory agent directly correlated with elevated CRP levels. I have seen patients consistently reduce their CRP levels after dropping belly fat. A driving factor for storing excess abdominal fat in the first place is a high-stress, pro-inflammatory lifestyle. Yes, the belly, thighs, and trunk are common fat storage areas for most people, including South Asians, but belly fat represents a more specific metabolic problem.

Raised HDL: HDL not only disposes of excess cholesterol accumulated at the blood vessel wall, a process called reverse cholesterol transport, but this healthful type of cholesterol also reduces insulin resistance and, consequently, inflammation. HDL reduces insulin resistance by means of a protein called Apoprotein A-I (Apo A-I), which increases uptake of glucose by your cells.

Reducing carbohydrate intake is one of the best ways to raise HDL. In fact, one study done in Chennai, India confirmed that total carbohydrate intake and glycemic load were inversely proportional to HDL levels.[11] I have had far more success raising HDL in my South Asian patients by cutting carbohydrates than I have by implementing any other lifestyle intervention.

Quitting smoking, increasing exercise (both cardio and strength), and consuming alcohol in moderation (if you have no contraindications like liver disease, really high triglycerides, etc.) can also help raise HDL levels.

Should Anyone Be on Cholesterol Medications?

I know I've been critical about the overuse of cholesterol medications. However, individuals who have already had a vascular event (heart attack, stroke, blockage in a limb artery, etc.) can indeed benefit from prescription statins. These patients need all the help they can get when it comes to lowering their risk of yielding to a second potentially fatal event.

A growing number of studies and the 2013 guidelines support the notion that it's not the cholesterol-lowering effect but instead the pleiotropic effects of statins that are most important. Pleiotropic is a fancy word doctors use to indicate other benefits a drug may have in addition to its intended effect, which for statins is to lower cholesterol. The potential pleiotropic effects of statins include…

- Reduced inflammation

- Thinner blood, thereby preventing artery-blocking plaques from forming

- Stabilized plaques that reduce risk of rupture

I also prescribe statins and other lipid-lowering drugs to very high-risk patients who cannot carry out even a minimum level of recommended lifestyle changes. For example, I would prescribe a statin to an overweight patient with a strong family history of early heart disease and metabolic syndrome, especially if he/she smoked! As soon as lifestyle changes were implemented I would review the necessity of keeping this patient on cholesterol-lowering meds. If I'm on the fence, I might make a decision based on the advanced tests we just discussed. If the hs-CRP is high or if the patient's heart scan shows a high calcium score indicating plaque, I'll lean toward initiating a statin.

A smaller percentage of patients may inherit more severe forms of cholesterol disorders that lifestyle modification cannot treat sufficiently. These include patients with certain genetic mutations or enzyme deficiencies that can lead to very high triglycerides, very low HDL levels, and/or very high LDL levels. These patients need close physician supervision by a lipid expert, and medications are usually required.

Back to Vinod

Vinod was put on a typical regimen of heart medications and a low-fat diet as part of the standard post-heart attack protocol. He also incorporated exercise five days a week, enrolled in a program of mbsr (mindfulness based stress reduction), and achieved a modest weight loss of eight pounds. However, he still had excess belly fat and a triglyceride level that would not drop below 200 mg/dL.

It is very difficult to convince a heart attack patient that a low-fat diet may not be optimal for heart health (and may even be harmful) and that replacing so called "healthy carbs" with healthier fats is a better strategy towards reducing future heart attack risk. Vinod and I did agree that losing a few inches from his waistline and lowering his triglycerides would be a sign of progress. I asked him to bear with my dietary recommendations for one month, at which point we would check his triglycerides and waist measurement. Sure enough, his conscientious effort in prioritizing carb reduction without worrying about fat, while maintaining his exercise and mbsr, lowered his triglycerides to 95 mg/dL, the lowest level he had ever seen. He lost an additional eight pounds, mostly from the inflammatory danger zone of his waistline, and he reported feeling great.

Vinod's story is like that of so many other South Asians who have similar lab results and who continue to follow outdated nutrition guidelines that push a low-fat, low-cholesterol diet. I recently visited a close friend in the hospital after he had suffered a heart attack and looked, aghast, at his "heart healthy" breakfast tray: a bowl of oatmeal with raisins and brown sugar, a banana, a low-fat blueberry muffin, a slice of whole wheat toast, and a glass of orange juice. This traditional breakfast is the ultimate symbol of how we continue to march backwards in the fight against obesity and chronic disease, brainwashed by erroneous government-issued guidelines and bombarded by unhealthy food options everywhere we turn. For insulin resistant South Asian children and adults, this toxic food environment has an even greater impact on health. The good news is that most South Asians can realize dramatic improvements in their cholesterol and other health risk factors when they finally get their hands on the right information.

Summary

- High quality, natural, unprocessed sources of saturated fat and dietary cholesterol simply and unequivocally do not increase blood cholesterol and heart disease risk, especially when consumed in the context of a lower carbohydrate diet.

- Inflammation is a far greater cause of heart disease and chronic disease than is high cholesterol.

- Follow the six rules for interpreting cholesterol results to gain a better understanding of what your numbers mean.

- Use the Metabolic 6-pack from Chapter 1 as a better overall assessment of heart and chronic disease risk.

- Eat an antioxidant-rich diet to reduce inflammation.

- Increase activity and manage stress to further reduce inflammation.

For Professionals

I urge all physicians and patients to use the information in this chapter to broaden their understanding of lipid profiles beyond the simplistic LDL-centered view pushed for so many years by antiquated guidelines. The controversy and contradictions that appear in the 2013 guidelines should be evidence that prior approaches to interpreting and treating cholesterol disorders have been seriously flawed. It makes no sense to prescribe a cholesterol-lowering drug to a healthy patient who shows no signs of insulin resistance or inflammation. We need to stop reducing our patients to a single number (LDL, total cholesterol, etc.), when determining a prescription for health. Physicians must provide detailed instructions on diet and exercise in order to give patients the best chance of reducing risk. Putting patients on lifelong cholesterol medications after prescribing an ineffective, unsustainable lifestyle plan has become the norm in medical practice, and I regret that it was a part of my own practice when I first came out of training. We need to take advantage of the tremendous amount of resources available to help patients reach their goals naturally. Unfortunately, most of the handouts and resources we give patients are still focused on low-fat, low-cholesterol diets that usually end up doing one of the following:

- Worsening lipids and weight by replacing fat with more carbohydrates.

- Leaving lipids relatively unchanged, but leaving patients frustrated since their results are not proportional to the amount of effort and sacrifice they are expending. Inevitably this plan fails.

- Improving lipids and weight in patients who led previously unhealthy lifestyles.

Note: an improvement in lipids and weight is usually not due to lowering fat or cholesterol, but due to patients' dietary changes, such as eliminating sodas, fast foods, and high fructose corn syrup, and incorporating lifestyle changes such as exercise. This is a good outcome, but sends patients the wrong message and may cause future challenges with weight and lipid issues. Patients need to understand that dropping the sugar, excess carbs, and trans fats were the primary drivers for success, as opposed to cutting back on dietary cholesterol and saturated fat.

If you are a physician who still hesitates to recommend a low-carb versus low-fat approach, try the lifestyle plan in this book on a few of your patients who have the more important cholesterol abnormalities discussed (elevated triglycerides, low HDL, elevated TC/HDL ratio, etc.) and who have failed repeatedly at implementing lifestyle changes. Recheck the results in two to three months. Hopefully a few case examples in your own practice will make a believer out of you.

Treating cholesterol disorders correctly with appropriate lifestyle changes rather than with premature and often unnecessary medications is not just the right thing to do; it also makes the practice of medicine so much more rewarding. I've received more gratitude from patients as a result of this approach than I ever have for prescribing cholesterol medications. That's because medication pinpoints the reduction of a few numbers on a cholesterol report. Prescribing lifestyle changes that work not only improves numbers, but also physically and emotionally transforms patients into stronger, fitter, more confident individuals who thrive in every area of their lives.

- Avoid overemphasizing LDL and pay closer attention to triglycerides, HDL, and the ratios mentioned in the six cholesterol rules.

- Triglycerides and body fat decrease quickly when excess carbs are lowered in the diet. A rise in HDL levels should follow. Monitor these numbers to motivate patients.

- Triglycerides over 150 mg/dL and especially over 200 mg/dL are strongly associated with more dangerous type B LDL. Ignore the outdated "normal" reference range on most standard lab reports that make 150 or 200 mg/dL the cutoff, and instead aim for a goal level of less than 100 mg/dL.

- Educate patients as to how to track their cholesterol numbers. Encourage them to stop focusing on total cholesterol and instead focus on ratios like the total cholesterol-to-HDL and the triglyceride-to-HDL ratios.

- For employers performing biometric screenings, offer full lipid panels (total cholesterol, triglycerides, HDL, and LDL) when possible. Total cholesterol alone is not useful in determining cardiovascular risk in most South Asians.

CHAPTER 3

BLOOD PRESSURE:
THE PRESSURE IS KILLING ME

HIGH BLOOD PRESSURE, OR HYPERTENSION, rings the alarm that multiple systems in your body are out of balance. It is most likely caused by a combination of a poor diet, sedentary lifestyle, health-leaching habits like smoking and excess alcohol intake, and emotional stress. In fact, out of all the Metabolic 6-pack criteria, blood pressure is most intimately tied to stress. Some of my patients, who execute all the right nutrition and exercise changes, may still not reach optimal blood pressure levels due to internalized stress and anxiety. Genetics, represented by your family history, can also play a strong role in hypertension. An individual with a parent with hypertension is about twice as likely to develop high blood pressure. To date, researchers have identified 28 blood pressure genes, and some studies have found a higher prevalence of hypertension in individuals of South Asian, African-American, and African-Caribbean descent.

Regardless of your family history, it is possible to reverse, or at least minimize, the effects of high blood pressure by implementing an all-inclusive lifestyle plan before resorting to medications. Don't worry; I will provide a step-wise plan at the end of this chapter to help you lower your blood pressure without medications, but first let's start with a case of high blood pressure in a South Asian senior.

Case Study: Nirmala

Nirmala is a 74-year-old vegetarian woman who came to see me with her daughter. She complained of severe arthritis pain in both her knees. Her only course of treatment was 800 mg of ibuprofen three times a day for several months. It was obvious Nirmala was uncomfortable, as she kept massaging her kneecaps. However, the most startling discovery was that her measured blood pressure was 230/110. I repeated her blood pressure several times in both arms and got similar values. She denied any chest pain, shortness of breath, headaches, dizziness, or numbness or weakness in her arms or legs. Aside from her arthritis, she seemed bright and energetic. Upon further questioning, she did state that her doctor in India had recommended blood pressure medication, but she refused. She told me she felt fine and didn't need medication.

If, fresh out of medical school, I had seen a blood pressure reading this high, my own blood pressure would have skyrocketed as I panicked about all the associated complications I had read about in medical school...a dissecting aorta, a heart attack, a stroke, etc. Unfortunately, I've gotten quite used to blood pressures in this range. Nirmala exemplifies why high blood pressure is called a "silent killer." Most patients with dangerously elevated blood pressures may have absolutely no symptoms at all. Typically, I pick up on these values when patients come to see me for an unrelated complaint, like Nirmala's arthritis pain. If you recall from our discussion on cholesterol, many patients and some doctors have developed a case of "triglyceride desensitization" that accepts high triglycerides as the norm. Unfortunately, this same desensitization is often applied to high blood pressure. It is so common in the South Asian community that unless levels are extremely high and fall into the stage 2 hypertension range (with a top number above 160 and/or a bottom number above 100), high blood pressure is often disregarded.

UNDERSTANDING BLOOD PRESSURE

Nirmala's blood pressure is on the extreme end, but high blood pressure at any level is not a condition to ignore. A borderline blood pressure can affect your health as adversely as smoking a few cigarettes a day; when your blood pressure number goes up, it's as though you are adding more cigarettes and more risk. Even a mildly elevated blood pressure will have a cumulative toxic effect on the health of your blood vessels and virtually every organ in your body.

In this section, I'll explain what your blood pressure numbers actually represent and how they impact your risk of chronic health conditions. Once you understand the basics, you'll recognize how lifestyle factors like dietary salt, carbohydrates, and stress influence blood pressure.

What Diastolic and Systolic Values Represent

Your blood pressure reading consists of two numbers separated by a "/" such as "120/80," verbally referred to as "one-twenty over eighty." The top number of your blood pressure reading is called the systolic pressure and the bottom is the diastolic pressure. Systolic sounds like "pistolic," a mnemonic to help you remember that the top number represents the pressure in your arteries right after the heart contracts (or "shoots") blood into your arteries, much like a pistol. Your systolic pressure will always be higher than your diastolic pressure, which is the pressure in the arteries after the heart relaxes. So in essence, blood pressure represents how much force is exerted on the walls of your blood vessels. The higher the blood pressure, the more force exerted on your arteries; over time this pressure causes your blood vessels to wear away, much like the pipes in your home would if you were to keep your faucets continuously running at high pressure.

As discussed in Chapter 2, the plaques leading to heart attack and stroke form when there is damage to the inner blood vessel lining or ECL (endothelial cell lining). Elevated blood pressure is one of the primary causes of ECL injury, triggering the familiar cascade of inflammation and blood clotting that lead to heart attack or stroke. The repercussions of high blood pressure affect your eyes, kidneys, brain, heart, limbs…every organ of your body is enmeshed in a network of blood vessels and therefore vulnerable!

Let's break it down:

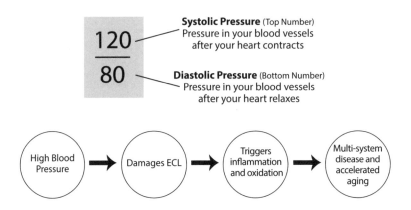

Systolic Pressure (Top Number)
Pressure in your blood vessels after your heart contracts

Diastolic Pressure (Bottom Number)
Pressure in your blood vessels after your heart relaxes

High Blood Pressure → Damages ECL → Triggers inflammation and oxidation → Multi-system disease and accelerated aging

The Mechanics of High Blood Pressure

Medical textbooks indicate that 5-10 percent of high blood pressure is due to some underlying cause such as thyroid disease, renal artery stenosis (narrowing of the kidney arteries), medication side effect, etc. The remaining 90-95 percent is due to "essential hypertension," which means we don't really know what is causing the high blood pressure.

Not enough emphasis has been placed on insulin resistance, which in my experience is the top cause of high blood pressure in my South Asian patients. Before I explain the link between insulin resistance and high blood pressure, let's talk about two major mechanisms that cause blood pressure to go up.

Wall stiffness: The walls of your blood vessels, particularly the arteries, should be nice and supple to accommodate the blood circulating through them. The more stiff they become, the more pressure is exerted against their walls, which results in higher blood pressures. The stiffness of your blood vessels depends on many factors, including various chemicals.

Chemicals that keep the blood vessels relaxed and open (dilated) are referred to as vasodilators, while those that keep vessels rigid and narrow (constricted) are called vasoconstrictors. For example, nitric oxide is a potent vasodilator (reduces blood pressure) produced in the body, while angiotensin II is a strong vasoconstrictor (raises blood pressure).

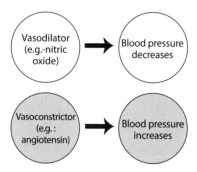

Blood vessel volume: The amount of blood in your blood vessels also determines your blood pressure. Think of a blood vessel as a garden hose. Keep filling the garden hose with more and more water, and the walls expand and the pressure within the hose rises. If the walls are soft and pliable, the hose may be able to accommodate this increased blood volume, but if the walls are stiff, then the combination can generate a tremendous increase in your blood pressure, as in Nirmala's case.

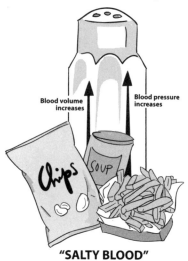

Salt (sodium) plays a key role in influencing blood volume. When you eat something extremely salty, you tend to crave water. Your blood vessels react the same way. When they sense too much "saltiness" from excess sodium, they draw extra fluid inside, raising your blood volume and subsequently your blood pressure. Sodium and fluid regulation is actually an extremely complex physiological process involving several hormones in the body. Let's summarize:

"SALTY BLOOD"
Increased dietary sodium from processed foods

Maintaining normal blood pressure is an intricate balance of regulating your body's vasoconstrictors, vasodilators, sodium, and blood volume. Your lifestyle habits directly influence these factors.

Insulin Resistance and High Blood Pressure

The excess insulin from insulin resistance directly influences the underlying mechanisms for high blood pressure. Excess insulin is a vasoconstrictor that increases wall stiffness and fluid retention, both of which lead to a rise in blood pressure. Fluid retention is due to insulin's effects on the kidneys; excess insulin causes your body to hold onto more salt and water and lose essential potassium. The link between insulin resistance and hypertension may start early in life with the birth of low-birth-weight babies.

As we've seen, insulin is a major determinant of body fat storage and a prime cause of obesity. Excess body fat increases your heart's work, since the heart has to deliver a greater volume of blood to these abundant areas of fat tissue. As your heart's workload increases, so do your heart rate (pulse) and your blood pressure. Not to mention, abdominal fat cells produce a wide range of chemicals that increase inflammation. Belly fat also releases angiotensinogen II, which we've learned is a potent vasoconstrictor that raises blood pressure. Let's visually check out the chain reaction insulin resistance sets into motion:

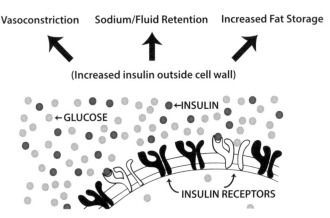

What is the Ideal Blood Pressure?

There is considerable confusion over what number represents normal blood pressure. In my opinion, a normal blood pressure is a level that does not increase your risk of having a heart attack, stroke, or other medical condition. Normal is classified as a top number below 120 and a bottom number below 80. Studies show that for every 20-point increase in the systolic and 10-point increase in the diastolic above a blood pressure of 115/75, your heart attack and stroke risk double. So, a blood pressure of 135/85 has double the risk compared to 115/75, and a reading of 155/95 quadruples the risk of heart attack or stroke. Now you can imagine where Nirmala's blood pressure of 230/110 would put her if left untreated. Despite feeling no symptoms, she was utterly vulnerable to a health disaster. The current classification of high blood pressure is listed below.

Blood Pressure Stage	Systolic (top number)	Diastolic (bottom number)
Normal	less than 120	**and** less than 80
Prehypertension	120-139	**or** 80-89
Stage 1 hypertension	140-159	**or** 90-99
Stage 2 hypertension	160 or more	**or** 100 or more

Notice that even prehypertensive blood pressures are above the threshold optimal blood pressure of 115/75. In other words, pre-hypertension doesn't just put you at a higher risk for hypertension; it puts you at a higher risk for heart attack and stroke. Do keep in mind that the ideal blood pressure number can vary depending on the individual. For example, some seniors may require multiple blood pressure medications to achieve a blood pressure of 120/80. This overload of prescriptions may be riskier than accepting a higher blood pressure goal of say 140/90. Always discuss your individual blood pressure goal with your doctor.

Monitoring Your Blood Pressure

If you have ever had a single abnormal blood pressure, I recommend you track your own blood pressure on a periodic basis, checking more frequently if it's high. Studies show that your home-recorded blood pressure is a better indicator of heart attack risk than the one mea-sured in the office, assuming you are performing the test correctly. You might be nervous in a doctor's office and generate a higher than normal reading. "White-coat hypertension" is one form of stress-in-duced hypertension in which blood pressures are always elevated in the doctor's office due to concerns about health issues. If you deliver a high reading in the doctor's office, measure your blood pressure at home using the following guidelines:

- Wait at least 30 minutes after consuming food, coffee, or nicotine (if you smoke, please quit!).

- Empty your bladder before checking your blood pressure (a full bladder can elevate blood pressure).

- Ideally, try to sit calmly for 5-10 minutes before checking.

- Don't talk or fidget while checking.

- Position your arm at heart level by resting it on a table or other flat surface.

- Use an arm cuff rather than a wrist cuff, and be sure it is large enough. The inflatable part should be at least two-thirds the circumference of your arm. A cuff that's too small typically will give a higher reading.

- Take two to three readings in one sitting, waiting at least one minute between readings. The initial blood pressure tends to run higher when you first sit down, so repeating the readings allows for better accuracy.

- Use a reliable manufacturer like *Omron* and periodically take your cuff to your doctor's office to verify accuracy. A slight discrepancy between your monitor and your doctor's is expected.

- Try to monitor at different times of the day so you know your average morning, mid-day, and bedtime blood pressures.

If you are a techie, consider purchasing a blood pressure monitor that uploads your numbers onto a digital device so that you can keep an online log and share with your doctor. The manufacturer *Withings* makes an arm cuff that connects directly to your Iphone/Ipad and allows you to track your blood pressure along with other factors, such as your weight and nutritional data. If you have family members in India or abroad who don't have ready access to a home blood pressure monitor, buy one for them and teach them how to use it. This may be the most important gift you can take on your trips to see loved ones.

DIETARY MANAGEMENT OF
HIGH BLOOD PRESSURE

The link between diet and blood pressure has been held together by the salt shaker for far too long. Although sodium (salt) does play a role, especially in the form of processed foods, the balance of sodium and potassium is far more important in the battle against high blood pressure. Most people don't even think about how their intake of carbohydrates can influence blood pressure, primarily through the action of insulin. The unfounded fear of all forms of dietary fat causes people to avoid consuming even healthy blood-pressure-lowering fats. Let's review each of these factors in detail, as well as additional dietary changes you can make to help lower blood pressure without medication.

Your Sodium-Potassium Ratio (SPR)

When couples come to see me, a spouse may complain, "my husband puts too much salt on his food." The problem is not the salt, but what the salt is being sprinkled on, which may be a plate full of rice, lentils, and Indian flat breads. Most of the sodium in your diet does not come from the salt shaker, but instead comes from the processed, packaged, and restaurant foods that have become dietary staples. In essence, sodium is a surrogate marker for processed, packaged foods in your diet.

In addition to the abundance of sodium obtained through unnatural foods, the other overlooked factor is the lack of the mineral potassium found in natural, plant-based foods. Potassium is a mineral that helps relax stiff blood vessels and allows your kidneys to remove excess sodium in your body. Plant-based sources rich in potassium include spinach, broccoli, avocados, oranges, nuts, and seeds. My average South Asian patient consumes far fewer of these foods than other ethnic groups do. Often it's one or two overcooked vegetable curry dishes (sabjis) and no additional raw vegetable or fruit snacks.

The simple act of replacing packaged foods with fresh, real foods will tip your sodium-to-potassium ratio in the right direction.

The sodium-to-potassium ratio (SPR) is more important than the amount of sodium added from the salt shaker.[1] SPR represents the ratio of processed (sodium) to plant-based (potassium) foods in your diet. Now, you don't have to measure grams of sodium and potassium directly, as this would be impractical and inaccurate. The simple act of replacing packaged foods with fresh, real foods will tip your SPR in the right direction. Don't forget that this ratio is made worse by carb-driven insulin elevations, since insulin makes your body hold onto more sodium and lose more potassium.

The other potent "S" ingredient in processed foods is "S"yrup, as in high fructose corn syrup (HFCS). This heavily processed sweetener is present in a huge percentage of processed foods found in virtually every grocery story. Among the many ways HFCS is harmful to your health is the double whammy damage it does to your SPR. First, HFCS directly increases sodium retention through its effects on the kidneys. Second, because it spikes insulin levels perhaps more than anything else you may eat, you experience increased vasoconstriction, fat storage, and further salt and fluid retention.

Look carefully at each meal and snack you eat and try to determine how you can improve your SPR. Can you add more vegetables to your plate and minimize the excess carbs? Can you replace that packaged salty snack with a serving of vegetables, fruits, nuts, and/or seeds?

Once you've successfully cut out processed foods, cut back on carbs, and incorporated plant-based meals, you may want to add some salt for flavor and satisfaction. The drop in insulin levels from lowering carbohydrates makes your body lose more sodium and water. Staying well hydrated and replenishing some of this lost sodium can help prevent fatigue and may curb cravings for salty, crispy processed snacks later on.

Let's not forget that some people are extremely salt-sensitive, so if you try everything I suggest and still have elevated blood pressure, you may need to further restrict your added salt and limit your daily intake of sodium to less than 1.5 to 2 grams. Be advised that excess sodium can interfere with the effectiveness of blood pressure medications.

Cutting Excess Carbohydrates

Excess carbohydrates in the South Asian diet are potent stimulators of high blood pressure. Nirmala ate a typical South Asian vegetarian diet that was actually more abundant in grains than in vegetables, what I call a "grainatarian diet." The grainatarian diet incorporates a low "net" intake of vegetables and fruits; the same amount of fruits and vegetables has less benefit when consumed alongside an excess carbohydrate diet, especially from grains. That's because grains contain "anti-nutrients" like phytic acid which block your body from absorbing essential nutrients such as vitamin D and iron. Anti-nutritive effects of grains neutralize many of the beneficial blood-pressure-lowering effects of fruits and vegetables. Nirmala ate minimal fat and made a conscious effort to lower added salt based on her prior doctor's recommendations. However, the excess carbs led directly to increased insulin levels, which had the following blood-pressure-raising effects:

- Increased weight due to insulin-triggered body fat accumulation and fluid retention

- Unfavorable SPR due to increased sodium retention and potassium loss

- Increased insulin-mediated vasoconstriction and sodium/fluid retention within blood vessels

The reduction in blood pressure often occurs very quickly once patients decrease carbohydrate intake. With carb intake and insulin levels lowered, stored body fat is broken down into free fatty acids available to burn for energy during exercise. I guarantee you will feel like being more active because you will literally have more energy pumping through your bloodstream (in the form of fatty acids as well as glucose) when you moderate carb intake and insulin production!

With improved dietary habits, your body loses not only excess fat but also excess water retention weight (thanks to moderated sodium levels). The loss of water weight is particularly noticeable in women, as hormonal changes often cause fluid retention.

What About Legumes?

Legumes are often prescribed as a heart and blood-pressure-friendly food. They are also staples of the South Asian diet. The good news is that legumes are a great source of the blood-pressure-lowering minerals, potassium and magnesium. The disadvantage is that, despite their nutritional value, they are predominantly carbohydrates and as such increase the overall insulin load you are trying to moderate.

The blood-pressure-raising effects of insulin far outweigh the benefits of obtaining potassium and magnesium through legumes. If—and this is a big if—you consume legumes in moderation and keep them within the carbohydrate goal range recommended in Chapter 6, then they are likely an acceptable element of your diet. Be sure to consume legumes with vegetables and/or meat rather than with rice or a chapati in order to avoid a double dose of carbohydrates. A nice vegetable dal dish maximizes the vegetable portion and minimizes the lentil portion. Feel free to add ghee or olive oil to improve richness and satiety. When preparing legumes, it is best to purchase them raw, then soak and sprout them. Buying raw and preparing appropriately will lower the concentration of an anti-nutrient called lectin, and enhance the nutritional value.

Incorporating Healthy Fats

In addition to cutting excess carbohydrates and sodium, incorporate healthy fats into your diet. Emphasize the following two blood-pressure-lowering fats:

Monounsaturated fats: These fats are a core component of the heart-healthy diet and include foods such as olive oil, nuts, seeds, and avocados. Nuts, seeds, and avocados are also excellent potassium sources! One study showed that 40 grams (4 tablespoons) daily of extra virgin olive oil for just four months cut blood pressure in half in hypertensive individuals taking medication![1]

Omega-3s: The predominant source of omega-3 essential fatty acids is oily, coldwater fish (especially wild-caught salmon, mackerel, herring, sardines, and anchovies). Some studies have shown the modest blood-pressure-lowering effect of omega-3s.[3] If you aren't inclined to consume these types of fish regularly, omega-3 fish oil supplements are an option. However, there is conflicting data on safety and the overall effectiveness of taking omega-3 supplements for overall cardiovascular health. Until the data is more definitive, try to obtain your omega-3s from natural food sources.

Adding Magnesium

Every organ in your body needs the mineral magnesium. It is a vital cofactor to numerous chemical reactions in the body that lead to energy production, and it helps regulate levels of potassium, calcium, vitamin D, copper, and zinc. That's right, a deficiency in a mineral like potassium, which we learned is important for blood pressure control, is often secondary to a deficiency in magnesium. It is estimated that the majority of people are to some degree deficient in magnesium. Why? Because modern day soil is depleted of magnesium and other nutrients like zinc, phosphorus, vitamin B-6, and vitamin E.[4] You won't catch magnesium deficiency on a standard magnesium blood test because only about one percent of your body's magnesium stores are in the blood, while the rest sit in other storage sites like your tissues and bones.

Eating copious amounts of plant-based foods in the form of vegetables, fruits, nuts, and seeds does provide magnesium, but for many people not enough. If you have tried optimizing your diet, managing stress, and increasing activity levels but are still experiencing elevated blood pressure, a magnesium supplement is worth a try. A reasonable dose is 400 mg daily for men and 300 mg daily for women. Magnesium citrate powder is a well-absorbed form of magnesium that is stirred into water. Topical magnesium oil allows even better absorption through the skin. Additional benefits of magnesium supplementation include potentially reducing heart palpitations, improving sleep, and reducing anxiety. Many patients report an overall "calming" effect after taking magnesium for four to six months, which may also help with stress-induced hypertension. Talk to your doctor before starting any supplement program, as magnesium supplements may not be safe for certain medical conditions.

Addressing Vitamin D Deficiency

We discussed the possible link between vitamin D deficiency and insulin resistance in Chapter 1. There appears to be an association between low vitamin D and high blood pressure as well. In fact, a study made up of African Americans with low vitamin D levels found that taking a vitamin D supplement lowered blood pressure.[5] We will discuss vitamin D deficiency in more detail in Chapter 11, along with recommended doses.

BEHAVIORS THAT RAISE BLOOD PRESSURE

We've examined at length how dietary factors influence blood pressure, but even if you optimize your dietary habits by following every shred of advice dispensed in this book, you can still run into problems if you don't properly manage the everyday stress of modern life. Another serious risk factor for high blood pressure is sedentary lifestyle patterns. First, you are lacking the exercise that serves as a great balance to the many desk-oriented careers that promote sustained periods of inactivity. Second, the physical decline associated with insufficient exercise can inhibit your ability to withstand common stressors of modern life, such as germs, polluted air, sweet foods you happen to indulge in from time to time, as well as the occasional physical activity you do engage in, weekend warrior style, but are not sufficiently prepared for. Finally, there are the substances such as prescription drugs, tobacco, recreational drugs, caffeine, alcohol, and even nutritional supplements that can adversely affect blood pressure.

The Stress Factor

Blood pressure typically increases in response to environmental stress. For our ancestors, this had an adaptive benefit. When faced with physical stressors like fighting or fleeing danger, the boost in blood pressure would increase the delivery of blood and oxygen to working muscles.

In the face of famine and dehydration, stress-induced vasoconstriction helped keep blood pressure high enough to deliver oxygen and nutrients to the brain and vital organs until we were able to find sustenance. If we were bleeding from a wound, vasoconstriction would act like an internal tourniquet and prevent us from bleeding to death.

Today, the nature of stress is very different in that our stressors are mostly chronic (never-ending—like the flood of emails into your inbox) instead of intermittent. Hence, the adaptive response of blood pressure increasing under stress becomes maladaptive by promoting hypertension.

Not everyone has stress-induced hypertension. Some people have very resilient blood vessels that are immune to blood pressure elevations unless the stressor is extreme, such as a life-threatening event. Others are so sensitive that even the slightest intrusive thought can be a hypertensive trigger.

If you have been diagnosed with high blood pressure or cardiac risk factors, I strongly recommend you monitor your blood pressure at different times of the day and in different situations to see if you have stress-induced hypertension.

BREATHING AWAY HIGHER BLOOD PRESSURES

You can monitor stress-induced hypertension by paying attention to your breathing. Notice how you breathe when you are relaxed versus when you are anxious. Normally, anxiety provokes more rapid, shallow breathing. Sensations range from not being able to take a deep breath in, to an almost suffocating feeling.

Your autonomic nervous system regulates stress. It is divided into the sympathetic (stress response) and parasympathetic (relaxation response) components. When stress is under control, your parasympathetic system is dominant, and the sympathetic system takes a back seat. Heart rate variability (HRV) is an excellent indicator of whether your parasympathetic system is in control. When you are in a calm, relaxed state, your breathing and heart rate work rhythmically in a fashion that produces increased HRV, while stressful situations produce low HRV states. Meditation and yoga, especially practices that incorporate pranayama or diaphragmatic breathing techniques, can help lower blood pressure. In essence, controlling stress often means controlling your breath, which in turn leads to beneficial effects on heart rate and blood pressure, mediated through your autonomic nervous system. We'll discuss effective stress management techniques in detail in Chapter 8—I've even recommended a useful app that can keep your HRV in check!

Sedentary Lifestyle

Marathon sitting sessions at the computer are detrimental to blood pressure and overall health. Prolonged sitting not only makes it more difficult to shed pounds due to fewer calories burned (excess body weight is a major cause of hypertension), but also promotes fat storage by disturbing important appetite-regulating hormones such as leptin. As a first measure, try to increase the frequency of movement breaks you take during a workday, and gradually add steps to your day (you can track steps with a simple smartphone app) with an eventual goal of 8,000-10,000 steps daily. Transition to a standup workstation in the office. Chapter 7 offers advice on incorporating "active work" in the office and at home. Even light to moderate activity in intermittent bouts (multiple short walks, etc.) delivers antihypertensive effects by lowering levels of the stress hormone cortisol, and raising levels of nitric oxide, a powerful blood vessel relaxer.

Substances

Some blood-pressure-raising factors to look out for are listed below.

Medications: Nirmala's intake of NSAID painkillers (ibuprofen, naproxen, etc.) may be contributing to higher blood pressure. Other medications that can raise blood pressure include, but are not limited to, cough and cold decongestants and certain migraine medications.

Supplements: Surprisingly, certain herbals, nutritional supplements, homeopathic remedies, and Ayurvedic medications can potentially contribute to hypertension. Many weight loss supplements commonly contain blood-pressure-raising stimulants. If you have high blood pressure, talk to your doctor about which supplements to quit in order to see if your blood pressure drops.

Caffeine: Excessive caffeine may directly raise blood pressure in some individuals. Too much caffeine can also contribute to stress and anxiety, which indirectly raise blood pressure, especially in stress-sensitive hypertensives. Experiment with curtailing caffeine use and track improvement. Avoid caffeinated sodas, since they have both a stimulant and insulin-triggering effect.

Alcohol: One serving of alcohol daily is fine for women and no more than two servings for men. Self-experimentation is recommended so you can assess the impact of alcohol on your blood pressure.

SIX STEPS TO LOWERING BLOOD PRESSURE

We've discussed many different recommendations for reducing blood pressure, and fortunately only a few lifestyle changes are necessary to incorporate most of these changes. If you feel overwhelmed and can only prioritize one or two items at a time, I suggest tackling the following steps in sequential order. If you are committed to a comprehensive attack on your high blood pressure, then by all means incorporate these steps simultaneously.

Step 1: Get your Metabolic 6-pack numbers measured (don't use a panel from a year ago!) and also include a vitamin D test. If your vitamin D is low, immediately start taking supplements and getting more sun exposure on large skin surface areas of your body.

Step 2: If any of the Metabolic 6-pack numbers are abnormal, reduce your carb intake by following the lifestyle plan in Chapter 6. In the process, be sure to increase your intake of healthy fats. Recall the potentially powerful effects of adding just four tablespoons of extra virgin olive oil to your daily eating plan. Reducing body fat and insulin resistance, along with adding heart healthy fats to your diet, can have an immediate favorable impact on your blood pressure and overall cardiac risk. Even if you don't fulfill any of the metabolic criteria, following this step should still improve your overall health and keep you at a safe distance from adverse 6-pack numbers.

Step 3: Increase your daily activity levels and incorporate brief exercise sessions as outlined in Chapter 7. Ideally, I would like you to combine Steps 2 and 3, since they work synergistically. Even if Step 2 reduces your blood pressure to a normal range, at some point you must incorporate exercise to reduce the risk of nearly every other disease known to mankind. If you are already physically active, add some more resistance training or interval training to your regimen.

Step 4: If your blood pressure is still too high, you need to determine the impact of life stress on your readings. Use a blood pressure monitor at home and at work, and keep an online or handwritten blood pressure diary. This can be eye opening. If you show signs of stress-induced hypertension, be sure to read Chapter 8, which will give you many practical tips on managing and monitoring stress.

Step 5: Reduce your SPR further by eating more plants and fewer processed foods. There is always room to improve on this ratio. Chapter 6 discusses the 6-S approach (Salads, Smoothies, Sauces, Soups, Snacks, Substitutions for grains) to maximize the nutritional value of your diet and minimize your SPR. Do not underestimate the antihypertensive effects of increasing your consumption of plant-based foods and reducing your intake of processed ones.

Step 6: Consider supplements. If you haven't already, and your doctor approves, I suggest adding magnesium supplements to your diet.

If you fail to control blood pressure with this type of approach, by all means adhere to your doctor's recommendation to medicate high blood pressure. The side effects of high blood pressure far outweigh the potential harms of most blood pressure medications. However, don't be one of the millions of people who use medication as a crutch. Follow your medication protocol, but redouble your lifestyle modification efforts as if your life depends on it, because it does! If you make considerable improvements in your weight and overall health at a later time, you can discuss with your doctor the possibility of cutting back on medications or eliminating them altogether.

> *Don't be one of the millions of people who use medication as a crutch. Follow your medication protocol, but redouble your lifestyle modification efforts as if your life depends on it, because it does!*

A Practical Approach for Nirmala

Controlling blood pressure is probably the most difficult of the Metabolic 6-pack factors to treat with lifestyle alone. The stronger the genetic risks and the older you are, the greater the likelihood that medication may be necessary. Nirmala's age, coupled with the fact that she had severe, uncontrolled hypertension for years, meant she needed a combination of medication and lifestyle changes to manage her numbers. If she had regular blood pressure screenings and her hypertension was caught earlier, she likely would not have needed medications and we could have protected her ECL from years of damage. The good news is that we caught it before she had a heart attack or stroke.

We were also able to minimize her medication use. Nirmala had stage 2 hypertension and current treatment guidelines recommend starting with two medications. Three to four medications would have been typical for her level of blood pressure elevation. Nirmala was able to drop 12 pounds by reducing excess carbs, incorporating an abundance of plant-based foods, and increasing her daily steps. She only needed one medication to get her blood pressure to goal range, while losing some body fat and increasing activity levels improved her quality of life. In fact, she no longer needed ibuprofen since her arthritis pain became minimal thanks to the combination of reduced weight on her knees and anti-inflammatory lifestyle habits. Since high dose anti-inflammatory medications like ibuprofen can cause kidney damage and bleeding ulcers and worsen hypertension, especially in seniors, dropping that medication alone significantly reduced Nirmala's future risk of developing a significant medical complication. Since she lived with her son's family and was in charge of most of the cooking, her healthy changes trickled down to the entire family.

Summary

- High blood pressure is a "silent killer" that normally does not cause symptoms.

- Get a screening blood pressure at least annually and monitor more frequently if there are any abnormal values.

- Insulin resistance, worsened by excessive carbohydrate consumption, is a major cause of hypertension in South Asians.

- Do not underestimate the impact of stress on high blood pressure.

- Sedentary behavior can raise blood pressure levels.

For Professionals

- Counsel patients on the link between carbohydrates, insulin resistance, and hypertension. Most hypertension handouts do not emphasize this link.

- Go beyond "limit sodium in the diet" to focus on optimizing the sodium-to-potassium ratio by reducing processed foods and increasing natural foods.

- Make stress management a key part of blood pressure control.

- Recognize vitamin D deficiency as a potential contributor to high blood pressure.

- Have patients track home blood pressures and share results with you during visits and online.

CHAPTER 4

YOUR BODY:
WIDTH OVER WEIGHT

LET'S START BY REDEFINING THE meaning of fat. When I use the word "fat," it's not in the derogatory "fatso" or fat-equals-lazy way. Fat, for the purpose of this discussion, means you are carrying around enough extra fat to pose some sort of health risk.

Take a moment to ask yourself the question: "Am I fat?" This is not always an easy question to answer due to conflicting opinions. You may think you're fine or just a little overweight, your wife may think you are significantly overweight, and your mother and other extended family members likely think you're too skinny. If everyone lives under the same roof, lifestyle changes become even more confusing—your spouse pushes you to eat healthier and exercise, while your mother (or mother-in-law) tempts you with extra food portions to keep you looking "healthier" (aka fatter). Add the fact that the majority of people around you are either overweight or obese and you may feel like you are one of the slimmer trees in a forest of fatness.

On the flipside, movies and media push men and women to strive for lean, toned bodies with very little body fat. In the past, there was a definite Hollywood-Bollywood differential between the noticeably thinner Hollywood leading men and women and their Bollywood counterparts. That gap has closed; Bollywood stars now sport the extreme physical ideals of Hollywood film celebrities. Many of my healthy weight South Asian patients, particularly women, experience negative body image issues because of this new standard. Go easy on yourself! Most people don't have celebrity chefs, daily personal trainers, and plastic surgeons to help them naturally or surgically achieve that "perfect body." Living up to a Hollywood, photoshopped ideal often perpetuates cycles of unhealthy dieting followed by binge eating, and creates a situation of chronic stress. Your challenge is to filter out this harmful external noise and set some healthy, realistic goals for weight loss, specifically fat loss.

> *Living up to a Hollywood, photoshopped ideal often perpetuates cycles of unhealthy dieting followed by binge eating, and creates a situation of chronic stress.*

WHY WORRY ABOUT FAT?

We used to think fat cells were just inert storage containers that took excess calories from our foods—carbohydrates, fats, and even protein (which when consumed in excess gets converted into glucose)—and stored them (as triglycerides) inside fat cells. We now know that fat cells have a different impact on your body depending on their location. One type of fat is called abdominal fat, also known as belly fat or visceral fat (since it commonly lines your inner organs). The fat in your arms and legs is called peripheral fat. If you were to look at peripheral fat under a microscope, you wouldn't see much going on. However, if you examined visceral fat, you would see all kinds of inflammatory hormones and chemicals in action. In fact, experts now classify visceral fat cells as an actual endocrine organ (like your thyroid or adrenal glands) that pumps out an assortment of substances that contribute to chronic diseases.

Visceral fat makes a notable contribution to heart disease. One important study looked at the cumulative effects of visceral fat cells and found that a longer duration of obesity, particularly abdominal obesity, correlated with a higher risk of developing atherosclerosis, marked by coronary artery calcification (CAC), a diagnostic test that detects heart attack causing plaques. Every few years, researchers measured the waist circumference and BMI of over 3,000 non-obese, young white and African American adults between the ages of 18 and 30. They then measured CAC 15, 20, and 25 years later. CAC was found in nearly 40 percent of those with over 20 years of overall or abdominal obesity, and the risk increased significantly with each additional year of obesity.[1] Keep in mind that these weren't South Asians and these subjects were not obese in young adulthood. The fact that obesity is now so prevalent in young children and teens means these plaques will be developing at an even younger age.

Let's take a look inside a belly fat cell to get a sense of how belly fat leads to heart attacks and why I worry so much about the epidemic of abdominal obesity in South Asians worldwide.

BELLY FAT CELL

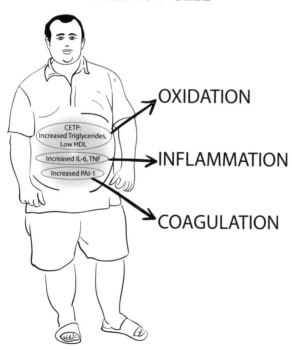

- CETP is a protein that promotes the formation of small dense LDL particles that lead to increased oxidation.
- IL-6 and TNF are chemicals called cytokines that stimulate inflammation. IL-6 also causes elevations in hs-CRP, which is one of our Metabolic 6-pack criteria that measure inflammation. Recall how lowering belly fat often reduces hs-CRP levels.
- Increased PAI-1 is a protein that promotes increased blood clotting.

So there you have it. An innocent looking fat cell produces all the substances needed to trigger a fatal heart attack—oxidation, inflammation, and coagulation!

The South Asian Body: Bulging Bellies and Meager Muscle

There are two primary defining features of the typical South Asian body regardless of gender. We've already discussed excess belly fat and its consequences. The other is the relative absence of muscles, most notably in the arms and legs. This combination of excess fat and reduced muscle mass is medically called sarcopenic obesity. (Sarcopenia specifically refers to the loss of muscle.)

Many South Asian men living in the US and other Western countries, including yours truly, grew up being called names like "chicken legs" by our more muscular non-South Asian peers. I consistently notice less muscle development in the legs, arms, chests, and backs of South Asians compared to most other ethnic groups. I've even discussed this lack of muscle with corporate fitness trainers at the high-tech companies where I lecture. One told me point blank, "Asian Indians are rarely seen in the free weight sections of the gym. Even when they do lift free weights, they opt for the lowest resistance possible. I've never seen an Indian do squats, other than my private clients."

The consequences of sporting insufficient muscle mass extend far beyond the aesthetic.

Worsening insulin resistance: Insufficient muscle mass strengthens the link between abdominal obesity and insulin resistance. Muscle cells have a receptor called Glut-4, which helps deliver glucose from the blood and into the muscle cells. More muscle means more Glut-4 receptors, lower blood glucose, and lower levels of the fat-storing hormone insulin. So indeed strength training is good for your "Gluts"—your gluteus maximus (buttock muscles) and your Glut-4 receptors! When my patients shift from chronic cardio workouts to a balance of strength and cardio, lifting heavier weights and adding some muscle, I often see further drops in triglycerides, blood sugar, and waistlines, and a bump up in HDL—encouraging signs of reduced insulin resistance!

Arthritis, osteoporosis, and other musculoskeletal pains: Muscles help take the load off of joints, thereby slowing the natural wearing away of cartilage. As cartilage deteriorates, painful and chronic inflammation ensues, leading to joint disorders such as arthritis. The action of muscles pulling against bone makes your bones stronger and denser, which helps prevent osteoporosis. Lack of sufficient resistance exercise or general weight-bearing muscular exercise (yes, even walking helps) accelerates all manner of joint and bone problems. In addition, conditions like tendonitis and back pain commonly result from a lack of supportive musculature. This also causes the classic hunched forward posture seen in so many South Asians.

Sports injuries: My South Asian clients seem to present more frequently with weekend warrior-type injuries from activities such as badminton, running, skiing, or even routine yard work. The risk of such injuries is greatly increased when the patient lacks strong leg or core muscles, or good general flexibility. There is no better way to get stiff and weak than coupling marathon-sitting sessions at the computer with insufficient exercise.

Difficulty with weight loss: Weight loss struggles are especially prominent in South Asian women who have a significant deficiency in strength relative to other ethnic groups. My South Asian female patients who exercise usually take walks on flat terrain, but forego any form of weight training. Recall the double trouble of increased fat and reduced muscle and how this deleterious duo worsens insulin resistance and fat gain. South Asian women already start off with more body fat than men do, and are at a distinct disadvantage when they do little to add precious muscle to combat insulin resistance.

Thanks to poor dietary habits, insufficient exercise, and genetic predispositions, South Asians typically have a poor fat-to-muscle ratio. Notice I said "ratio" as opposed to absolutes. A skinny South Asian who lacks muscle tone is by no means immune from heart disease risk factors. A poor ratio of fat to muscle is a recipe for insulin resistance and many other chronic health disorders and disabilities.

Consider the concept of organ reserve, which indicates how well your vital organs are able to function above and beyond normal if called upon for the effort. Your organ reserve is a strong predictor of longevity. It is closely related to the amount of functional muscle mass you have, because muscles help organs function optimally. For example, feeble elderly folks have poor organ reserve and as a result can die from pneumonia because their lungs are too weak to expel mucus and clear the infection. A well-muscled, active person, on the other hand, calls upon his or her organs to perform beyond capacity every time they conduct a workout. Consequently, as the various organs and systems of the body keep up with the demands of an active lifestyle, the aging process is delayed and longevity is promoted.

In order to improve your fat/muscle ratio, you must refine your eating habits and exercise regularly. The importance of eating and exercising optimally goes beyond just looking good to directly influencing your disease risk and predicted lifespan. If you eat the wrong diet but lift weights, you'll resemble my South Asian patients who have muscular limbs but inflated bellies. If you eat a diet low in carbohydrates and high in antioxidants but do not engage in some form of resistance training, your waistline will shrink, but your arms and legs will remain flabby and put you at risk for the aforementioned health conditions and much more!

In their quest to lose weight/fat, many South Asians neglect to add muscle. They focus on the diet aspects and may add some activity or cardio, but rarely incorporate any resistance training. To make things even more challenging, one small study suggests that the muscle South Asians do have is metabolically inferior. Researchers took muscle biopsies of South Asians after exercise and compared them to the muscle biopsies of age-matched and BMI-matched exercisers of Caucasian heritage. South Asian muscles used energy less effectively and burned fats less efficiently—two key features of insulin resistance.[2] This means we need to be even more committed to adding muscle to make up for these genetic inefficiencies. It's imperative to make strength-training a part of your lifestyle plan. Many of my patients who have hit a "wall" with their weight or measures— including cholesterol, blood sugar, and blood pressure results— make breakthroughs once they incorporate strength training.

Skinny-Fat: The Iceberg Effect

About ten percent of a typical iceberg is visible above water while the rest of its mass is below water, completely invisible to a passing ship. The body fat composition of many South Asians is similar to that of an iceberg. On the visible surface, "above water," you may not see much body fat, especially if you hide the fat with a loose shirt or kurta (long and baggy, collarless Indian shirt). However, the "underwater" fat that lines your internal organs and is stored inside fat cells in the form of triglycerides is the truly dangerous visceral fat.

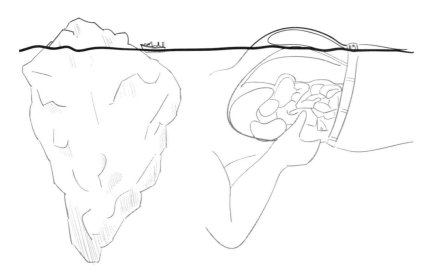

The impulse to overfeed family members and guests and shower them with excess carbohydrates, especially sweets, is an ingrained gesture of warmth and hospitality that goes beyond rationality.

What's really troubling about visceral fat is that it creates the perception that your body size is normal, or even underweight by the woeful standards set by the South Asian population. If only your mother had x-ray vision and could see that your fat cells were overflowing with triglycerides. If she could actually see the fat that's infiltrating your liver and surrounding your digestive organs, would she still call you too thin, or would she scale back her efforts to overfeed you? I'd like to think she'd convert to a healthier mindset and food options, but perhaps not. The impulse to overfeed family members and guests and shower them with excess carbohydrates, especially sweets, is an ingrained gesture of warmth and hospitality that goes beyond rationality. You might be diabetic, but your mother may still serve you a plate full of white rice and sweets after dinner.

Let's take a look at a case study that shows how a South Asian with a normal body weight still falls prey to heart disease risk and metabolic health issues.

Case Study: Kumar

Kumar is a 35-year-old patent attorney who came to see me for a routine physical exam. A slender Indian male, Kumar bragged about being the same weight since his college days. At the time of the exam, he was 5 foot 10 inches tall and weighed 155 pounds, putting his BMI (body mass index) at 22. He had comprehensive labs done in India a few years ago and they found something "abnormal" with his liver function. Given his reported history, I ordered basic labs, including a blood sugar, cholesterol, and liver panel test. His initial lab results showed normal blood sugar levels, and his cholesterol panel was notable for the South Asian pattern of elevated triglycerides and low HDL. His liver function tests showed an

---

elevated AST and ALT. (The AST and ALT are known as trans-aminases, which are markers of liver inflammation.) I ordered a second round of labs to look for other possible causes of his liver inflammation, including tests for viral hepatitis and an hs-CRP test for blood vessel inflammation, which returned elevated. He denied alcohol use and did not take any med-ications or supplements that could affect his liver test. I or-dered an ultrasound of his abdomen, which showed diffuse fatty infiltration of his liver. Kumar was shocked that he was stashing away extra fat in his liver even though he was so skinny! We immediately implemented a lifestyle plan that re-moved excess carbohydrates from his diet, and an exercise plan that encouraged strength training and an overall increase in activity levels. We were able to normalize all of his lab tests within six months through a significant improvement in body composition.

Kumar grew up as the skinny kid in the neighborhood and is still the slimmest among friends and co-workers. However, as you can see from his initial labs—particularly his triglycerides and liver tests—he had plenty of fat stored under the surface, surrounding his digestive organs and invading his liver. The ultrasound only confirmed what we already knew from his lab results: his liver was a secret compart-ment for stored extra fat, and he had been living blissfully unaware under the deceptively "healthier" guise of a skinny-fat South Asian.

The medical term for skinny-fat is MONW (metabolically obese, normal weight), which describes someone like Kumar who has met-abolic evidence of obesity, but whose weight falls within the nor-mal range. Many South Asians simply cannot rely on weight or body mass index to assess disease risk, and need to focus instead on their Metabolic 6-pack, which combines the more specific waist measure-ment with additional metabolic factors. Their body fat is hidden deep, lining the internal organs and infiltrating the liver.

The liver test I ordered for Kumar is an additional recommended test for most South Asian patients. Liver inflammation that stems from fat infiltration is quite common in South Asians and is called non-alcoholic steatohepatitis (or NASH). We've known for a long time that excess alcohol consumption can cause fatty liver, but NASH arises in South Asians who have never touched alcohol, but have visceral obesity and insulin resistance. These South Asians don't have an alcohol addiction, but instead have a carb addiction that fuels their fatty livers. You might intuitively think having a "fatty" liver means you need to cut fat out of your diet, as many doctors and even educational resources on fatty liver might recommend, but excess carbohydrates are the primary culprits. Adding alcohol on top of obesity and insulin resistance can make existing liver inflammation even worse.

Many of my skinny-fat South Asian patients truly feel they are "healthy" because they are slimmer than their peers, and continue to indulge in more overeating and less exercise. They have given in to the misperception that they have been handed the "lucky gene" that allows them to over-consume calories without suffering any health consequence. Here's the reality of that misperception: one study found that adults who were of *normal* body weight at the time of their diabetes diagnosis had a higher future death rate than those who were *overweight or obese* at the time of diagnosis![3]

So does that mean that all you skinny prediabetics or slender, newly diagnosed diabetics should start overeating and putting on extra pounds so that you can live longer? Definitely not. What the study does tell us is that there is something at least as metabolically abnormal with someone who is skinny-fat as there is with someone who is "fat-fat." One theory holds that fat-fat people generally have more muscle because of the excess fat they have to carry around. This extra cushion of fat acts like a set of heavy weights: lifting weights all day long may, in theory, lead to muscle growth, especially in the legs. Since muscle tissue protects against insulin resistance, perhaps the extra muscle outweighs some of the harms of the extra body fat. A skinny-fat person with excess visceral fat but less muscle tissue is less protected. Keep in mind, this is just one study and we'll need further studies and more research to validate and better understand these findings.

Regardless of whether you're skinny-fat or fat-fat, the metabolic signs of obesity represented by the Metabolic 6-pack (high tri-glycerides, low HDL, elevated blood sugar, etc.) are more accurate indicators of the harmful effects of obesity than how much fat you see or how much you weigh. Losing some fat is often necessary if you show any signs of insulin resistance. If you're concerned about losing too much weight, you should focus on adding more muscle. Remember, this is a two-part problem...too much fat and too little muscle compound insulin resistance. Whether you're fat-fat or skinny-fat, you need to lose fat and add muscle.

We need to start thinking twice—as a community, as parents, and as family members—before we throw around comments about someone being too skinny and needing to eat more. We should avoid telling someone they are too skinny when we have no clue what's going on under the surface.

BODY MEASURES (WEIGHT/BMI, WAIST MEASURES, STRENGTH MEASURES)

Let's set some goal measurements before discussing our lifestyle plan.

Weight and BMI: Body weight measurement is a blunt tool that doesn't always give you all the information you need. The BMI (body mass index) takes weight measurement one-step further by factoring height into the equation. There is obviously a world of difference between an individual who is 160 pounds and 5 foot 10 inches and someone who is 160 pounds and 5 foot 4 inches.

To calculate your BMI take your weight in kilograms and divide it by your height in meters squared. If using pounds and inches, multiply your weight in pounds by 703 and divide it by your height in inches squared.

BMI formula (using kg and meters)	=	$\dfrac{\text{weight in kg}}{\text{height in meters}^2}$
BMI formula (using pounds and inches)	=	$\dfrac{\text{weight in pounds x 703}}{\text{height in inches}^2}$

BMI does not account for muscle mass, which throws off the accuracy. A body with a normal or low amount of fat and lots of muscle would have an abnormal BMI. On the other hand, your BMI may be normal or low, but you could be skinny-fat like Kumar. If you are tracking BMI, be sure to use the Asian-adjusted BMI scale shown below. Studies show that insulin resistance and heart disease occur at a lower body weight for South Asians and Asians overall.[4]

South Asian BMI Ranges:
Underweight: 18.4 or less
Healthy: 18.5 to 23
Overweight: 23.1 to 25
Obese: Greater than 25

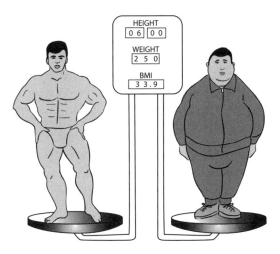

Although measuring weight is simple and something you can easily track, it is only one of the many measures of health you should be monitoring. Measuring abdominal obesity is more accurate. For example, many South Asians have slender limbs with very little muscle, but a protruding belly. These individuals most likely have a normal weight and BMI, but abnormal waist measurements.

Waist measurements: The INTERHEART study, involving 52 countries and over 27,000 participants, consistently ranked waist-to-hip ratio (WHR) a better indicator of heart attack risk than BMI.[5] Unfortunately, most doctors don't check WHR. Measuring WHR takes longer, and there is more room for error when not measured in a specific, repeatable way each time. Also, patients tend to cheat by sucking in their bellies. Although WHR is the most accurate way to assess if you're carrying excess belly fat, I've included a few other ways for you to measure belly fat as well. The first two are more precise, and the others include quick and easy subjective measures.

1. Waist Circumference (WC): Measure your WC before measuring your WHR. Below are the proper steps to measuring your waistline.

- Measure yourself at the same time each day using a flexible tape measure.

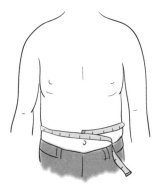

- Wrap the tape around your unclothed abdomen at the level of the belly button. The bottom of the tape measure should be about even with the top of your right hipbone. Don't wrap the tape too tightly, and keep the tape parallel with the floor.

- WC goal for men is less than 90 cm (or 35 inches) and for women less than 80 cm (or 31 inches). Your WC should be about half your height. Just as taller trees have wider trunks, taller humans naturally have wider waists to provide stability. If you are 70 inches tall (178 cm), your WC should be less than 35 inches (89 cm).

2. Waist-to-Hip Ratio (WHR):

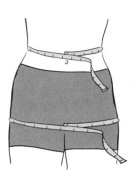

- Use a flexible tape measure to measure the circumference of the widest part of your buttocks.

- Divide your waist measurement by your hip measurement to obtain your WHR.

- If you are male and your WHR is greater than 0.90, then you may be at an increased risk for a heart attack. If you are female, the cutoff for increased risk is 0.85.

Beyond the WC and WHR, you can use the following rough measurements to assess risk.

3. Feet test: I created this simple test to provide a quick and dirty estimate. Stand up straight and tall, keep your stomach relaxed (no tummy tucking or inhaling!), and look straight down. If you can't see your toes, you have a high amount of excess abdominal fat. If you can see about half your feet, you have moderate abdominal fat. If you can see most of your feet, including the front part of your ankle, you've got normal to low amounts of visceral fat. I call this a rough measure because what if you have a big belly and oversized feet, or no belly and really small feet? You still want to back these estimates up with the more specific measures discussed above.

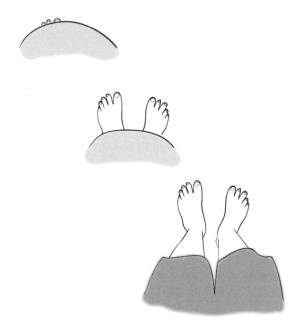

4. Loose pants test: We all love this one. When your pants feel loose or you have to move down a couple notches on your belt line, you must be doing something right! There's nothing like fitting into an old pair of pants or a dress from your younger years. You are literally reversing the aging process when this happens!

I want to emphasize that these measurements serve as guidelines and not absolute goals. For example, I've had male patients who went from a 44-inch waistline to a 38-inch waistline, and even though that's above the target outlined above, it was enough to reverse their Metabolic 6-packs and make them feel healthy and energetic. I'm not going to keep cracking the whip to get those last three inches off if it means sacrificing happiness and increasing stress. On the other hand, I've also had patients whose waist measurements fell in the normal range, but whose labs indicated skinny-fat characteristics like high triglycerides, low HDL, and fatty liver. These patients clearly need to implement lifestyle changes regardless of their relatively slimmer waist size.

Muscle measurements: You can monitor your progress with muscle development by assessing strength, muscle circumference, and lean body mass.

1. **Assess strength:** The stronger you are, the more insulin sensitive muscle you're packing on. You may only be able to do 10 push-ups now, but once you've moved up to 20 you've increased muscle mass and are moving the needle on insulin resistance downward. Whatever resistance exercise you perform (and there are many suggested in Chapter 7), keep track of how much weight you're lifting and how many repetitions you're doing. There are many terrific online tools and free apps, like *Fitness Buddy*, that allow you to choose from a huge database of exercises, track and graph progress, and watch short instructional videos to help you perfect each exercise. *Runtastic* has some great apps that use the accelerometer in your smartphone to motivate you to do more squats, push-ups, and pull-ups. Don't perform the same exercises with the same weights; add variety and pile on more heft as you progress.

2. **Measure muscle circumference:** Measure the circumference of your upper arms, thighs, calves, and chest using a flexible tape measure. As your muscles grow and develop, the circumferences should increase. This may not be the case if you carry excess fat on your arms and/or legs. Over time, you will instead notice a leaner, more defined musculature, possibly resulting in a lower circumference than when you started, which indicates less fat and greater lean muscle mass. This is progress, even if the circumference of your biceps hasn't increased.

   Tracking your strength or the look of your muscles with photos provides a more objective view. I realize this may seem like an exercise in vanity, but there's nothing more telling than before and after photos taken in minimal clothing to really show off body composition changes. Going from flabby arms and legs to toned, well-defined muscles is best captured on film. So don't be shy! Whip out your camera or camera-phone and start taking some "before" shots for comparison.

3. **Follow lean body mass (LBM):** For those who like more precision with specific numbers, you can track your lean body mass, or LBM. LBM comprises your non-fat body mass, which includes your muscles, bones, blood, internal organs, skin, etc. The formula is:

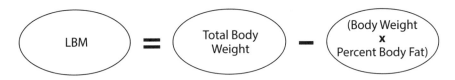

   For example, if you weigh 200 pounds and measure 20 percent body fat with skin calipers, then your LBM would be 200 pounds – (200 pounds x 20%) = 200 – 40 = 160 pounds of LBM. Your overall goal is to lose body fat, not muscle, so strive to lose the weight without losing LBM.

WAYS TO MEASURE BODY FAT PERCENTAGE

There are a number of ways to measure body fat. The more accurate techniques are costly and less convenient, whereas more economical, portable measures can have a significant range of error. Although I don't push patients to get body fat tested, it has been useful for my skinny-fat patients who don't realize what a high percentage of body fat they're carrying around. If you're in denial about extra body fat, you should consider testing.

I've often found that people can get a little obsessive about their body fat once they start measuring it. Keep the focus on achieving a body weight that optimizes your health by reversing your metabolic risk numbers and preventing chronic disease. Anything beyond that may be a personal or cosmetic goal, but be sure you are not chasing an unrealistic number that's going to create chronic stress. Let's look at some of the different techniques for measuring body fat.

Skin fold caliper testing: This is a fat-pinching device designed according to a simple concept...the more fat you can pinch off your belly with the caliper, the greater your body fat percentage. If done correctly and measured consistently over the same part of your body, it can provide a rough estimate of body fat and help track progress over time.

> *Keep the focus on achieving a body weight that optimizes your health by reversing your metabolic risk numbers and preventing chronic disease.*

Bioelectric impedance analysis (BIA): Many weigh scales have incorporated this technology. Because muscle contains more water, it conducts electric currents better than fat does. The BIA scales use this property, along with height and weight, to calculate percent body fat. This test is much easier to conduct than is a skin caliper test since you just step onto a scale and read a number, but your level of hydration can influence accuracy. Try to measure at the same time of day and under consistent nutrition and hydration conditions.

Hydrostatic weighing: This highly accurate test involves submerging an individual in a tank of water. Since fat is less dense and more buoyant, a body with more fat will weigh less under water than a body with more dense muscle. This test is more costly than the previous two and needs to be done at a special center.

DEXA scan: You may recognize this test from its more common use, as a bone density measure for osteoporosis. Like hydrostatic weighing, it also gives a very accurate body fat percent reading and must be done at a specialized center for a higher cost. The other advantage is that it offers fat localization, so you can see which areas store more fat, in case it isn't obvious.

A Lifestyle Cure for Kumar

Let's revisit Kumar to see about a treatment plan. Kumar is a typical MONW (aka skinny-fat) South Asian. Even though Kumar had a "normal" BMI weight of 155 pounds, I recommended a few more pounds of weight loss and a consistent strength-training program. Such lifestyle recommendations can be an uphill battle with spouses and parents who protest that skinny-fat South Asians like Kumar are already too skinny, but he needed to treat the underlying metabolic abnormalities with some fat loss. Kumar expressed cosmetic concerns about being underweight, so we shifted focus to adding more muscle by lifting heavier weights rather than lifting heavier spoons of rice and carbs, as these will only add more insulin-resistant fat.

Kumar simultaneously tracked his waist circumference along with his weight. Fortunately, he had a gym at work and enrolled in personal training sessions. I prescribed a lower carbohydrate-eating plan and strongly recommended he do squats with his trainer in order to add muscle bulk in an effort to reduce insulin resistance and inflammation. It took Kumar six months, but he was eventually able to normalize his liver tests, cholesterol, and hs-CRP levels as a consequence of reducing visceral fat and adding some insulin-sensitive muscle.

Interestingly, he shared with me that several family members were not happy with the additional weight he had lost. For example, his spouse complained that she looked even more overweight when standing next to him. In their eyes, an already underweight South Asian just got skinnier. They couldn't see beyond the visible weight loss and acknowledge the more significant benefits of reduced insulin resistance and inflammation. Not all families are like this, but such reactions exemplify the importance of setting personal goals based on proven risk measures, rather than cultural stereotypes and familial expectations.

Summary

- Abdominal fat is a major cause of inflammation and chronic disease in South Asians.

- Visceral fat is directly correlated to heart attack risk because it releases chemicals that promote oxidation, inflammation, and coagulation.

- Sarcopenia (lack of muscle) is very common in South Asians and may contribute to insulin resistance.

- Body weight and BMI are less accurate than waist-based measurements (WC, WHR) when it comes to assessing risk for heart disease and other conditions.

- A skinny-fat South Asian with a normal body weight and waist measurement may still have abnormal metabolic markers.

- Reverse the dangerous combination of increased body fat and reduced muscle by removing excess carbs and incorporating strength training into your exercise program.

For Professionals

- Emphasize to patients the correlation between adiposity and chronic disease, including heart disease.

- Use measurements of waist size in addition to a South Asian adjusted BMI range when determining ideal body size. If it's impractical to do in the office, provide patients with instructions on measuring at home.

- Remember that MONW ("skinny-fat") is very common in South Asians.

- Emphasize the importance of adding muscle as a way of combating insulin resistance and aim for an overall goal of lowering the fat-to-muscle ratio.

- If patients are resistant to gym-based strength training prescribe apps like Runtastic's squat, push-up, and pull-up apps.

- Lowering body fat through carbohydrate reduction and increased physical activity can help improve inflammatory markers like an elevated hs-CRP and liver transaminase levels.

CHAPTER 5

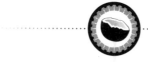

THE SOUTH ASIAN STRUGGLE
WITH FAT AND WEIGHT LOSS

MOST OF MY PATIENTS, and most people in general, struggle to lose excess body fat. In many cases, diligent efforts are made to control caloric intake, exercise regularly, and avoid unhealthy foods, but even with these combined measures, people still fail to shed pounds. Weight loss struggles can be attributed to three prevailing myths:

Myth #1: Weight is gained when you eat more calories than you burn
Myth #2: Eat low-fat foods and you'll lose excess weight and fat
Myth #3: Exercise alone helps you lose weight

Most of my patients struggle to lose weight and improve health because they construct their efforts around these three myths. Eating greater portions of the right foods will control your weight more effectively than eating smaller portions of the wrong foods. Eating even a moderate amount of low-fat, high-carb options not only sacrifices your weight loss efforts, but also results in cycles of compensatory overeating and chronic stress. Likewise, a singular focus on increasing exercise and activity levels in the absence of making correct dietary changes will not help with fat loss. Before implementing the exercise strategies presented in Chapter 7, I recommend first putting an effective eating plan into action.

Although exercising without changing your diet will still exert beneficial effects on overall health and stress management, it won't help you burn fat effectively. Take a look at the empirical evidence: many recreational runners, cyclists, and gym attendees are overweight despite a diligent commitment to exercise. Even some serious athletes, such as ironman triathletes or marathon runners, struggle with excess body fat despite training for 10, 15, or even 20 hours per week!

Researchers now believe that this type of extreme calorie burning stimulates a compensatory increase in appetite. If you ignore those hunger signals and starve yourself while working out faithfully, you'll likely experience a reduction in your metabolic rate—your body's response to the perceived life-threatening combo of excessive exercise and not enough fuel. A low metabolic rate means your body has a greater tendency to store energy (weight gain) than to burn it (weight loss). Shifting your metabolism through dietary changes, however, lays the foundation for exercise to whittle away the fat.

Let's examine a typical case of an overweight South Asian woman struggling to lose fat.

Case Study: Sumita

Sumita is a 38-year-old woman who came to see me about her weight loss struggles. Her Metabolic 6-pack was normal, other than an elevated waist-to-hip ratio. She recounted how slender she was before the birth of her two children. "I could eat anything I wanted, hardly exercise, and not put on a pound. Now I go to the gym five days a week, skip breakfast, eat salad for lunch, and eat chapatis (Indian breads), lentils, and sabji (curried vegetables) for dinner. Still, my weight does not budge. What am I doing wrong?"

Sumita's diet is typical of that of many patients who cannot shed a pound despite eating less and exercising more. Others have tried fad diets, Ayurvedic treatments…even home remedies recommended by family members, such as drinking lemon water first thing in the morning followed by a spoonful of ghee. In nearly all cases, these approaches result in temporary weight loss at best. Permanent weight loss comes down to understanding the role carbohydrates and fats play in weight gain, weight loss, and ultimately weight maintenance.

UNDERSTANDING CARBOHYDRATES AND FATS

Confusion about two major macronutrients, carbohydrates and fat—and the subsequent dietary choices this confusion encourages—leads to adverse changes in body composition and overall health. It's critical that you understand what happens to your body the moment a spoonful of rice, a piece of bread, or a dollop of ghee or coconut oil enters your mouth and activates digestion and metabolism. The biggest misconceptions are:

- Dietary fat leads to increased body fat

- Dietary cholesterol leads to blood vessel cholesterol and plaque formation

- "Healthy" carbohydrates such as whole grains counteract these negative effects

Nothing could be further from the truth than these three statements! I'll simplify the science of carbohydrates and fat, so you'll understand how it's possible for fats like ghee, coconut oil, or butter to not directly result in weight gain, and how carbohydrates like rice, breads, and wheat play a central role in the accumulation of excess body fat.

Carb Trafficking

Carbohydrates are essentially chains of glucose molecules (often referred to as "complex" carbohydrates) that are broken down into individual glucose molecules (often referred to as "simple" carbohydrates) during digestion. For the purpose of this discussion, I'll be interchanging the term "carbohydrates" with "carbs" and "glucose" with "sugar." After carbs are broken down into glucose, the glucose travels through your body, providing energy and carrying out essential metabolic functions.

We've ridden the insulin train and cruised the cholesterol boat, how about we take a drive in the carbohydrate car? Let's think of glucose molecules as cars that have three major destinations in the body—the liver, muscle tissue, or fat cells. Picture these glucose cars at a busy three-way intersection, trying to decide which way to go.

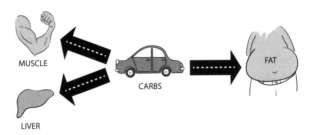

Ideally, you want most of this glucose traffic to head towards the muscle where it can immediately be burned as fuel or stored as glycogen in the liver and muscle cells.

The critical question is, who's directing all this traffic? The answer is insulin. Insulin, the master hormone produced by the pancreas, is the key determinant of where glucose traffic ends up in the body. One of insulin's primary jobs is to move excess glucose out of your bloodstream and into muscle or fat for storage. This is important because high glucose levels are toxic in the bloodstream. Over time, high blood glucose causes damage to vital organs like the eyes (retinopathy), kidneys (nephropathy), and nerves (neuropathy). Glucose enters the liver without the help of insulin, but once it gets inside, insulin stores it as glycogen, if there's room. If there's no room, the liver starts making fat.

The next question is, if you've got plenty of insulin around to direct traffic, how do you get more of the traffic to move away from fat and towards muscle? Glucose traffic is driven by three factors:

1. **Capacity:** Does the site have enough parking spaces for more glucose, or is it already filled with stored glucose (glycogen)?

2. **Permissibility:** Will the site let glucose enter?

3. **Demand:** Does the site, particularly muscle, need the glucose (how active are the muscles)?

Most South Asian bodies have a serious parking problem. If you've ever driven down the busiest streets of downtown Delhi, Mumbai, or New York desperately looking for parking, then you can imagine how your glucose molecules feel. South Asians consume so many excess carbs that liver glycogen and muscle glycogen parking spots are filled to capacity. The liver generally has space for about 100 grams of glycogen, while muscle can hold another 300-500 grams (range depends on fitness and activity level—athletes can store more than sedentary folks). If there's no room to park in liver or muscle, there's one very accommodating parking lot left in town with plenty of space...your fat cells! They'll gladly take on this overflow traffic, causing your fat cells to expand, which means you become fatter.

Even if there is space to park in the muscle and liver lots, there's still the question of permissibility. The actual term for this is insulin sensitivity, which is the opposite of insulin resistance. Insulin's your parking voucher that you present at the gate to the muscle and fat parking lots. If the gates, which are actually the insulin receptors on your muscle cells, are insulin sensitive, then the voucher is accepted and glucose traffic is allowed inside. If they're insulin resistant, your voucher will not be accepted and the gates will not open.

If you're already overweight, and especially if you have any of the Metabolic 6-pack criteria that indicate insulin resistance (high triglycerides, low HDL, etc.), there's a good chance that glucose from your high-carb meals isn't getting inside your muscle cells. Guess which destination will accept your insulin parking voucher? It's those darn fat cells. When you are insulin resistant, the muscles stop responding to insulin first. Meanwhile, the fat cells remain wide open because they are still insulin sensitive. Over time, the fat cells will also tire out and become insulin resistant, at which point your extra glucose cars will have no place to park and your blood sugar levels will move skyward, worsening diabetes and a whole host of diabetic complications and chronic health conditions.

So far we've focused on muscle and fat. What about the liver? Even though you don't need insulin to usher glucose into the liver, once the glucose gets inside, you do need insulin to decide what to do with it. If there's parking space, insulin will store the glucose as glycogen to be used for future energy. If there's no space, insulin will convert the glucose into fat in the form of triglycerides. Triglycerides are either exported into the bloodstream, causing your triglycerides to go up, or deposited directly into the liver, causing the all too common fatty liver syndrome in South Asians. For high-carb-consuming South Asians who have run out of glycogen parking spaces, staple carbs like rice and chapatis fatten up your body (inflated fat cells), your bloodstream (high triglycerides), and your liver (fatty liver).

Finally, we come to the issue of demand. What if you don't exercise and typically spend more than 10 hours a day sitting? Here's what's happening behind the scenes: all those parked cars in your muscle (glycogen) never get broken down into glucose for energy use. Those cars will only start moving out when you start moving more. Remember, your muscle has 300-500 grams of parking space, and if you don't regularly exercise and stay physically active, you're never going to empty out those glucose stores and make room for the carbs you are consuming on a daily basis.

When you ramp up your exercise, including frequent and comfortably paced movement, as well as brief, high-intensity exercise that burns tons of glucose, you create open parking spaces in your liver and muscle cells every day. You become insulin sensitive, because the liver and muscles love to restock with energy for future work efforts. The next time a glucose car comes driving by, the insulin sensitive liver and muscle cells will grab those glucose molecules and put them in their parking spaces as glycogen before they can travel to fat cells.

Let's use two different scenarios to look at how all three of these factors (capacity, insulin sensitivity, and demand) interact.

Scenario 1: Typical, inactive South Asian who eats excess carbs and is insulin resistant.

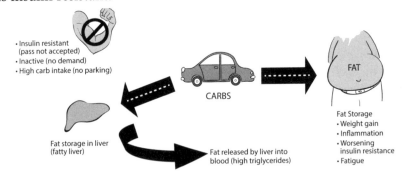

Notice how the muscle has no parking available and no demand in the form of energy exertion. Under these conditions, it won't accept the insulin parking pass and is, therefore, insulin resistant. Excess carbs either go to fat (increased body fat), or go to the liver, which switches into fat-producing mode because there's no room for liver glycogen. The fat in the liver either accumulates (fatty liver) or is dumped into the bloodstream, elevating triglycerides and increasing heart attack risk.

Muscle normally soaks up 60-70 percent of the glucose you eat, and if glucose can't get inside muscle, your blood sugar is going to substantially increase. In response, your pancreas pumps out even more insulin in a desperate attempt to lower your blood glucose. As a result, the excess insulin drives nutrients even more aggressively towards fat storage in fat cells and fat production in the liver. As a result of a high-carb diet, inactivity, and insulin resistance, Sumita, and most other South Asians, are fighting a desperate uphill metabolic battle.

Scenario 2: Someone who is insulin sensitive, active, and consumes fewer carbs.

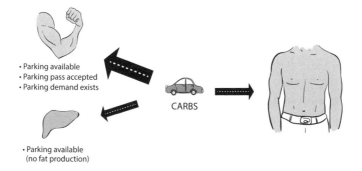

- Parking available
- Parking pass accepted
- Parking demand exists

CARBS

- Parking available
(no fat production)

This is the ideal scenario. By reducing excessive carb consumption and staying physically active, you open up plenty of available parking spaces in the muscle and liver, so that your muscle can burn glucose for energy. Traffic is diverted away from fat, and your waistline inevitably becomes slimmer. With sufficient parking available, your liver does not need to shift into fat production, and you no longer suffer from fatty liver and elevated triglycerides.

Fast Carbs Versus Slow Carbs

There are two major types of carbs. All carbs are comprised of chains of sugar molecules (of assorted lengths) linked together like building blocks. Simple carbs are made from two or fewer sugar molecules, while complex carbs are made from longer chains of three or more sugars. Given their simpler structure, simple carbs are quickly broken down (digested), causing a rapid rise in blood sugar levels, while complex carbs are harder to digest and cause a slower rise in blood glucose. In deference to their relative rates of absorption, let's refer to simple carbs as "fast carbs" and complex carbs as "slow carbs."

Abrupt increases in blood sugar levels from fast carbs cause insulin levels to spike, leading not only to fat storage, but also to an immediate drop in blood sugar, which exacerbates hunger and triggers even more high-carb eating. In comparison, slow carbs cause a gradual rise in insulin levels, which lessens fat storage and keeps hunger at bay. Remember, your brain relies on glucose for energy; when blood sugar levels spike and then drop from eating too many fast carbs, your mood and energy levels do the same. Let's summarize:

> Fast carbs lead to a fast rise in blood sugar, a steep climb in fat-storing insulin, and rapid swings in blood glucose, manifesting as fluctuating hunger and energy. Slow carbs (in moderation) cause a steadier rise in blood sugar and a more controlled release of insulin, which keeps hunger and energy more stable.

Here are some examples of the two types of sugars:

Simple (fast) carbs: Glucose, fructose (fruit sugar), lactose (dairy products), sucrose (table sugar)—found in sweetened beverages (like soda, energy drinks, sports drinks, and even fruit juices)—candies, sweets, condiments (like jelly and jam), assorted processed, packaged, and frozen foods (like popsicles, ice cream, breakfast cereals, fruity snacks in a wrapper, and even fancy energy bars).

Complex (slow) carbs: Lentils, beans, starchy vegetables (think potatoes), whole-grain cereals, breads, pastas, brown rice, and grains (like barley, millet, buckwheat, amaranth, quinoa, etc).

South Asian bodies are locked into a mode of constant fat storage due to the continued ingestion of high-carbohydrate meals that stimulate excessive insulin production.

Fructose, the sugar found in fruit, is a fast carb that can cause your blood sugar to spike. Many patients indulge in excessive intake of fruit to satisfy their sweet tooth while they restrict more traditional desserts. Unfortunately, abundant fruit intake can cause significant weight gain since fructose promotes increased insulin levels and subsequent fat storage. Unlike glucose, which acts on various cells in the body (muscle, brain, etc.), fructose is primarily metabolized in the liver where it contributes to the production of triglycerides (fat). Fruits do have nutrients and fiber that offset the fast absorption effects of empty sugars, but if you're insulin resistant and sedentary, tropical fruits such as bananas, mangos, and pineapples can still pose a problem. Be it fast fructose, or slower whole grains, excess carbs in any form will increase hunger, drop energy levels, and promote increased fat storage due to elevated insulin.

As you might imagine, a constantly fluctuating energy and appetite throughout the day is not healthy or productive. In fact, your body perceives blood sugar fluctuations (caused by high-carbohydrate meals) as stressful events and activates the familiar fight-or-flight response. After all, a brain and body running short of energy has been a matter of life or death throughout human evolution. When the fight-or-flight stress response kicks in again and again, its related hormonal mechanisms become exhausted, and you experience what is best described as burnout. This state of burnout leads to additional sugar cravings and overeating, especially at the end of long days fueled by poor meal choices.

Too Much Insulin is the Enemy

Insulin in optimal amounts plays an important role in converting dietary nutrients into energy that our cells can use to carry out vital functions and to recover from exercise. However, most South Asians have far too much insulin and stored energy. South Asian bodies are

locked into a mode of constant fat storage due to the continued ingestion of high-carbohydrate meals that stimulate excessive insulin production. For external proof, look to the epidemic of abdominal obesity in your fellow South Asians.

Think of insulin as an "insulating" hormone. Many animals produce layers of extra body fat before winter to serve as insulation from
extreme conditions. Extra body fat on humans, however, increases
the risk of chronic conditions like heart disease and diabetes, rather
than providing a survival advantage (we have heaters and clothing
for that!). We can summarize this effect as follows:

Insulin provides excess <u>insulation</u> through fat cell <u>inflation</u>.

To make matters even worse, this extra body fat, especially around
the belly, produces chemicals that further worsen insulin resistance.
The fatter you get, the more insulin resistant you become and the
easier it is to pile on even more body fat. If insulin resistance is not
addressed early on, the chronic overproduction of insulin will cause
the pancreas to eventually tire out and stop producing adequate levels of the hormone. With inadequate insulin mechanisms in place,
your blood sugar continues to climb, worsening diabetes and its associated complications (eye disease, kidney failure, nerve damage, etc.).

Transitioning From Sugar Burner to Fat Burner

Reducing excess carbohydrates in your diet not only reduces insulin
levels and potentially reverses insulin resistance, but it also gives you
the opportunity to shift your body from fat-storing to fat-burning
mode. When insulin levels are lowered, stubborn body fat is broken
down into fatty acids that are released into the bloodstream for energy.
Fatty acids are the good version of fat in the blood and a tremendous
source of energy for the body. When you lower insulin levels through
reduced carb consumption and use fatty acids rather than glucose for
fuel, you feel energetic and less hungry.

Think of it this way: when you eat food, your body can use two
major types of energy, sugar or fat. In other words, there are sugar
burners and fat burners. South Asians tend to be sugar burners.
Because excess insulin has been tucking fat away for years, many South

Asian bodies have forgotten how to burn fat for fuel and rely instead on sugar (in the form of regularly timed, high-carbohydrate meals). The good news is that once you reduce your dietary carbs and insulin levels, you will free up years of stored fat deposits for use as energy.

Significant changes can occur within a few short weeks of carb reduction, such as a drop in weight, a reduction in food cravings, and an increase in energy. How quickly this happens depends on various factors such as genes, hormones, stress, and sleep. Don't get impatient if you don't see immediate results. Most of us have been sugar burners for the majority of our lives and have sustained significant metabolic damage accordingly. What this means for some is that success with fat loss, and programming your metabolism to prefer fat for fuel, may take weeks instead of days, or in some cases months instead of weeks. When you sit back and think about it, it's remarkable that we can shift into fat-burning mode within such a relatively short time, especially considering the decades of damage caused by modern South Asian dietary practices.

What About Dietary Fat?

You may be surprised to learn that fat alone does not raise insulin levels. That's right—fat in the absence of excess carbs and insulin is not fattening. However, if plenty of insulin is hanging around due to a high-carb diet and/or insulin resistance, then fat will hitch a ride on insulin and head straight into your fat cells, where it's stored as triglycerides.

Does this mean you can freely consume all forms of fat if you keep your carbs low? Definitely not. You still need to identify good fats and bad fats in your diet.

Saturated fats, which mainly come from animal sources (meat, milk, and butter), are the most misunderstood type of fat. These fats have been erroneously referred to as "bad fats." After analyzing a 20-year review of 21 studies that collectively followed 350,000 people, researchers concluded:

> "There is insufficient evidence from prospective epidemiologic studies to conclude that dietary saturated fat is associated with an increased risk of CHD, stroke, or cardiovascular disease (CVD)."[1]

After all, saturated fat comprises our cell membranes and is involved in many critical hormonal and cellular functions.

Other fats with outstanding health benefits include monounsaturated fats and omega-3s. Monounsaturated fats, like those found in olive oil, avocados, and nuts and seeds, not only have no impact on insulin levels, but also have health-promoting benefits. They are a core part of the Mediterranean diet and have repeatedly been shown in studies to reduce the risk of heart disease and chronic inflammation. Similarly, omega-3s, especially from marine sources such as salmon, mackerel, herring, and sardine, have anti-inflammatory and heart healthy benefits.

Omega-3s are the healthier of the two types of polyunsaturated fatty acids (PUFAs). The other PUFA is omega-6, found predominantly in vegetable oils. Even though omega-6s may not raise insulin like carbohydrates do, they are still potent inflammatory agents. Manufacturing vegetable oils such as canola oil, corn oil, and safflower oil requires a high degree of chemical processing, unlike harvesting more natural forms of saturated fat such as butter, ghee, and coconut oil. Omega-6s are also not as heat stable and become easily oxidized when cooking. Recall how oxidation and inflammation are major contributors to heart attack causing plaques.

When it comes to PUFAs, focus on optimizing your omega-6-to-omega-3 ratio. Most experts agree that an ideal ratio of omega-6-to-omega-3 is 3:1 or less, reflective of our primitive diet. Our current state, with abundant vegetable oil infiltrating nearly every food we eat, has pushed these levels up to 16:1 or higher. This imbalance has been implicated as an underlying cause of many inflammatory, chronic health issues.

As for unhealthy fats, nothing's worse than trans fats, aka "hydrogenated" or "partially hydrogenated" fats. Unlike saturated fats, trans fats are chemically altered agents that are extremely hazardous to ingest. These fats are used in processed foods to increase shelf life. They definitely perform that task well, but they also reduce human shelf life by causing oxidative damage and inflammation immediately upon ingestion. The most definitive consequence of consuming trans fats is the repercussion on heart disease risk.

A 2006 comprehensive review of studies on trans fats published in the *New England Journal of Medicine* showed a strong connection between trans fat intake and coronary heart disease (CHD) risk. Study authors concluded: "On a per-calorie basis, trans fats appear to increase the risk of CHD (coronary heart disease) more than any other macronutrient, conferring a substantially increased risk at low levels of consumption (1 to 3% of total energy intake)."[2]

A surprising number of packaged and frozen snacks in grocery stores are made from these harmful oils, including many Indian crispy snacks, sweets, and baked goods. Vanaspati is a cheap ghee substitute. This partially or fully hydrogenated vegetable oil is used widely in Indian restaurant foods and found in many Indian processed snack foods. Be sure to read labels and avoid anything with the words "hydrogenated" or "partially hydrogenated." Do keep in mind that there are natural trans fats in foods like grass-fed meat and dairy products that have not been shown to be harmful. For purposes of our discussion, we can summarize that chemically altered fats (trans, hydrogenated, partially hydrogenated) should be completely avoided.

Let's review the main dietary fats:

Saturated fat: Found mainly in animal sources (meat, milk, butter), but also in coconut products (oil, butter, flakes, milk). Saturated fat is an efficient source of energy with assorted health benefits, and is only problematic when consumed with excess carbohydrates.

Monounsaturated fats: A healthy fat found in olives and extra virgin olive oil, avocados, macadamia nuts, and almonds.

Polyunsaturated fats: Omega-3s are healthy fats found in certain oils and coldwater fish (the best source). Omega-6s need to be limited (vegetable oils are the leading offender) due to inflammatory effects. Aim for an omega-6-to-omega-3 ratio of 3:1 or less.

Trans fats/partially-hydrogenated fats: Chemically altered fats that are completely unfit for human consumption.

Why is Sumita Struggling with Fat Loss?

Now that you've seen how carb-driven-insulin increases are the culprits behind fat storage, let's apply this principle to Sumita so you understand how this process works in real life. What if Sumita were to eat a chapati, or a bowl of rice topped with ghee or butter? The excess insulin triggered by the chapati or rice would convert both dietary fat <u>and</u> dietary carbohydrates into triglycerides and deliver them both to the fat cells.

> *The excess insulin triggered by dietary carbs converts both dietary fat and dietary carbohydrates into triglycerides to store in fat cells.*

This double whammy causes fat cells to swell and waistlines, hips, and buttocks to expand. In an effort to be healthier, Sumita—still unaware that carbohydrates are the primary culprits—reduces the amount of ghee spooned onto her rice, or cuts back on the oil or butter used to panfry her chapatis. What she doesn't realize is that the rice and chapatis are the main problem, not the fats! The following image illustrates how carbs directly initiate the process of fat storage via insulin, and how fat (ghee) passively follows the carbs into the fat cells.

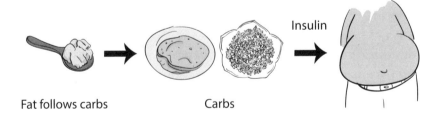

Fat follows carbs   Carbs   Insulin

If the ghee were instead spooned onto a plate of non-starchy vegetables or protein, there would not be enough insulin to usher the ghee inside fat cells. Instead, the ghee would become free fatty acid circulating in the bloodstream and available to Sumita as a source of energy.

Eating fat won't make you fat without insulin, which comes from eating excess carbs.

Essentially, you cannot store any ingested calories as fat without insulin acting as a guide. In the absence of excess carbs, if Sumita were to eat a bowl of ghee on a particular day and nothing else, she would not get fat. She would be putting an excellent source of energy into her bloodstream for immediate use, and she would get really full, really fast, precluding her from eating more food for many hours afterward. Since there are great benefits to be obtained from nutrient-dense carbohydrates like vegetables and fruits, you certainly don't need to go around eating just fat in the name of weight control. However, it's important to recognize the scientific fact that eating fat won't make you fat without insulin, which comes from eating excess carbs.

Insulin Resistance Makes Fat Loss More Challenging

A small amount of dietary carbohydrates can tip the balance in favor of fat storage over fat burning, depending on how insulin resistant you are. Let's say Sumita, an insulin resistant woman, goes out to lunch with her friend Ann, an insulin sensitive woman who maintains an ideal body weight. They both order chicken curry and rice, but the meal only triggers fat storage in Sumita, not Ann. Why is that?

Recall that one of the primary consequences of insulin resistance is increased insulin production in an effort to overcome resistant muscle cells. Since Sumita is insulin resistant, due primarily to excess body fat, her insulin levels are already elevated before she takes a bite of curry. Ann's insulin levels, on the other hand, are stable. After the meal, Sumita's insulin levels shoot way above the threshold required for fat storage. Since her muscle cells are barred up tight due to insulin resistance, and her liver and muscle glycogen parking lots are full due to chronic carbohydrate overconsumption, her lunch flows predominantly to her fat cells.

Ann, on the other hand, gains no fat at all. She is lean, insulin sensitive, and eats an optimal amount of carbs compatible with her active lifestyle. Her baseline insulin levels are nice and low, she's got plenty of muscle and liver parking space since she burns her glycogen regularly with physical activity, and her muscle cells are sensitive enough to take on the nutrients from her lunch and fuel her more active lifestyle.

> *When you exercise and reduce body fat, you become what I call "insulin resilient." Then, you can occasionally indulge in less-than-healthy foods and not store fat."*

You can exclaim, accurately, that Ann was born lucky. But that's definitely not the whole story. Her eating style and activity levels have allowed her to adapt to a fat-burning metabolism. Sure, genes do play some role in influencing your level of insulin resistance, but I assure you the majority of cases can be attributed to dietary and exercise choices—the predominant factors that influence whether your body chooses to burn fat or store fat! As fitness and nutrition expert Mark Sisson states in *The Primal Blueprint*, "If you are carrying excess body fat it's due to the combination of your genetic predisposition to store fat combined with the amount of insulin you produce in your diet." It's not fair to leave your waistline up to chance.

Fat-storing Sumita and fat-burning Ann also illustrate how the same meal has completely different outcomes depending on an individual's level of insulin resistance. If Sumita were to gain more fat, her body would become even more insulin resistant, because fat, especially abdominal fat, releases substances that promote insulin resistance. A smaller meal with fewer carbs would still prompt fat storage, because she is starting off with such drastically high levels of insulin. The more body fat you accumulate, the more insulin resistant you are and the higher your pre-meal insulin levels. Your body is primed to store fat before your first bite, and even small amounts of carbs can push you into a state of fat storage.

Conversely, ten years ago, when Sumita was younger, lighter, and less insulin resistant, she could eat a full plate of rice and not gain fat. Back then she was more like Ann. When you are insulin resistant, even so-called healthy carbs like fruits, lentils, and whole grains can all of a sudden become fattening carbs, which explains why so many of my South Asian patients experience tremendous weight gains year after year despite eating what they think is a healthy diet of grains.

Fortunately, it is possible to reduce your level of insulin resistance very quickly through exercise and body fat reduction. Making lifestyle changes designed to promote insulin sensitivity will make you less susceptible to storing fat. After your body composition improves and insulin resistance lowers, the same foods that used to make you fat may have little effect on fat storage. Once you become less insulin resistant and more insulin sensitive, you will be less likely to gain weight, even when you occasionally indulge in less-than-healthy foods. I call this "insulin resilience"...something Ann has and something Sumita can achieve with the right dietary decisions.

The Mind-Insulin Connection

Insulin release is not just triggered by glucose in your bloodstream. The very aroma or thought of food can cause what is called a "cephalic" or "preprandial" (before meal) release of insulin. This is a quick shot of insulin before you've even touched your food, kind of like a racecar revving its engine before taking off full speed. For example, when you come home after a day of work, the smell of home-cooked food triggers your pancreas to pulse out a little bit of insulin. When you bite into your chapati, your already revved up pancreas pumps out even more fat-storing insulin hormone.

This phenomenon also explains why appetizers increase hunger. Apart from making your mouth water from saliva production, the anticipation of a plate of crispy samosas triggers the release of a small dose of insulin. This insulin release drops your blood sugar and intensifies your hunger. Animal and human studies have shown that this type of preprandial insulin response can lead to overeating.

OTHER FACTORS THAT AFFECT FAT STORAGE

There are other factors besides insulin that play a role in fat storage, such as genes, hormones, and chemicals in your body. If you inherit a tendency towards obesity, it doesn't mean there is no hope. Reducing your carbohydrates to the right level and exercising regularly may help you overcome, or at least minimize, the effects of any genetic propensities towards obesity.

> *Insufficient sleep elevates hunger hormones, suppresses satiety hormones, and promotes fat storage instead of fat burning.*

Gender also plays a role in where we store fat. Men tend to have greater fat storage activity around their abdomens. Women tend to have more fat storage activity below the waist, and around the hips and buttocks. Pregnancy and menopause are other conditions that may increase fat storage in women.

Poor sleep and high stress levels can also lead to weight gain due to their destructive effects on the stress hormones that impact fat metabolism. Cortisol—the central component of the fight-or-flight response—is a hormone released by the body when under physical or emotional stress. One of its effects is to cause excess fat deposition around the abdomen, especially when insulin levels are high. Insufficient sleep is not only associated with higher cortisol levels (and thus a greater propensity for fat storage), but is also associated with increasing levels of the hunger-stimulating hormone ghrelin, lowering your sensitivity to the fullness hormone leptin and reducing the amount of growth hormone (which promotes leanness by stimulating muscle growth and fat burning) our bodies produce. How's that for getting hit from all angles, just for staying up late to catch up on your favorite streaming movies and TV shows!

These additional hormones and conditions can make fat loss more challenging, but insulin is still the most important modifiable mediator of fat metabolism. Assuming you have high levels of insulin, if you are also under a lot of stress or not sleeping sufficiently, these additional factors will make matters worse. Prioritizing sleep and reducing stress helps you lose weight and reduces your risk of developing many other physical and mental health conditions.

WHY LOW-FAT DIETS SEEM TO WORK

I have come across patients and other members of the community who did achieve success on a low-fat diet. However, based on the science of insulin, I strongly believe that their success was not due to the low-fat nature of the foods, but instead due to the following factors which traditional low-fat and low-carb diets share:

- Both reduce overall glycemic load (nutrition term for the total glucose load in the diet) due to the elimination of junk carbs and HFCS

- Both increase vegetable and fruit intake

- Both encourage increased activity and exercise

- Both encourage stress management, which reduces fat-storing cortisol

- Both encourage consumption of healthy fats like olive oil, nuts, seeds, and fish

If you achieve success, optimize your Metabolic 6-pack numbers, and feel more comfortable and satiated eating a low-fat diet, then great. Stay on track with that success. I wrote this book in an effort to get you healthier, and if a low-fat diet gets you there, then more power to you. I do want to mention that we should reevaluate your success after a year or two, because almost all dieters who follow the traditional approach of calorie restriction and low-fat eating have difficulty sustaining initial positive results. Let's face it, humans love to eat, they love to indulge, and they are averse to deprivation of any kind, for any length of time, especially food.

What the *South Asian Health Solution* is presenting is an alternative approach that has been proven to work for years instead of mere weeks or months. The program works because it eliminates all the acknowledged difficulties that accompany mainstream diets: there's no calorie restriction, no calorie counting, no obsessive, difficult-to-adhere-to eating guidelines. Instead, you guide your eating habits by personal preference and enjoyment, and simply choose from the incredibly broad categories of foods that humans have adapted to over the course of evolution.

●

ESTABLISHING A NEW NORM

I've had patients and doctors ask me, "Aren't you just promoting a low-carb diet?" "Low carb" assumes you are currently eating a normal amount of carbs, while "diet" implies a temporary change rather than one that lasts a lifetime. If I thought our community was eating a normal amount of carbs, I wouldn't be writing this book—most of the health issues discussed so far would be the exception rather than the rule.

> *"Low carb" assumes you are currently eating a normal amount of carbs, while "diet" implies a temporary change rather than a life change.*

How many of your South Asian friends and co-workers have slim waistlines, normal cholesterol panels, and no family history of heart disease or diabetes? If you accept conditions like diabetes, early heart disease, accelerated aging, obesity in adults and children, and chronic fatigue as normal, then yes, South Asians are eating a normal amount of carbs.

I realize that much of what I said in this chapter goes against everything you've read and learned about a healthy diet. Why am I so passionate about this innovative approach? Because I was someone who followed the standard nutrition guidelines for years, and still saw my triglycerides hover between 200-300 with a low HDL. I was a normal BMI South Asian with metabolic syndrome. In 2011, I significantly reduced my net carb intake and witnessed a dramatic improvement in my Metabolic 6-pack criteria. Before I discovered this approach, I preached the traditional Western diet strategy to patients and lecture attendees. On the heels of my personal success, I put my patients on a similar plan. I have been blown away by the results, which is something you don't say very often in the world of medicine, and I am convinced that we need to rethink the way we eat and get back to what really constitutes "normal."

Sumita's Solution

On average, when you consume more than 200 grams of net carbs daily, no matter how healthy the carbs or how low your caloric intake, your body will enter fat storage mode with no hope for weight loss. To burn fat effectively, you may need to lower your intake of net carbs to 50-100 grams or less. With this information in hand, let's take a look at one of Sumita's typical dinners, consisting of one chapati, one cup of lentils, and one cup of sabji (vegetables). The rough nutritional breakdown of such a meal is as follows:

Sumita's Dinner	
1 Rotiland brand chapati	24 g net carb, 4 g protein, 5 g fat, 160 cal
1 cup cooked lentils	30 g net carb, 10 g protein, 1 g fat, 200 cal
1 cup cooked aloo sabji (potato curry)	40 g net carb, 2 g protein, 5 g fat, 150 cal

We've got a potent fat-storing meal on our hands! At first glance this looks like a very nutritious, low-calorie, low-fat meal that runs just over 500 calories. However, Sumita consumed 94 grams of net carbs—the average daily net carb quota for someone of her weight to burn fat. She fulfilled this quota in a single meal! Despite being low in fat, this is a meal that will cause Sumita to store more body fat than she would eating a 12-ounce steak with a side of vegetables.

How do we transform Sumita's meal from a fat-storing disappointment to a fat-burning win? We cut her down to a single chapati made with a high protein flour such as coconut or almond flour, reduce her lentil servings by adding more vegetables, replace the potato in her sabji with non-starchy vegetables like cauliflower and spinach, and add a side of yogurt to further boost her protein intake. We'll discuss these types of fat-burning food substitutions further in the next chapter.

These meal changes reduce the amount of insulin that enters Sumita's blood after she is done eating. In the ensuing hours, her body will shift from storing fat to burning fat for energy. Remember, when you consume excess carbohydrates, your body preferentially burns glucose for energy, while the fat remains stored. Often we refer to this as "stubborn fat," but it's not just the fat that's stubborn. It's the prevailing cultural momentum that influences you to center your diet around carbohydrates. This dietary pattern ultimately prevents your body from choosing to burn fat over glucose.

Restaurants and grocery stores don't make the shift to fat burning very easy on you. Most of the "low-fat" foods in your local grocery store are high in carbs to make up for the reduction in fat. Food manufacturers are well aware that adding addictive carbs to products increases hunger, causing you to eat more and buy more...a very unhealthy, but effective sales method.

I realize I may have painted a hopeless picture of our struggle with insulin and fat loss, especially considering that even the smell or thought of food can cause a release of insulin. My intent is not to discourage you, but to help you understand how your daily food choices impact whether your body burns or stores fat. Hopefully you'll now look at food in a new light. Next time you come across a potato samosa, see it for what it really is—a deep fried carb layer wrapped around a starchy potato filling—an insulin bomb waiting to explode! Armed with this knowledge, my patients have successfully made food choices and added exercises that have freed them from the vicious sugar-burning insulin cycle.

Sumita now enjoys a sense of control over her eating habits and body composition. At her six-month follow-up appointment, now 15 pounds lighter, Sumita tells me she can keep up with her kids, looks forward to exercise, and reports a newly discovered enthusiasm and optimism for life. The next two chapters will give you a detailed nutrition and activity plan to help you achieve the same type of success experienced by Sumita and so many other South Asians who have taken control of their diets and lifestyle choices.

Summary

- The three major weight loss myths are common barriers to weight loss (weight is gained when you eat more calories than you burn, eat low-fat foods and you'll lose excess weight and fat, exercise alone helps you lose weight).

- Insulin is the hormone that controls fat metabolism.

- Carbohydrates cause more fat storage than fat or proteins do.

- Increasing body fat makes you more insulin resistant and thus more susceptible to fat storage after a given meal.

- Reducing body fat makes you more "insulin resilient," with less potential fat storage after a given meal.

For Professionals

- Explain the three myths to patients struggling with weight loss.

- Identify excess carbs as a critical factor in weight gain and progressive insulin resistance.

- Allow patients to incorporate healthy fats back into the diet and remove the stigma about saturated fat when they commit to cutting excess carbs.

- Be sure to emphasize eliminating all trans fats, which can be found in many South Asian restaurants and processed snack foods.

- Motivate patients with the concept of "insulin resilience." Let them know that dropping body fat and gaining muscle will not only maintain weight loss, but also allow occasional dietary deviations without contributing to significant weight gain.

CHAPTER 6

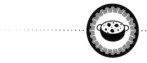

CARBS APPROACH TO BURNING FAT

HEALTHFUL DIETARY CHOICES hold the key to burning fat and reversing insulin resistant risk factors. I developed the **CARBS** acronym to help you identify the major South Asian fat-storing foods to avoid next time you're at the grocery store or a party staring down a long row of dangerous delicacies. Without even knowing it, many South Asians choose the very foods that trigger fat storage the most. I realize that cutting back the foods on this list may seem daunting, but I assure you that I've had South Asian patients from all walks of life achieve tremendous success in doing so. Many have shared that the best part of this dietary modification is that it is an eating plan they can follow for life, rather than another short-lived, failed diet.

THE "CARBS" APPROACH FOR SOUTH ASIANS

The major fat-promoting CARBS:

C = **Chapatis:** Includes all Indian flatbreads, and breads in general, even those made from wheat

A = **Aloo:** Includes mainly potatoes and other starchy vegetables (peas, corn, winter squashes)

R = **Rice:** Includes rice and grains (barley, millet, semolina, sorghum, etc.)

B = **Beans:** Includes lentils, chickpeas, and kidney beans

S = **Sugar:** Includes syrup and assorted sweet-tasting foods and beverages

Food Finance: How to Track Your CARBS Bank Balance

One of the hardest parts about making proper dietary changes is that most recommendations are vague and non-specific. They're based on subjective pictures of portion plates or suggestions like cutting back on your fat or replacing unhealthy carbs with healthy carbs. I find that most of this information is ineffective and impractical. I'm going to make this process much easier for you.

I know most South Asians are good at math and managing money, so I'm going to teach you how to apply your disciplined spending behavior and accounting skills to your eating plan. You'll understand why you are in your current health predicament and enjoy a sense of control over your body composition that will allow you to quickly bounce back from inevitable hurdles like vacations, trips to India, and family dinners with relatives who love to show affection by serving carbs!

I'm giving you a single unit of currency, called the NC (net carbs), which accounts for your total grams of carb minus your total grams of fiber. We're subtracting fiber because it mutes the insulin effect of carbohydrates and provides some health benefits. Some people just track carbs, but I prefer NC because it helps to prioritize more nutrient-dense foods like vegetables, which are low in carbs and high in fiber. When you eat vegetables, the NC count is virtually nil, and you benefit from additional antioxidants and rich micronutrients. Now that's what I call a food bargain...maximal nutrients at a low NC cost! "Expensive" foods are those that provide little to no nutrients at a high NC cost, such as white rice.

NC = TOTAL GRAMS CARB – TOTAL GRAMS FIBER

Bargain Foods ($) **=** Low NC and maximal nutrients in return (vegetables, nuts, seeds, etc.)

Expensive Foods ($$$) **=** High NC and little to no nutrients (white rice, noodles, flour, etc.)

I strongly encourage keeping close track of your NC initially so you can learn which high cost foods to eliminate and which bargain foods to add to your nutrition portfolio. After a while, you will intuitively start making the right food choices. If you occasionally veer off course, simply start tracking again until you re-enter your fat-burning zone.

There are many online food trackers to help you reach your goals. To track net carbs, I use MyFitnessPal.com, a free nutrition tracker with an extensive food database that includes virtually every South Asian food on the planet. MyFitnessPal.com allows you to set a custom carb target and track your progress. At the end of each day, the tool tallies up the total grams of carb you've consumed, along with the total grams of fiber. From there, subtract the fiber from the carbs to get your NC. Don't worry about the other nutrients right now, just focus on NC during your initial foray into online food logging.

Your Daily NC Allowance

You start with a given allotment of NC every morning. Knowing your daily NC goal helps you make smart food choices throughout the day. Notice how I'm not focused on calories or grams of fat. If you keep your NC within range, you will avoid the painful process of measuring portion sizes and estimating calories. Choosing nutrient-dense, filling foods that have little to no effect on insulin, that burn fat, and that sustain energy throughout the day, will gradually become habit. So, what is your daily NC?

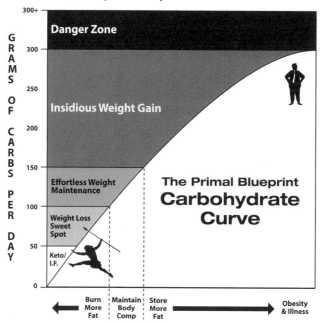

The Carbohydrate Curve, adapted from Mark Sisson's book, *The Primal Blueprint*, illustrates how the more grams of carbohydrate you eat, the deeper into fat storage you move. This curve counts total grams of carbohydrates, so we'll modify the ranges a bit to match our focus on net carbs.

My experience confirms that a NC of 100 grams is generally the zone at which insulin drops to a level that terminates persistent fat storage and activates fat burning. Note: since you are subtracting fiber from total carb amount, your daily net carb count will almost always be lower than your gross carbs if you are eating the recommended fiber-rich, plant-based foods. If you are eating less desirable, empty carbohydrates without fiber (all too common in processed foods) your total carbohydrate and net carbohydrate intake will be similar.

Some insulin resistant patients may need to keep their NC in the 50-100 gram zone initially until their body composition shifts to a more insulin sensitive state. At that point, 100-150 grams of NC will sustain weight loss and health goals. For most of my patients, 100 grams is the NC range at which all or most of their Metabolic 6-pack numbers become normal. If, however, you engage in vigorous physical activity for an hour or more, your muscles will require additional carbs. Intensive exercise is analogous to earning extra money because it increases your daily NC allowance. Don't be too liberal in your NC allotment—light activities like casual walking or housework won't earn you extra NC.

Safe Starches

Starches, including whole grains, contain toxins and anti-nutrients such as phytic acid. Anti-nutrients inhibit your body's absorption of key vitamins and minerals. Safe starches like white rice and potatoes do not contain toxins and anti-nutrients after cooking. Although they are considered "safe," they still carry a very high NC content, so if you are overweight, insulin resistant, highly inactive, or all of the above, then I recommend eliminating or significantly limiting these safe starches and staying within your daily NC allotment. If you reverse insulin resistance, achieve a better body composition, and stay physically active, you may be able to incorporate some safe starches into your diet, particularly as a post-exercise snack or meal.

A Few CARBS Precautions Before Starting

I'd venture to guess that most of you have eaten a carbohydrate-heavy diet over the course of your lifetime. My average South Asian patient consumes 300+ grams of NC daily! Since your body may have developed a certain degree of dependence on carbohydrates, you may experience some withdrawal effects, such as weakness and mild dizziness. Please read the precautions below.

Replace lost fluids and sodium: When you transition out of a high-carbohydrate diet, your body may lose excess fluid and salt. This can sometimes cause dizziness or weakness. Be sure to stay well hydrated and don't worry about restricting sodium while cutting carbohydrates, unless your doctor recommends a strict low-sodium diet based on medical conditions like CHF (congestive heart failure). The Duke University Medical Center's "No Sugar, No Starch" diet recommends consuming 2 cups of broth (vegetable or meat-based) each day, but this diet also recommends less than 20 grams of carbs per day for effective weight loss. If you are at 100 grams daily of net carbs, you may only need a cup of broth to balance sodium and fluid levels, or alternatively you can add some extra salt to your foods. Hypertensives should keep an eye on blood pressure when adding extra sodium to their diets.

Diabetics beware: If you are diabetic and on insulin or glucose-lowering oral medication like a sulfonylurea, then you must carefully cut back on your carbs while diligently checking your blood sugars. Decreasing carbohydrate consumption too abruptly can result in life-threatening hypoglycemia (low blood sugar), so be sure to discuss with your physician or a diabetes-certified nutritionist.

Vigorous exercise: Most South Asians don't engage in vigorous exercise for over 60 minutes, so adding more NC to your bank balance is probably not warranted. This is especially true if you are carrying excess body fat. However, if you do any intense level exercise for over an hour, like running, team sports (soccer, basketball, etc.), or cross-training, then you can add some additional carbs 30-60 minutes after your workout. For example, incorporating safe starches like a sweet potato or a serving of rice post-workout should be fine. Your muscles will need their glucose stores replenished, but remember: casual strolls or walks don't count as intense!

C = Chapatis and Breads

Indian flat breads—like chapatis, phulkas, naans, puris, and parathas—are Indian staples, but unfortunately, they are also major sources of fat-storing insulin. Many of my patients have switched from rice to whole-wheat chapatis without realizing that their consumption of chapatis is still a problem. Cutting rice does not give you license to binge on wheat. Wheat may actually do more harm if you are even mildly sensitive to gluten, which many people are. Not only do flat breads made of wheat supply excessive carbohydrates, but today's wheat is also a genetically engineered product that can send blood sugars skyward and trigger inflammation due to proteins like gluten. Often, wheat is a worse digestive offender than the spicy, greasy foods that typically get blamed. In fact, when many of my South Asian patients cut wheat from their diets, their digestive complaints, including bloating, gas, acid reflux, and bowel irregularities, disappear. Due to reduced inflammation, chronic joint aches and pains may also resolve.

Excess body fat is commonly reduced as a result of cutting out or scaling back on wheat intake. In his bestseller, *Wheat Belly*, cardiologist William Davis makes a compelling case for wheat as the primary culprit behind a number of chronic health conditions…from obesity, diabetes, and heart disease to arthritis and dementia.

I'm not suggesting that every South Asian eliminate all flatbreads and wheat, but instead recognize that chapatis, breads, and other wheat-based foods may be major contributors to fat storage, digestive issues, and other chronic health problems. At the very least, try to trim portions as much as you can.

I've listed some typical carbohydrate values for common Indian flatbreads on the next page. I used Trader Joe's brands when available since I know the nutrition labeling is relatively accurate and consistent. However, NC really varies based on brand so check package labels. Although the NC values for some wheat bread products may not be alarming, the type of starch in wheat, known as amylopectin A, has been known to increase blood sugar levels dramatically. According to Dr. William Davis, eating two slices of whole wheat toast can raise a patient's blood sugar more than eating a Snickers candy bar! Doesn't happen in everyone, but does happen often enough to render wheat a possible suspect in your health issues.

- 1 Trader Joe's Malabari Paratha = 47 g (nearly half your daily allowance!)

- 1 Trader Joe's Naan = 35 g

- 1 Rotiland Chapati = 24 g

- 1 Masala dosa = 30 g

- 1 slice whole wheat bread = 15 g

Substitutions: Almond flour and coconut flour are two excellent high-protein, low-carbohydrate substitutions for wheat that will help economize your NC count. Many of my patients are initially concerned about coconut flour and almond flour because of fat and calories, but remember that fat and calories play much less of a role than insulin does. I assure you that wheat contributes to far more adverse health effects than these nut flours do, unless you have an allergy to almond or coconut. Trader Joe's sells almond meal ("Just Almond Meal"), which is made up of crushed almonds with the skin intact. I have used this product successfully for many recipes, including pancakes and bread. If you prefer something closer to the consistency of flour, then try almond flour, which is made with pulverized almonds without the skin. I've incorporated almond flour into many of the recipes included in the appendix.

- 1 Coconut flour chapati = 3 g

- 1 Almond toast slice = 1 g

- 1 Almond flour pancake = 2 g

- Romaine lettuce (as bread substitute) = 0 grams

For sandwiches, I suggest using lettuce wraps (lettuce in place of bread) whenever you can. Most fast food and deli restaurants serve lettuce wraps upon request. When eating Mexican food, you can make lettuce wrap tacos with meat or vegetarian filling and a small amount of black beans. Most quality Fresh-Mex restaurants like Chipotle and Baja Fresh offer burrito bowls without the tortilla. Be sure to hold the rice. Add a small amount of beans if you are craving something heartier. In both cases you can add guacamole, cheese, and some sour cream to make the meal more satisfying.

If you must have your masala dosa, experiment with a low-carb batter by cutting back on the rice portion and using mostly lentils mixed with nut or coconut flour. Add some non-starchy vegetables for the filling to limit overall carbs. Chopped cauliflower is a wonderful substitute for potatoes in dosa fillings.

A = Aloo and Starchy Vegetables

Although vegetables are generally low NC due to low-carb and high-fiber content, potatoes are higher on the starch count, meaning higher blood sugar and insulin levels, and should be limited. Potatoes are abundant in many South Asian diets either as stand-alone curry dishes or as fillings in dosas, aloo parathas, and crispy samosas. Indian bread stuffed with potatoes is a double carb load; just one serving can make up nearly half your daily allowance.

Below are some NC costs of common starchy foods.

- Aloo sabji (1/2 cup) = 20 g

- 1 Aloo paratha (Deep Brand) = 40 g

- Corn (1/2 cup or 1 ear) = 15 g

- Peas (1 cup) = 20 g

- Acorn, pumpkin, and butternut squash (1 cup) = 20 g

Substitutions: Cauliflower is a great substitute for potatoes and has 20 times less the NC! For any Indian mashed potato dishes, try mashed cauliflower instead.

- Cauliflower sabji (1/2 cup) = 1 g

- Virtually any crunchy, leafy vegetable can serve as a healthier alternative for curried vegetables. Choose a variety of different colors to maximize antioxidants and reduce inflammation

- Sweet potatoes are a better alternative than white potatoes, but still relatively high in carbohydrates, so reserve for a post-workout snack

- Spaghetti, zucchini, and summer squash are less starchy squashes with one cup accounting for about 5 g of NC

R = Rice and Noodles

Rice is another core Indian staple. I have witnessed some of the most dramatic reductions in weight, triglycerides, and blood sugar follow either the complete elimination of rice, or at least a significant cutback. Rice is one of the worst food investments you can make if you are sedentary and/or insulin resistant, as most South Asians are. You pay a very high NC cost and get virtually nothing in return. Rice behaves no differently in the body than table sugar, and for all intents and purposes eating a plate of white rice is like eating an unsweetened plate of sugar. Don't believe me? A meta-analysis (collection of studies) showed a significant increase in type 2 diabetes risk with higher rice consumption, especially among Asians.[1] According to the study, the average daily rice intake in the Chinese population was 625 grams—exorbitantly higher than our NC goal of 100 grams! This high NC accounts for just the rice without all the other carb sources. Combine this level of intake with a highly sedentary lifestyle and the export of Western fast food and junk food, and you now have an obesity and diabetes crisis in China. A traditional South Asian diet is comparable. You'll see from the NC costs listed below why South Asians suffer from a predominantly rice-fueled belly. If you reverse insulin resistance and implement an active lifestyle, then controlled portions of rice, especially after exercise, may be acceptable. Unlike grains, rice is considered a "safe starch" because it does not contain anti-nutrients like phytic acid, which impair absorption of key minerals.

When South Asians need a break from traditional foods, they often opt for East Asian cuisine or Italian, in which case noodles and pasta act as substantial carb sources. One very popular brand of ramen noodles that South Asians stock in their pantries is "Maggi 2 Minute Noodles." See the NC below for the fat-free Maggi chicken noodles and prepare to fall off your chair! These noodles are anything but fat-free, with a single serving accounting for more than half of most individual's daily NC allowance. Again, keep in mind that reported carb values vary significantly between brands, but no matter how you look at it, when you eat rice or noodles, you pay a high NC price!

- 1 cup cooked white rice = 40 g

- 1 cup cooked Indian brand basmati rice = 76 g

- 1 cup cooked Trader Joe's <u>brown</u> basmati rice = 68 g

- Maggi 2 Minute Noodles—Chicken 99% Fat Free = 56 g

- 1 cup cooked spaghetti = 40 g

The accuracy of nutrition labeling on some Indian brands is questionable. I listed brown rice also to point out that although the NC is less than that of white basmati rice, it is still very high. If you make the switch from white to brown, you still have to restrict portion sizes.

From everything you've learned thus far about carbs and insulin, which food do you think would store more fat, a bowl of basmati rice (70 grams of NC) or a bowl of ghee (0 grams of NC)? I don't suggest eating a bowl of ghee, but want to make the point that "low-fat" rice is far more fattening than "high-fat" ghee. Many foods that contain less fat trigger more body fat storage due to their effects on insulin, while high-fat foods like ghee or coconut milk typically do not cause fat storage when combined with a carb-controlled diet. You may have heard the saying "fight fire with fire." In the context of a lower carb eating strategy, you are often fighting body fat with dietary fat as a replacement for carbs.

Substitutions: Using shredded or chopped vegetables as substitutes for rice and grains is one of the most potent fat-burning substitutions you can possibly make, since the NC difference between rice and a shredded/chopped vegetable is substantial. It's also an excellent way to introduce a few extra servings of vegetables into what is normally a plant-deficient South Asian diet. I have had the most diehard rice-eating South Asians reluctantly make this change, but when they saw their bellies shrink and their triglyceride and blood sugar levels plummet, they were sold! The majority of converts have never turned back to rice and some only eat it once or twice a week.

- Cauliflower rice = 4 g (white rice has about 10 times the NC of cauliflower rice—now that's what I call a bargain!)

- Shredded cabbage = 4 g

- Shirataki rice and noodles = 1 g

- Spaghetti squash = 6 g

- Other alternatives include shredded/chopped broccoli, carrots, or broccoli slaw (which comes packaged in most grocery stores)

If your daily NC stays within the target zone and you incorporate these low NC substitutions, you can then add rich-flavored curries made with coconut milk, ghee, and other healthy fats since you are keeping insulin levels low. Try my spaghetti squash recipe in the appendix, and feel free to add meat and cheese if you wish to make the sauce more filling and satisfying.

B = Beans and Lentils

Beans and lentils (dal) are excellent sources of fiber, protein, and multiple micronutrients. You are still paying a relatively high NC price but, unlike rice, you at least get something in return. If you pour the typical serving of beans or lentils on rice, or serve with a few chapatis, then you've turned the meal into another potent double carb load. Add an aloo sabji and you get what I call the "triple carb threat" with a serving of Indian bread, legumes (beans and lentils), and potatoes all in one meal. I didn't even count dessert! This combination of foods meets or exceeds your entire daily NC allowance, which means you are either bankrupt or possibly in debt after just one meal.

The key with legumes is to use a small amount of bean and add lots of volume with low NC vegetables like cauliflower, spinach, carrots, etc. Add some ghee to make it more rich and satisfying, and avoid the temptation to eat legumes with rice or an Indian flatbread. Instead, use one of the bread substitutes like a coconut-flour chapati, or if you're a non-vegetarian, eat legumes with a meat or fish-based curry.

Keep in mind that, unlike rice, beans, lentils, and legumes do contain anti-nutrients like phytic acid, which can impair absorption of minerals; the traditional practice of soaking legumes overnight or sprouting them can reduce the amount of anti-nutrients. Nuts also contain high levels of phytic acid, but since they are usually eaten between meals and in smaller quantities than staple legumes, their anti-nutrient effects are less significant.

There is quite a bit of variability among different brands and types of lentils (toor, mung, etc.). Most legumes cost around 30 grams of NC: 40 g total carbs – 10 g fiber = 30 NC. I've listed the average NC for lentils and other legumes below.

- 1 cup cooked dal = 30 g

- 1 cup kidney beans = 30 g

- 1 cup chickpeas = 30 g

There are a variety of other types of lentil and bean dishes that can pile on excess carbohydrates and exceed your daily quota; beware of South Indian rasam and sambar, along with the use of besan (ground chickpea flower) as a thickener and coating.

Substitutions: Many of my patients cook rasam, a South Indian soup made from tamarind juice, with little to no lentils and add vegetables instead. One cup of pure rasam without lentils contains about five grams of net carbs. Reduce the amount of legumes to keep you within your daily NC allowance and add volume with vegetables, protein with foods like paneer and even nuts (e.g. vegetable lentils with toasted almonds and fennel), and richness by topping your lentil dish off with extra virgin olive oil, ghee, or coconut oil. Try to avoid compounding your carb load by pouring over rice or dipping in chapatis and other Indian flatbreads.

S = Sugar, Syrup, and Most Sweet-Tasting Things

Sugars and all things sweet is the most obvious category to avoid. Even brown sugar is a culprit. I once had a diabetic patient who was making Indian sweets from brown sugar, believing them to be healthier!

A more hidden source of dangerous sugar is a form we've come across before—high fructose corn syrup (HFCS). HFCS is a chemically modified sweetener that is cheaper to manufacture than pure sugar. It is also sweeter than sugar, making it the drug of choice... excuse me—the sweetener of choice—in sodas, sweets, and many packaged foods. The metabolic effects of HFCS are nothing short of devastating, with an increasing number of studies showing its strong association to diabetes and obesity, and its impact on brain chemistry, rendering it highly addictive. Read nutrition labels and avoid HFCS at all costs. Other sources of liquid sugar aside from sodas include juices, designer coffee drinks, mango lassis, and fruit smoothies.

Overconsumption of fruits can deliver high levels of fructose into your bloodstream, which in turn can lead to fat storage. Since the general health recommendation is to "eat more fruits and vegetables," most South Asians opt for far more fruits than vegetables. The NC cost of most fruits is higher than that of vegetables. Tropical fruits such as mangos, bananas, and pineapples provide a fairly large sugar load. Blended smoothies made up of mostly fruit are another large source of fruit sugar. Fruits that trigger less of an insulin response are berries, cherries, apples, and pears.

Now, I wouldn't call fruits an expensive NC food because you do get fiber, antioxidants, and other important micronutrients in return, but I would definitely track these foods and make sure they are not putting you outside your daily NC allowance. Try to make a habit of snacking more on vegetables, nuts, and seeds, and indulging with a couple of fruit servings, preferably berries.

I'm not trying to scare you away from enjoying fruit, and I am not discounting the wonderful nutritional benefits that fruit offers. I'm asking you to take a big picture view of your total carbohydrate and net carbohydrate intake in order to address the most pressing health concerns in the South Asian community. Prioritize carb management by eliminating the nutritionally deficient grain foods and sugary foods mentioned, and you can be less concerned about enjoying your daily mango than someone who casually allows cultural traditions and modern life momentum to push their daily carb intake into the danger zone.

Take a look at the high NC costs of the following:

- 1 medium banana = 24 g

- 1 raw mango = 30 g

- 1 cup pineapple = 20 g

- 3 dates = 50 g

- 1 cup prunes = 60 g

Substitutions: When looking to lower carbohydrates and regulate the insulin response, think berries.

- 1 cup blueberries = 15 g

- 1 cup raspberries = 7 g

- 1 cup strawberries = 10 g

As you can see, berries are about half the NC cost of bananas and mangos, with raspberries the best budgetary option. Every cup of berries delivers an incredible amount of antioxidants, which makes for a great investment. If you enjoy mangos, I suggest carving off a few wedges to top off a salad or a bowl of yogurt rather than eating them whole like many South Asians like to do. Dried fruits (dates, prunes, mangos, etc.) are favorite snacks that South Asians often deem healthy, but dried fruits can have as much sugar as candy!

PRIORITIZING CARBS FOR THE CARB CHALLENGED

Ideally, it's best to cut all CARBS foods so you can experience maximum benefits. Should this goal be too overwhelming, refer to the following ranked priority list for which food groups to cut first:

1. **Cut sugar, sodas, and HFCS first:** Read all package labels and avoid these ingredients. Don't compromise. Cut it all out!

2. **Rice or wheat is the next to go:** Both can have adverse effects on health. Generally, I've seen more improvements in insulin resistance after cutting back on rice. You can strategize based on your symptoms. If you have significant digestive issues or inflammatory conditions such as arthritis, tendonitis, inflammatory bowel disease, etc., I suggest cutting wheat first while portion controlling your rice.

3. **Wheat or rice:** Cut whatever you didn't cut in #2. If you cut rice first and haven't reached your goals, cut wheat next.

4. **Cut back on potatoes:** Restrict consumption of potatoes if they are a major portion of your diet.

5. **Portion control your legumes:** This includes beans, lentils, etc.

I've seen a range of different responses to efforts to cut CARBS, which is a testimony to the individual genetic variations of insulin resistance. For some patients, cutting a single category, like sugar/sweets or rice, is sufficient to achieve health goals. For more insulin resistant individuals, it's necessary to cut most, if not all, the CARBS foods. The good news is that as your body composition changes to less fat and more muscle, you become more insulin sensitive and enter a state of "insulin resilience." This means foods that used to make you fat now have less of a fat-storing effect. Many patients report that their annual trips to India, which typically caused 10 pounds of weight gain, now cause little to no gain at all. And once they dial in their fat-burning NC target number after returning, they lose that post-vacation weight in just a few days. It is truly liberating to have this type of control over your body composition.

All this may sound overwhelming to a South Asian who has been eating excessive carbohydrates his or her entire life. Food (carbs in particular) is truly addictive, which makes it even more important for you to monitor your intake. What if your teenage son came home from college and said he was addicted to a drug that made him fat and put him at risk for heart disease and diabetes? Would you respond by saying "Yes, I know that drug is addictive and difficult to quit, so don't worry about it. Just keep taking it." Of course not! You would provide emotional support and come up with a plan to get him off the drug so he could live a full, happy, and productive life. Do the same thing for yourself. Acknowledge that you have a food/carb addiction problem, realize that it is causing significant health consequences, and then implement a plan to get those CARBS under control.

FATS

Now that you have some useful strategies to help you cut back on carbs, let's turn our attention to fats. Include the following saturated fats and heart-healthy monounsaturated and omega-3 fats in your diet.

Extra virgin olive oil: A heart-healthy monounsaturated fat that is not as heat stable as saturated fats, so don't use extra virgin olive oil for high-temperature cooking. Avoid cooking at or above its smoke point (when the oil starts emitting smoke), typically between 325°F and 375°F. Low-temperature vegetable sautéing is fine. Enjoy extra virgin olive oil on salads, vegetable dishes, dressings, and sauces, or pour it over eggs and curries. The highest quality extra virgin olive oil is domestically grown, extra virgin, and "first cold-pressed only," meaning the seed has been pressed once without heat. Buying local products with this designation (extra virgin, first cold-pressed) ensures minimal processing and maximum purity. Search finer supermarkets such as Whole Foods; Trader Joe's offers great California oil at a moderate price.

Omega-3: An essential fatty acid that helps subdue inflammation. Fish is your best source of omega-3, especially salmon, mackerel, herring, and sardines. Plant sources include seeds (flax, chia, pumpkin), walnuts, leafy green vegetables, and marine algae.

Ghee: Not to be feared but embraced, this traditional South Asian fat is loaded with anti-inflammatory health benefits. Ghee is very heat stable, so you can cook with it at high temperatures. The highest quality ghee is organic, grass-fed, and non-homogenized.

Coconut oil: An excellent source of high-energy, medium chain triglycerides (MCTs), coconut oil is the most heat stable cooking oil at high temperatures. Buy organic, virgin coconut oil.

Butter: A much healthier fat than vegetable oil, the highest quality butter is organic and grass-fed. Butter is one product you should consider buying organic since many hormones and chemicals present in conventional butters are well preserved in butterfat, and thus more apt to cause harm to your body. Grass-fed also ensures a higher vitamin content.

Other acceptable oils: Avocado, walnut, macadamia, dark roasted sesame oil, and high omega-3 oils (borage, cod-liver, krill, salmon, etc.) can also be consumed in moderation.

Other healthy fats: Avocados, nuts and nut butters, seeds and seed butters, and other coconut products such as coconut milk and coconut butter are healthy fats.

I know you've been told fats like ghee and coconut oil are bad for you, but this is because conventional health advice is dispensed in the context of a high-carbohydrate diet. A high-carb diet can turn any good fat into a bad one, since the excess insulin ushers the fat into the fat cells, thereby leading to increased fat storage and high triglycerides. South Indians, especially in Kerala, have a very high incidence of heart disease. We used to blame the prevalence of cardiovascular illness on coconut oil and ghee, but it is in fact the excess carb consumption that is the main problem. I've witnessed many South Indians cut their excess carb intake, keep their fats, and achieve their Metabolic 6-packs.

When my patients cut back carbs to the recommended levels, formerly feared foods like eggs, butter, ghee, and coconut oil have more beneficial than harmful effects on their health as proven by subsequent fat loss, reduced inflammation, and improvement in Metabolic 6-pack risk factors. In fact, premier athletes and CrossFit enthusiasts are combining lower-carb lifestyles with organic ghee and coconut oil in their training regimens. I have seen many fitness aficionados in my office and I can assure you that their metabolic numbers are typically stellar, as is their physical appearance.

When you start adding these fats to your diet, don't rely on intuition or your gut feeling to determine if you're eating within the recommended carb target zone. Patients significantly underestimate how many carbs they consume daily. I've had patients liberally add fat to their diet while still consuming carbohydrates at a level of 150-200 grams or greater. This is a recipe for disaster since high insulin levels end up transporting both fat and excess carbohydrates into fat cells, thereby promoting increased body fat and worsening cholesterol levels.

PROTEIN

Meat and fish are obvious staple sources of protein, but I want to provide plenty of other protein choices for vegetarians as well. I would not be able to sleep at night if I wrote a book addressed only to South Asian meat-eaters and marginalized those who, for personal, religious, or moral reasons, choose to eat meat-free diets. Both vegetarians and meat-eaters can freely choose from the protein-rich sources below.

Eggs: Please keep eggs a part of your diet if that is an option. Many of my vegetarian patients cut out eggs due to fears about high cholesterol. Eggs are one of the densest foods on the planet, particularly the yolks. Forget this nonsense about just eating the egg whites. Enjoy the entire egg so you can benefit from the protein in the whites and the multiple nutrients and healthy omega-3 fats in the yolk. In fact, one study showed that whole egg consumption (including the yolk) improved all cholesterol parameters and insulin resistance in subjects on a carb-restricted diet, even more so than a yolk-free egg substitute did.[2]

That toast, low-fat muffin, bagel, or high-fiber cereal you've been eating will raise your cholesterol and body weight more so than a couple of eggs. Eggs also keep you fuller, longer. Shake things up with an egg curry dish for lunch or dinner.

Nuts, seeds, and their respective butters: Nuts and seeds are packed with power in the form of protein, vitamins, minerals, fiber, and healthy fats. They are an excellent snack choice when eaten in raw form. Avoid honey or sugarcoated nuts or trailmix that includes other high-carb mix-ins like dried fruit or chocolate chips. Nut butters such as almond or macadamia, and seed butters such as sunflower seed butter, provide versatile spreads that can be applied to cut fruit and vegetables. Nut and seed butters should not contain additional ingredients other than salt and can be easily made with a high-grade food processor.

Dairy: Milk, yogurt, paneer, and cheese are acceptable, but not necessary sources of dietary protein. If including dairy, stick to organic, pasture-raised, and grass-fed to eliminate the hormones, pesticides, and antibiotics found in commercial dairy products.

Quinoa: If you must include a grain-like substance in your diet, choose quinoa, which technically is not a grain, but instead a seed related to leafy green vegetables like spinach. It is high in protein (contains all nine essential amino acids) and is a good source of nutrients, including calcium, phosphorus, and magnesium. Quinoa is a reasonable option for vegetarians looking for more protein sources, but do be aware of its relatively high NC.

Almond flour or coconut flour breads and baked goods: Substitute with these flours as much as possible. Coconut flour is high protein and requires more eggs for recipes, packing in a double protein punch.

Lentils and beans: Legumes are a good source of protein, but beware of their NC cost and volumize with vegetables. A bowl of lentils should be three-fourths vegetables and one-fourth lentils.

Protein shakes: Choose a whey protein shake that is low carb and high quality. Whey is one of two major groups of protein found in milk. Use regular or coconut milk as your base, and you can add a nut butter like almond butter for an additional protein boost. Add limited fruit and mostly vegetables to keep carbs low.

Soy: Choose fermented soy products such as tempeh and miso. Be wary of most tofu products, which are unfermented and genetically modified, and carry potential toxicities and health risks.

High protein vegetables: Don't forget that vegetables like asparagus, broccoli, Brussels sprouts, and cauliflower contain protein. Most of my vegetarian South Asian patients consume insufficient amounts of vegetables, far less than my typical Western vegetarian patients.

So there you have it—a nice long list of several protein options. Vegetarians can mix these options to maximize protein even further, like making cauliflower fried rice with eggs (if allowed), nuts, high protein vegetables, and tempeh. How about a protein power smoothie with low-carb whey powder, vegetables, almond butter, and a handful of berries? Or a coconut flour pancake topped with sliced almonds and Greek yogurt? I can keep going, but I'll let the real South Asian chefs reading this book take it from here. Bottom line is that vegetarians with the right information and some culinary creativity can absolutely make dramatic body composition changes and achieve their Metabolic 6-packs.

"6-S STRATEGY" TO EAT MORE VEGETABLES

Meat-eaters and vegetarians pretty much all agree that vegetables are an essential part of a healthy diet. Regardless, most South Asians need to significantly increase their intake of vegetables. A diet high in veggies is linked to reduced heart disease, cancer, and virtually all other chronic illnesses. One or two overcooked sabjis daily is not sufficient. To incorporate the "6-S" strategy (Salads, Smoothies, Soups, Snacks, Substitutions for grains, and Sauces) you will need a high-speed blender and a food processor. I'm guessing you spend plenty of money on smartphones, tablets, laptops, and assorted other technology and personal possessions, so make your health a priority and invest in a high quality product that can serve as both a blender and a food processor. VitaMix brand blending machines (available at Costco) are lauded as the gold standard and cost several hundred dollars. Cuisinart offers versatile blending machines that allow you to attach a food processor blade or a jar for liquid drinks. Find the best product in your budget, but definitely stay away from the twenty-dollar drugstore blenders that might break after whipping up just a few delicious smoothies.

Salads: Eat nutrient-dense salads. You can do better than a few slices of cucumber on lettuce! Pick dark greens as your base, such as spinach, kale, collards, chard, and mustard greens. Darker greens typically have more nutrients. Next, mix in a variety of multi-colored vegetables (carrots, peppers, tomatoes, etc.). Use nuts as your crispy add-ons instead of croutons, tortilla strips, or Asian crunchy noodles. Avoid sweetened dressings and choose simple vinaigrettes and creamy dressings.

Smoothies: Avoid fruit-based smoothies with mangos, bananas, pineapples, etc., which are basically sugar-loaded milkshakes. Smoothies should be primarily vegetable-based with some berries to add sweetness. Other mix-ins include coconut milk, almond milk, almond butter, or a low-carb Greek yogurt. If you exercise vigorously, you may want to consider a high quality whey protein powder to add to your smoothies. Keep track of the NC for all your ingredients, as they add up quickly in smoothie recipes.

Soups: Keep chicken or vegetable liquid broth or bouillon cubes handy at all times. Leftover vegetables can be easily turned into soup in just minutes, and you never need to worry about rotting vegetables in your refrigerator drawers ever again!

Snacks: Eat at least two raw vegetable snacks a day. Pack baby carrots, sugar snap peas, mini-peppers, cherry tomatoes, or whatever other portable vegetables you enjoy. When you come home from work with raging hunger pains, dip crispy vegetables into a tasty, creamy, low-carb dip that's either homemade or store-bought. Trader Joe's has a great selection of low-carb dips like hummus, Greek yogurt guacamole, cilantro and chive yogurt, and ranch dressing.

Substitutions for grains: We've discussed grain substitutions in detail, but a reminder that foods like cauliflower rice and shredded cabbage can add generous helpings of vegetables to your diet.

Sauces: Use your blender or food processor to make vegetable and citrus-based sauces and marinades for vegetables, meat, and fish. Make your own fresh pasta sauce. Prepare in bulk and freeze.

I suppose "Sabji" could have been our 7th "S" but most Indians are already eating plenty of sabji. My main advice is to avoid overcooking your sabji, which drains precious nutrients, and get creative by using a variety of different vegetables in your sabji dishes.

BREAKFAST:
THE UNHEALTHIEST MEAL OF THE DAY?

Forget everything you've heard about how breakfast is a necessity for weight loss and optimal health. For most of my patients, breakfast is the meal that counts for the greatest number of carbs, all in the name of "high fiber" or "whole grain." I used to eat a breakfast of steel-cut oats, a banana, and a cup of berries every single morning. That meal alone delivered over 50 grams of net carbs (over half my entire daily allowance) and I hadn't even left home yet! A glass of orange juice, a banana, and whole wheat toast sounds pretty healthy, but that too will drain some precious NC funds early in the day.

Indeed, there are many negative aspects of a traditional breakfast. Breakfast typically delivers a substantial carb load and can actually make you hungrier. Cortisol levels are high in the morning and can increase insulin secretion after a carb-loaded breakfast, which causes a drop in blood sugar and triggers intense hunger a couple of hours later (the 10 am hunger pains). Eat a "healthy" breakfast, and you impair fat burning. When you wake in the morning, your body is more optimized for fat burning than at any other time of the day. A high-carb breakfast immediately ruins this fat-burning potential!

The concept of optimal fat burning in the morning is important to understand, as we have been heavily programmed to believe that consuming carbs right away is essential to health and to a fast metabolism. Assuming you didn't have a heavy late-night dinner, evening snack binges, or sleepwalk your way into the pantry, your body is pretty much in a fasted state when you wake in the morning. That's why they call it "break-fast"! In a fasted state, if you were to get some exercise or simply function for a few hours without ingesting any calories, your body would actually tap into its fat stores for energy.

Here are some of my favorite breakfast options:

Fasted workout: A fasted workout—eating nothing before your morning workout—unlocks your "inner pantry," tapping into your fat stores for energy. There's no need to look for breakfast in your fridge or pantry. You've got plenty of fuel locked away inside your fat cells, so turn to this for breakfast whenever possible! Notice how, after a morning workout, your appetite is moderated for a while due to the hormonal and metabolic effects of a fasted workout. By all means, eat something when you feel hungry, and appreciate the sensation of actually being hungry in advance of a meal. Using Tabata exercise techniques, you can complete a quality fasted workout in less than 15 minutes if you're pressed for time (see Chapter 7). If you feel light-headed or dizzy during fasted workouts, try eating a smaller breakfast of protein and fat, and then see if you can gradually taper down to a fasted workout.

Nothing: Many patients confess they are less hungry when they skip breakfast. Strange as it may seem, those 10 am screaming hunger pains actually go away when breakfast is skipped. Eating carbohydrate-dominant meals activates the vicious cycle of hunger and food dependence that most people would rather avoid. I find that I feel much more focused and alert when I avoid eating breakfast, especially a carb-heavy breakfast. Of course, if you do wake up feeling hungry and can't fit in a workout, choose from some of the following more satiating options below.

Eggs: Omelettes, soft-boiled eggs, scrambled eggs, and egg curry are all wonderful ways to prepare one of the healthiest, most versatile foods. Remember that eggs do not worsen your cholesterol or contribute directly to heart disease risk, unless you combine with an abundant amount of carbs. Replace that side of toast with vegetables!

Almond meal/flour or coconut flour pancakes: These are the flour substitutes I use to make "BLS" (Bread-Like Substances)." BLS for us medical folk stands for "Basic Life Support" or CPR training. I have renamed this acronym "Bread-Like Substances" to help curb my intermittent urges as a recovering breadaholic. I strongly suggest every South Asian learn to use these flours as substitutes for white and wheat flours. You get used to the taste and consistency, and adding some fresh berries, a little cream, a dollop of yogurt, and a spoonful of raw honey makes for a very satisfying baking bonus.

Almond meal oatmeal: I used to eat oatmeal and a banana for breakfast almost every morning. The minute I removed this go-to breakfast from my diet, I dropped 14 pounds almost effortlessly. Many of my patients have experienced the same effect. However, I do miss the consistency of oatmeal and can't eat eggs everyday, so I will occasionally stir up some almond meal, mix in some almond or coconut milk, and add a handful of berries and a touch of honey.

Low-carb Greek yogurt with berries and nuts: I typically use the plain *Fage* brand of Greek yogurt and avoid the liquid sugar syrup pocket they call "fruit." You are better off adding real fruits like a handful of fresh berries and some nuts for extra protein. Since I'm not as concerned about fat content given my low overall carb intake, I get the richer, more filling 2% or full-fat version rather than the 0% fat option—keeps my belly full and my brain satisfied. Be sure to read the ingredient labels on low-fat versus full-fat yogurts and dairy products. The lack of fat gets replaced by all kinds of mysterious chemical fillers that are far less natural and far more harmful than the fat that has been removed.

Dinner leftovers: That's right. Why shouldn't you eat that chicken drumstick, lamb curry, or sabji from last night? There's no rule saying you have to eat "breakfast foods" for breakfast. The leftover lamb curry will likely be less fattening and more filling than cereal, toast, or some other high-carb breakfast choice, assuming you're not pouring the curry over a plate of white rice.

YOUR WORKPLACE CAFETERIA: FRIEND OR FOE?

As part of my role managing health and wellness programs for Silicon Valley companies, I tour cafeterias and offer suggestions for healthier nutrition. I'm overwhelmed by the abundance of international options, cooked up to feed a diverse workforce. Many of these food halls have a separate section featuring Indian food. There's no doubt that providing this type of food access is a luxury and convenience, but it can also be a major health risk. Employees often watch their weight balloon 10 to 15 pounds within their first year of work. Free access to food and a highly sedentary lifestyle are a recipe for weight gain and worsening insulin resistance. Many employers are now making a conscious effort to offer more nutritious selections, but unfortunately many of these foods are mislabeled "heart healthy" due to a low-fat designation or a reduced cholesterol content with no attention whatsoever paid to carbohydrate amount. Cubicle adjacent micro-kitchens stock low-fat "100-calorie snacks," which may be low calorie, but usually contain sugar and excess carbohydrates. Conscientious employees selectively consume these so-called healthy foods and watch their insulin resistant signs, such as triglycerides and belly fat, increase. Catered meals, such as pizza, pasta, noodles, rice, and subway-style sandwiches, are extremely high in carbohydrates. Ultimately, we want all employers to offer alternatives that help lower insulin and fat storage. For now, use the nutrition principles outlined so far, and if healthy choices are limited at your workplace, then bring in your own meals and snacks. With the right knowledge in hand and a focus on lowering excess carbohydrates, employees can easily take advantage of the wide selection of healthy foods and assemble meals and snacks that facilitate fat burning and prevent heart disease. Reducing these risk factors is not only good for health, but also increases energy and productivity in the workplace.

INTERMITTENT FASTING

Most South Asians are familiar with the practice of fasting. If you've never fasted, you likely grew up in a household with a parent or grandparent who fasted on certain day(s) of the week as a mark of devotion to a deity or perhaps in honor of a departed family member. As fasting trends in the mainstream, health enthusiasts are adopting intermittent fasting as an effective method of fat burning. Do an online search for "Intermittent Fasting" (IF) and you'll see this practice promoted on various health and fitness websites.

Intermittent fasting typically consists of one or more weekly fasts lasting twelve hours or more. For a typical South Asian eating 300+ grams of carbohydrates daily, the thought of any form of fasting may seem impossible due to insulin-dependent cycles of intense hunger. However, once you shift your body into the fat-burning zone for four to six weeks, you will naturally notice hunger diminish thanks to the more filling proteins and healthy fats in your diet. Skipping meals will not only feel easier, but also you will find yourself accidentally forgetting to eat since you won't be distracted by extreme hunger pains. The old advice about eating three meals and two scheduled snacks each day is really designed for carb-addicted individuals as a way to suppress intense hunger and compensatory overeating.

> *The old advice about eating three meals and two scheduled snacks each day is really designed for carb-addicted individuals as a way to suppress intense hunger and compensatory overeating.*

Once you adapt to fat burning, you will no longer be constrained by these types of ill-conceived rules, but instead will be able to instinctively respond to less frequent periods of hunger. Initial studies of IF have been conducted mostly on animals, but the results are striking. Lifespan increases of fifty percent and improved brain function are just two of its studied effects. For example, research on calorie-restricted mice conducted at the National Institute on Aging in Baltimore showed boosted levels of BDNF (brain-derived neurotropic factor), a chemical that helps protect human brains from Alzheimer's disease. Think of your own family members or religious figures like yogis who perform regular fasts. Typically, they are in excellent health, look youthful, and remain mentally sharp throughout their lives.

The additional benefit of IF is that for the first time it puts you in complete charge of your hunger and food intake. Practicing intermittent fasting cues you in to how infrequently you need to eat and how food itself is a major source of fatigue. I know it seems counterintuitive since we refer to food as "fuel," but pay attention to how your energy and alertness levels feel before and after a meal, especially after a carb-heavy meal.

Many of my South Asian patients who eat a high-carb diet already skip breakfast, so they may claim they are already doing some form of "Intermittent Fasting." While it may be true that they go for extended periods without eating, the intended benefits are ruined when they engage in high-carb compensatory overeating hours later, particularly in the evenings. This type of binge commonly consists of pre-dinner South Asian crispy snacks, a high-carbohydrate dinner, and post-dinner sweets. Also, since their metabolisms are not adapted for fat burning, the fasting will not trigger any significant fat loss. Instead, the body slows down fat burning and metabolic rate in general, and releases stress hormones into the bloodstream that promote the breakdown of hard-earned lean muscle tissue into glucose. This occurs in response to the perceived starvation of a carbohydrate-dependent eater not eating overnight and then skipping breakfast. Simply put, the wonderful benefits of intermittent fasting are only available to those who have optimized their fat-burning abilities by eating a moderated carbohydrate diet, exercising appropriately, managing all forms of life stress, and getting adequate sleep for a sustained period of time. Once you have built some momentum with a low carbohydrate-eating pattern, you can consider incorporating IF as a healthy lifestyle practice and a very effective fat-burning method—especially if you have hit a plateau with fat loss. I have included some tips to help optimize your IF efforts.

Skip breakfast: Your sleeping hours count as fasting hours, so skipping breakfast is an easy way to get in 12+ hours of fasting. It should also encourage you to get more sleep since sleeping is the most effortless and pleasurable form of fasting. Try gradually pushing your lunch later if you can. A later lunch also helps prevent the common pattern of binge eating when you come home from work.

Bulletproof coffee: If you are hungry upon waking, drink your coffee or tea with some heavy cream to make it filling, or you can add a spoonful of coconut oil which is readily converted to energy and promotes satiety. Adding coconut oil to your morning beverage is a popular practice among Primal/Paleo enthusiasts, who have nicknamed the drink "bulletproof coffee."

Cleanse: Engage in one IF session a month to see how things go and then add more sessions whenever you can. I sometimes intermittent fast as a "cleanse" after one of my occasional days of dietary indiscretion.

Be spontaneous: Follow your body's instinctive signals and base it on demand. I often fast on days when I need exceptional focus and attention.

Be scheduled: Pick one or two days out of the week and fast with conviction, as is part of South Asian tradition and so many other cultures around the world. Fast for a Hindu god, Buddha, Allah, world peace, a lost loved one, or whatever person, spirit, or ideal inspires you.

IT'S ALL IN THE ROOTS

Think about much of the advice given in this chapter, especially the emphasis on eating healthy fats like ghee and coconut oil, consuming more natural vegetables, and performing intermittent fasting. Let's embrace traditional Indian herbs and spices like turmeric, cardamom, ginger, and cilantro that have anti-inflammatory, health-promoting properties, while letting go of the unnatural chemicals and additives found in processed foods. Traditional South Asian practices performed by our more physically active, sunlight-exposed ancestors ensured optimal physical and mental health well into the golden years. I still recall the incredible mental clarity of my grandparents and how smooth and unwrinkled their skin was even when they were beyond 80 years of age.

Our generation has no hope of reaching this type of optimal health in later years if South Asians continue on their current path. As you'll learn in Chapter 11, South Asians are experiencing accelerated aging and chronic disease as early as their thirties and forties!

That's not to say that everything older generations did was optimal for health. Some of my relatives who have now passed were overweight due to excessive carbohydrate and sweet consumption. Many of them smoked, and virtually none of them did any preventive health screenings. Our answer is not to completely replicate the lifestyles of our recent or distant ancestors, but to instead combine the best of the old with today's breakthroughs in areas like preventive health, nutrition, and exercise science. Past practice coupled with current advancements offers each of us the best chance of preventing chronic disease and fulfilling our genetic potential.

"RICE FOR RICKSHAW WALAS ONLY"

One of my childhood memories during my summer trips to India was standing on the balcony of my father's old house in Kolkata, looking down at the rickshaw "walas" (rickshaw pullers) who congregated in the alley below for meals, showers, and social gatherings. These were the days of original human-pulled rickshaws, before the modern auto rickshaw. Every meal these walas ate consisted of a giant mountain of rice and lentils. The rickshaw wala physiques were mostly emaciated or lean. If they had adequate access to protein, there's no doubt they would have had ideal, muscular physiques. I was mesmerized by their superhuman strength, carting around overweight families for long distances or carrying enormous bundles of cargo. Rice and lentils were necessary to fuel these tremendous physical demands.

Today, human-pulled rickshaws are nearly obsolete and have been replaced by motorized rickshaws (auto rickshaws). As a result, auto rickshaw drivers are significantly more overweight than their predecessors because they continue to eat a carb-heavy diet, but the nature of their job has abruptly turned sedentary. Unless you are pulling rickshaws all day, carrying heavy pieces of luggage as does a porter in bustling Howrah train station in Kolkata, or laboring in the fields, your body doesn't require the tremendous amount of glucose fuel you are consuming in the form of rice, lentils, breads, noodles, etc. The South Asian belly is direct evidence of this unnecessary surplus fuel.

Large servings of rice and lentils act as high-energy foods designed for bodies in frequent motion. Our ancestors were constantly on the go, walking over 20,000 steps daily, engaging all muscles with daily physical labor, soaking in vitamin D from the sun, getting adequate sleep and rest between periods of intense work without 24/7 digital distractions, living in a more natural food environment uncontaminated by processed foods loaded with trans fats, high fructose corn syrup, and a plethora of other chemicals and additives.

If you can recreate anything close to this traditional lifestyle, then yes...you can probably handle the high glucose energy effects of rice, breads, and noodles with less trouble than a less active person can. Alas, it's still not healthy to fuel your active lifestyle with pro-inflammatory carbohydrates. The amount of glucose fuel you are putting in your body is meant for a racecar that is moving full speed around a track all day, not for an oversized mini-van parked in the garage most of the time. And yes, in our current state we are the oversized mini-van. The same foods, such as rice and noodles, have a completely different metabolic and physiological effect when consumed in today's artificial environment than when consumed in the natural environment we used to live in (and were meant to live in). I realize it is not practical in today's world to recreate this situation exactly, but it is possible and absolutely necessary to take a few steps back and incorporate at least some of these traditional principles, while adjusting our fuel source (carbs) downward to be more compatible with our current lifestyles and activity levels.

Summary

- In order to burn body fat, focus on tracking and controlling NC like a bank balance.

- Use the CARBS categories to remind you which major carb sources to avoid.

- Prioritize quitting sugar and rice, and be very wary of wheat, which can be a major source of fat storage and inflammation.

- Track your Metabolic 6-pack before and after making dietary changes to monitor effects.

- Be sure to add enough protein, and don't fear fat, which in the absence of excess carbs is energizing and healthy.

- Beware of breakfast sources that provide excess carbs. Early morning carbohydrate consumption can trigger fat storage and increase post-breakfast hunger. Don't fear eggs, especially when you cut back on carb intake.

- Consider incorporating intermittent fasting to accelerate fat burning.

For Professionals

- Help individuals set their NC target goals without calorie restriction.

- Once individuals are eating the recommended amount of carbs, be sure to stop pushing outmoded advice like, "eat breakfast every day" or "eat three meals and two snacks." Let your patients follow their own natural instincts and hunger signals.

- Track Metabolic 6-pack, especially triglyceride level, which is a good direct indicator of reductions in carb intake.

- Do not push low fat. Encourage healthy fats coupled with lower carbs to help keep individuals satiated and to improve compliance. Remember that low carb + low fat = low compliance.

- Provide adequate protein sources for vegetarians while encouraging sufficient fat intake.

- Keep in mind that many of the foods and snacks labeled "low-fat" in company cafeterias are contributing to employee obesity and chronic disease. Provide suggestions to make sure your patients are consuming enough protein, vegetables, and healthy fat options in these circumstances.

CHAPTER 7

EXERCISE: AN ENJOYABLE APPROACH TO FITNESS AND STRENGTH

MOTIVATING MY SOUTH ASIAN PATIENTS to increase activity and reduce sitting time has been one of my most challenging tasks as a physician. The entire global population has become more sedentary, but South Asians in particular are among the champion sitters, and this inactive tendency begins in childhood. South Asians are also the only patients I have encountered who ask me point blank if there is any way they can improve their health through diet alone without exercising. This mindset conveys their extreme aversion towards even basic forms of movement, let alone serious exercise programs. In this chapter, I'm going to provide some creative suggestions that will hopefully motivate even the most devout couch potato to get up, get out, and enjoy some physical exercise.

TOP THREE REASONS SOUTH ASIANS REFUSE TO MOVE

Before we delve into movement, let's first discuss the three main reasons for the extreme state of inertia in South Asians.

High-carb Diet

A high-carb diet promotes a chronic state of fatigue. Let's break it down:

Excess carbs = excess insulin = persistent fatigue

I suppose you could say that your aversion to movement isn't really even your fault! It's your diet's fault! Who wants to exercise when they're running on little to no energy? Even though you may be eating more than enough calories, a high-carb, insulin-raising diet pushes your energy into your fat cells, making it unavailable to fuel your brain and your muscles. Pay attention to how you feel in the hour or two following one of your typical high-carb meals, and you'll understand the relationship between what you eat and why you're not moving.

When high-carbohydrate meals are consumed and insulin floods the bloodstream in response, energy in the form of glucose and fatty acids is removed from the bloodstream and shunted into storage. Soon after you eat a hearty meal, your bloodstream is literally starved for energy and you feel like taking a nap instead of taking a lap around the block! If you consider yourself too lazy to exercise, you might be correct, but more from a biochemical perspective than from a personality perspective. This is great news because it means you can increase your everyday energy levels, as well as your motivation to exercise, simply by altering your dietary habits to produce less insulin. Let's face it: a meal foundation of rice, lentils, and Indian breads already exceeds the maximum allowable daily carb amount. Add on snack foods, sweets, processed foods, and sweetened beverages, and you are so far over optimal carb intake that you are essentially locked in an energy depleted, fat storage pattern at all times. You have plenty of fuel locked away in your fat cells and in your muscle and liver glycogen, but none available in the bloodstream to burn for energy.

When I convince patients to reduce their carb intake using the methods discussed in Chapter 6, they naturally feel more energy and less inertia. When insulin levels are moderated, fatty acids and glucose are easily mobilized from storage (or from ingested calories) into the bloodstream to burn for energy. Reduce your carb intake and you'll enjoy a bounce in your step during your daily routine, and when you start a proper workout, you'll feel strong and energetic instead of worn out. Consequently, a complete disinterest in activity and exercise suddenly transforms into an appreciation of and enjoyment in movement!

Sedentary Influences in Culture and Upbringing

Most of us do not come from families that place an emphasis on physical activity. A South Asian family's prestige often relies on the academic and financial success of its members. I still recall my trips to India: relatives and neighbors would introduce their children with a name, followed by an immediate tagline describing his or her school ranking. Something along the lines of, "this is my son Ramesh—he graduated 3rd out of 5,000 students in the College of Engineering at IIT." The same taglines are employed by South Asian parents in the US; how often have I heard, "this is my daughter Shilpa—she has a 4.2 GPA, scored a near perfect score on her SAT, and is on her way to Princeton."

Without a doubt, these are remarkable achievements that families should be proud of, but the South Asian cultural obsession with these types of success metrics undermines the importance of physical and emotional health and happiness. In fact, this cultural mindset creates excessive pressure that can compromise physical and emotional health. I'm talking about youth here, but these dynamics hold true for adults too. As a parent, I understand the importance of providing for my children and setting an example of hard work and career accomplishment, but during the relatively few formative years I have with my children, spending simple, joyous quality time is more important than anything else.

I must assert strongly that physical activity—especially the spontaneous, unstructured play that characterized childhood until the dawn of the digital age—is not a barrier to intellect, but instead a significant enhancer of cognition in kids and adults. There are volumes of proven scientific research that confirm exercise and activity improve all major brain functions and are linked to higher academic achievement in children. We'll discuss these findings further in Chapter 10.

Exercise Aversion

We've built a tremendous metabolic and cultural barrier to activity, worsened by Western society's overaggressive exercise recommendations. How can someone who sits for a living immediately transition to the recommended 150 minutes of exercise a week (which breaks down to 30 minutes, five days a week)? This is like asking a toddler to start running before he can barely walk. Pushing unrealistic exercise goals turns physical activity into a burden and a chore. Motivated by fear of disease, the most diligent few will exercise, but probably will not enjoy the pure exhilaration that comes from shifting to a more active lifestyle. A nagging spouse or family member that accuses you of being lazy and insists you get exercise only reinforces activity as an act of torture rather than a source of pleasure.

What's more, I know many motivated, well-meaning folks who have tried but failed to sustain an exercise habit. In virtually every case, they were misguided or misinformed, believing that exercise translates to pain, suffering, and extreme regimentation. These are the individuals who burst into the fitness center in January with big smiles and even bigger resolutions. They work diligently for weeks on end, drop a few extra pounds, and gradually deplete their reserves of physical energy, motivation, and spirit. By April, they are back on the sidelines, nursing physical aches and emotional exhaustion. Each time a failed effort of this nature occurs, resistance builds in the psyche and exercise becomes an even more formidable task the next time around. The human genetic code is averse to suffering, fatigue, and energy depletion. This is why a calorie-restrictive diet typically results in rapid fat accumulation once normal eating is resumed, and why many people who used to choose the front row of their exercise class now take the elevator over the stairs on a daily basis.

HOW TO MAKE EXERCISE HAPPEN

If you have the energy and the motivation, then by all means jump right in with a regular exercise program. Those of you (I'd guess the majority) who struggle with the thought of exercise, should focus most of your initial efforts on reducing insulin and shifting to a more energizing fuel source through dietary changes. I recommend initially spending more time in the grocery store scanning food labels and in the kitchen concentrating on meal and snack preparation, rather than in the gym trying to pump up your biceps.

Once you've laid the foundation for dietary changes, you should start to notice a sudden or gradual shift upward in energy levels. As soon as you do, add the new goal to increase general everyday forms of movement. Don't even worry about formal exercise yet—ban the word exercise from your preliminary vocabulary! Simply look for opportunities throughout the day to stand, to take a few extra steps, to stretch. Once you get some regular movement under your belt, pick one day out of the week to do something active that you enjoy. One day and something you enjoy! If you feel you can handle more, then by all means add on more days. Err on the side of making exercise an easily achievable goal so you don't overstretch your emotional will and burn out. This is key!

Here's a summary to help you gradually move towards greater movement:

1. **Free your fuel:** The energy you need to spur and sustain activity has been imprisoned in your fat cells for years. Lower your carbohydrates/insulin and liberate these precious energy stores. This shift takes about three to four weeks on average.

2. **Move a little:** Now let's put that fuel to some use! Forget the standard exercise guidelines and merely incorporate a few minutes of standing, walking, and core, functional movements. (By the end of this chapter you'll learn how to work all major muscle groups in less than 10 minutes without any equipment and before you've even left for work!)

3. **"Play" once a week:** Perform a physical activity you enjoy for at least 30 minutes once a week. Again, enjoyment is critical! We are trying to disconnect your negative associations with formal exercise and replace them with a new approach to activity that is more reminiscent of childhood memories of play. If you enjoy running on a treadmill, then you can

use that as your play, but ideally pick outdoor activities that involve some social connection. Options include…

- An outdoor hike or brisk walk with a neighbor or friend

- A team or individual sport, such as soccer, cricket, badminton, tennis, etc.

- A group exercise class (dance, yoga, etc.)

- An activity with your kids! Pick a sport you both enjoy, or engage in a simple game of tag

- Ideally try to connect #2 (gradual movement) and #3 (play)—chances are your gradual, intermittent movements will improve your soccer, badminton, dance, or whatever form of play you enjoy

A Quick Summary of Exercise Benefits

I've discussed the benefits of exercise throughout this book, but wanted to quickly summarize some of the key rewards before we start getting you fit.

Fat loss: Lowering carbs burns fat more effectively than exercising alone does, but exercise enhances fat loss and helps maintain weight loss long term. If you only eat a low-carb diet, then your fatty acid fuel will be liberated from fat cells but not used to fuel your brain and muscles. Fats that are not used tend to get stored back into fat cells. So, when it comes to fats you either use them (through exercise) or store them (by remaining inactive).

Insulin sensitivity: Recall how lowering your fat-to-muscle ratio is a critical component of taming insulin resistance. In Chapter 3 we discovered how a muscle cell has receptors called Glut-4 on its surface, which allow glucose to be transported out of the bloodstream and into the muscle cell, keeping blood sugar and insulin levels nice and low. Want proof? A study made up of South Asian diabetics showed that three days a week of progressive resistance training for only three months lowered blood sugars, lipids, and body fat, and increased measures of insulin sensitivity.[1]

Enhanced brain function: Exercise improves mood, increases memory, and helps your brain perform at its best by boosting several brain protective chemicals such as BDNF (brain-derived neurotropic factor).

Delayed aging: Aging is no longer a concern just for the elderly. An arthritic spine, insulin resistant conditions such as diabetes and heart disease, and reduced memory and cognitive function are all "older age" conditions that can appear much earlier in life due to sedentary behavior and poor diet. Exercise can protect you from accelerated aging.

Stress management: Exercise is one of the most effective stress management techniques around. Exercise moderates the stress hormone cortisol and enhances the release of chemicals that help you deal with the inevitable stressors you face at home and work. No matter how substantial the workload on your desk, a walk, hike, or other form of exercise is never a waste of time, but a battery-recharging event that will improve the quality of your work.

Role model: Kids of alcoholics and smokers have a higher risk of becoming alcoholics and smokers. The addiction to sitting is no different. If your child sees you as an inactive, out of shape parental role model, he or she will most likely become the same. No matter what you say or how many physical activities you add to your kid's schedule, the behavior you model has a bigger impact on their evolution than any other variable. This was one of the compelling points made in the bestselling book, *Freakanomics*: the sedentary trait gets passed on as easily as insulin resistance to future generations. Make fitness fun for your child and try to participate, rather than watching from the sidelines.

DON'T BE AN "ACTIVE COUCH POTATO"

The following is an excerpt from Mark Sisson's book, *The Primal Connection*):

Sitting is unnatural and uncomfortable for a species that has been standing, walking, and squatting for 2.5 million years. The human default resting position is actually squatting; it's only been in our very recent history that we've taken to marathon sitting. No wonder we contort and distort our bodies in vain attempts to avoid discomfort and pain while stuck in a chair!

So, what's so bad about sitting? For one, it weakens your gluteal muscles by deactivating them and putting them into a static stretch. Sitting also causes your hip flexors and hamstrings to shorten and tighten, gradually worsening over time. Unfortunately, strong glutes and good hip and hamstring mobility are critical to just about all manner of activity, from mundane daily tasks like picking up that paperclip off the floor to playing a demanding contact sport. If you are glued to the chair all day except for that lunchtime pickup basketball game or trail run, you can pretty much expect to get injured when you call upon your atrophied, imbalanced body for peak performance.

But far more sobering is the fact that scientists are now linking a sedentary lifestyle (defined as sitting for 23 hours a week or more) to diabetes, high blood pressure, cancer, cardiac disease, and premature death. [Note: One South Asian study found that sitting time increased blood glucose levels, independent of time spent exercising.[2] - R.S]

The physiology of inactivity theory suggests that prolonged sitting also causes weight gain by creating imbalances in critical metabolic hormones such as leptin, which regulates appetite and fat metabolism in the body. When leptin signaling is compromised, your brain craves more food, and your body defaults into a fat-storage hormonal pattern instead of a fat-burning hormonal pattern. All this has scientists and members of the medical community repeating the same tagline: "sitting is the new smoking."

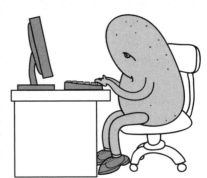

There's even a new medical term associated with chronic sitting: *active couch potato syndrome*, used to describe people who suffer from the same health risks as the absolute inactive despite a devotion to vigorous daily workouts—simply by virtue of the fact that they spend so much uninterrupted time sitting in long commutes, at desk jobs, and again when they get home and plop in front of the television, computer, or preferred digital device. While a devoted exercise regimen offers assorted benefits, it's simply not enough to protect you from the hazards of marathon sitting.

> *Due to a predominantly sedentary lifestyle, people who engage in vigorous daily workouts suffer from the same health risks as the inactive.*

Taking frequent breaks from sitting, even brief ones consisting of a minute or so, can measurably improve your health. The moment you get up and get moving down the hall or around the office courtyard, you kick into gear hormones that shift you into a fat-burning mode. As endocrinologist James Levine of the Mayo Clinic explains: "simply by standing, you burn three times as many calories as you do sitting. Muscle contractions, including the ones required for standing, seem to trigger important processes related to the breakdown of fats and sugars. When you sit down, muscle contractions cease and these processes stall."

Using this Chapter to Get Fit

Perhaps most of you have had difficulty getting in the groove of regular exercise. I understand the challenges of balancing work life and family life, as well as the lethargy that makes the thought of exercising seem impossible at times. So as not to overwhelm you further, I've only included the most fundamental moves. These are moves every person should be skilled at performing on a regular basis, regardless of fitness level. And there's no avoiding them, because you can do these exercises at home, in your hotel room, and even at work with some creativity. No need to join an expensive gym. You might even discover that you can get a better workout at home for free, all while spending time with your family!

Many of the movements I suggest have been inspired by a combination of yoga and the recommendations of fitness authority Mark Sisson, whose Primal Blueprint program presents the most balanced and sustainable approach to fitness I've ever encountered. After reading this chapter, I strongly encourage you to download his free e-book on exercise at http://www.marksdailyapple.com/subscribe-to-blog/ for more guidance. The e-book, as well as the Marks Daily Apple website, features many links to videos that demonstrate how to perform the core movements detailed below.

Along with core movements, I've included some modifications to make walking a more dynamic exercise that can be used to improve posture, and increase strength and aerobic fitness. Finally, we'll discuss some creative ways to incorporate movement into your busy work schedule, along with some tools to help you track your progress and keep you motivated. So let's get moving!

THE TREE APPROACH TO STRENGTH AND MOVEMENT

Many South Asians may feel like exercise is an unnatural practice, but it has been a part of our ancient tradition for thousands of years with the origination of yoga. In an attempt to revitalize this connection with our yogic roots, I'm using an approach inspired by the yoga "tree pose" called vrksasana. Thinking of your physical body as a tree is a great way to organize and prioritize muscle groups. It also serves as an inspiring metaphor, since a strong and sturdy tree is better able to withstand the physical and emotional storms we constantly face.

A strong tree starts with its roots (legs) and trunk (core). Many South Asians focus on their branches (arms) and underemphasize the most important parts of the tree. Think about how much weight you really lift in your everyday life. The heaviest object many of us lift on a regular basis is a smartphone! However, every time you stand or walk, your core and legs engage to stabilize and move significantly heavier loads, especially if you're carrying extra pounds.

Having strong branches but a weak trunk and roots, leaves the tree susceptible to damage from external forces, represented in the body as repetitive stress tendonitis, injuries, and premature arthritis. A stable tree, on the other hand, prevents injuries and allows you to perform everyday activities and recreational sports with much less effort and maximum enjoyment. For example, when you strengthen your roots and trunk, you'll find your yoga practice will dramatically improve as you step into deeper lunges and more powerful warrior positions. You'll be able to hold poses longer thanks to increased leg strength and core-assisted balance, which in turn allows you to focus on your form and breathing, rather than your aching thighs or fear of falling off balance.

Having a strong core and roots will dramatically improve your running, walking, and performance in recreational sports. If you have never participated in recreational sports for fear that you wouldn't be able to keep up, you will be motivated and inspired to do so once you gain this newfound strength and mobility. Often we are held back from certain activities not because we are out of breath, but because we start to feel the "burn" and fatigue in our legs. One of the most gratifying improvements I experienced was on vacation, when I discovered I could run through the sand with much less exertion and for longer distances as a result of increasing leg strength and mobility with simple body weight exercises I had been performing at home.

I truly believe that the best approach to strength and movement incorporates time spent outdoors, using our bodies as evolution intended. Many of my patients who regularly use cardio machines at the gym (treadmill, elliptical, etc.) still report difficulty with climbing stairs or complain of limited endurance with running or sports like soccer. Human-engineered cardio equipment can never compare to the workout of running or walking briskly outdoors, up hills and stairs, or through sand and dirt. You don't have to ditch your favorite elliptical machine, but try to replace some of those indoor workouts with outdoor ones. Moving outdoors and interacting with an imperfect natural environment offers a more complete full body workout because it uses full body, functional movements that your body was designed to perform.

Aging gracefully and remaining indepen-dent, without the assistance of a cane or walker, often depends on your ability to squat, an excellent marker for leg strength and mobility.

Roots (Legs)

I'm starting with your roots since legs are often the most neglected part of the body among fitness novices. We obviously underuse our roots when we sit. Even regular gym-goers will conveniently ignore legs and head straight to the upper body and arm machines. This is a backwards plan of attack, since weak roots lead to age-related balance problems and an increased risk of recreational sports injuries.

I realize leg exercises such as squats require more exertion, but they are also the most fulfilling once you make progress. Since the leg muscles are large, adding more mass to your legs also recruits more muscle cells and Glut-4 to help you combat insulin resistance. Even if you have limited exercise time at home or in the gym, start with your roots. Many of my female patients who have struggled with weight loss have benefited greatly as soon as they started squatting and strengthening their roots. Squats and lunges effectively work your trunk, while the additional modifications simultaneously work your arms.

The Squat

Squats are one of the most important functional movements. Squats are also a natural part of our tradition. It's the position we assumed before the days of toilets and modern chairs. Drive through urban villages in India and you'll see people of all ages squatting with ideal form as they line up alongside a road or congregate for social gatherings. Aging gracefully and remaining independent, without the assistance of a cane or walker, often depends on your ability to squat, an excellent marker for leg strength and mobility.

You don't have to relegate the squat to an exercise session. Make squatting a natural part of your life. The yoga squat is the familiar squatting position used naturally by generations of South Asians. Assume the yoga squat while watching your favorite television show or while eating from a plate perched on the floor or a low stool.

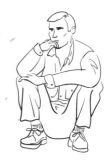

The regular squat (non-yoga squat) is a more intense movement. Women and men who struggle to lose additional weight despite lowering carbohydrates often experience breakthrough weight loss as soon as they start squatting, thereby adding significant leg strength to their activity program. Remember, adding muscle lowers fat-storing insulin and also allows your body to more effectively burn fuel.

How to perform a regular squat:

1. Assume a comfortable stance with feet shoulder-width, or slightly wider, apart and toes forward or pointed slightly outward. Extend arms straight out or crossed over your chest, forming an X. Keep your gaze forward throughout the movement so as not to strain your neck.

2. Lower yourself by extending your butt out and bringing your thighs to parallel (or just below parallel). Picture an upside down bucket behind you as you lower your butt onto the bucket.

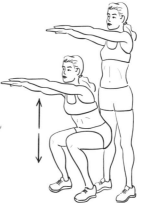

3. Your knees should line up on the same plane as your feet throughout the motion. Do not shift your knees forward past the tips of your toes. Don't allow your knees to buckle or bow inward. Keep your weight on your heels, not your toes. With each repetition, think, "butt in bucket, knees track with toes, weight stays on heels."

Once you've strengthened your roots, you can build on your foundation of squats with the following yoga poses:

Chair pose: Start with feet together and toes spread apart to help ground you. Slowly lower your body as if you're sitting into a chair while keeping your arms outstretched and parallel, reaching towards the sky and as close to your ears as possible.

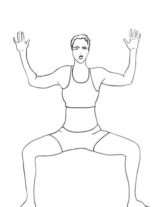

Goddess pose: Move into a wide squat with your thighs parallel to the ground and knees directly over your ankles. Lift your arms up with elbows bent at a 90-degree angle and palms facing out.

There is always room for advancement. Once you have mastered the squats above, move on to the advanced variations below.

Squats with weights: You can perform the basic squat motion while holding dumbbells at your sides. Other options for weights include a barbell, kettlebell, a sack of rice, or a weighted vest. Be sure to consult a trainer to guide you on proper form when using heavier objects.

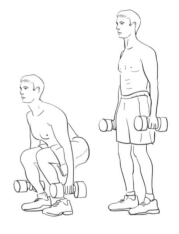

If any of the movements are too difficult, even a basic version, there are always modifications. Exercise newbies and seniors should start off with the modified squat variations below.

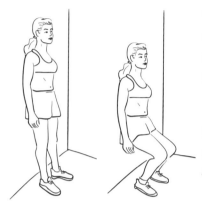

Wall squat: Use the wall for support. Only go down as far as you feel is comfortable, and never let your knees sink below parallel.

Pole squat: Hold on to a pole or other support object in front of you as you squat.

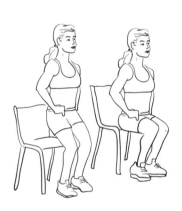

Chair squats: Sit and stand from a chair, using armrests for assistance if needed. As strength improves, try to depend less on the arms for support and eventually try a pole or wall squat.

One excellent app I use regularly is Runtastic's Squats Pro. This app uses my smartphone's accelerometer to count squats, putting me on a regimen to achieve specific goals, and reminding me every other day to do my squats. I've prescribed this app to many patients who have gone from being able to perform less than 10 squats to succeeding with over 100!

The Lunge

The lunge is another excellent movement for your roots. Unlike the squat, it is a unilateral exercise, meaning you exercise one side at a time. Focusing on a specific side leads to better balance and coordination, and also allows symmetry since you are isolating and working one side at a time, rather than allowing your stronger side to compensate for any instability. The lunge is also a highly functional movement, as it mimics an exaggerated walking or running stance, providing deep hip flexor mobility and maximal activation of your glutes. This is one of the best exercises for women who want to tone their thighs and buttocks. Start with no weights until you perfect your form and balance.

How to lunge (without weights, novice level):

1. Stand with feet shoulder width apart.

2. Take a big step forward with one leg, bending your front knee as far to parallel as possible.

3. Your forward thigh will be parallel to the ground while your back knee drops just above the ground. Both legs are at 90-degree angles in the lunge position.

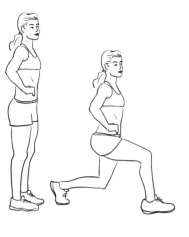

4. As with the squat, don't let your knees cross over your toes.

5. Hold for a beat, and bring your forward leg back to standing position. Repeat with the other leg. You can also perform walking lunges. Rather than stepping back to standing position, step forward with each lunge, alternating legs.

Once you can perform 20 repetitions of bodyweight lunges (stationary or walking) on each side with good form, you can move on to the intermediate level exercises.

Weighted lunges: Do the basic lunge exercise but now hold weights in your hands (dumbbells, kettlebells, etc.). You can hold the weights straight at your side, or you can do bicep curls each time you step into a lunge. Use enough weight to allow for 8-10 repetitions.

Twisting lunges: As you lunge forward, twist your trunk over your forward foot. So, if you lunge forward with your right foot, twist your trunk to face to the right. You can place your hands in a prayer position or even clasp them behind your head while you twist. Once you're comfortable with this movement, use both hands to grasp a single weight like a heavy ball, kettlebell, or weight plate.

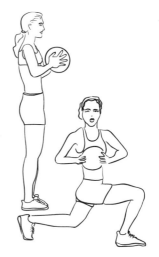

If you can comfortably do weighted and twisting lunges, then move on to Goddess-Warrior level, a series of lunges for the super fit! Do not attempt these lunges until you are comfortable with the basic and intermediate lunge exercises.

Rear foot elevated lunges: Assume lunge position and place your rear foot (toes curled under) on a stable, elevated surface like a bench or sofa arm cushion. Bend into the pose so your forward thigh is parallel to the ground and your back knee drops close to the ground. Do 10-15 repetitions. To make this lunge sequence more challenging, hold weights in both hands and/or prop your leg on an unstable surface, such as an exercise ball, to challenge balance.

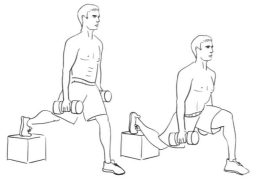

Upper body lunges: These lunges efficiently and effectively work your entire tree because the movements incorporate your upper body and arms. Three variations are on the next page.

1. **Lunge with lateral raise:** Start with your arms at your sides with a weight in each hand. As you lunge forward, raise your arms so they're parallel to the ground. If weights are too much for you, then lift arms without weights.

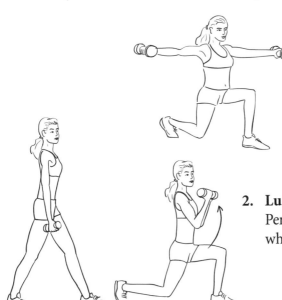

2. **Lunge with bicep curl:** Perform a basic bicep curl while you lunge forward.

3. **Lunge with bicep curl and shoulder raise:** Start with weights at your sides; perform a bicep curl at mid-lunge position, and then raise weights above your head at full lunge.

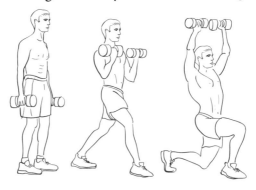

Lunges are a primary yoga movement. Get into the flow with the yoga lunge poses on the following page.

Warrior poses I and II: These poses are part of the Surya Namaskar (sun salutation) series, which we will flow through in a bit. In Warrior I pose the forward knee is flexed to 90 degrees and your front toes are pointing straight ahead. The rear leg extends back, while the rear foot angles in at about 45 degrees. Keep your hips facing forward (angling your back foot in helps turn your hips forward) and keep your heels aligned on the same plane. Arms remain parallel while reaching up towards the sky.

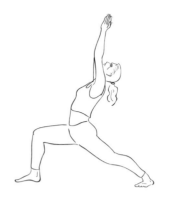

In Warrior II, your hips shift to face the side of the room. Your front foot remains pointed forward, but your back foot spins out to a 90-degree angle. Your front heel should align

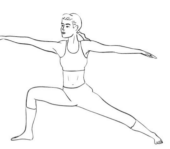

with the arch of your back foot so you will probably have to shift your front foot over a tad. Arms stretch long out to the side, parallel to the ground while you look straight over the forward hand.

Yoga twisting lunge pose: Enter a twisting lunge from Crescent pose. Front foot points forward while you bend into a 90-degree angle. Your back heel is up and only your back toes are on the floor. Twist your torso to the side, with your hands folded into prayer position. If you are lunging forward with your right foot, twist your torso to the right and hook your left elbow onto the outside of your right knee. When lunging to the left, twist to the left and hook your right elbow to the left knee.

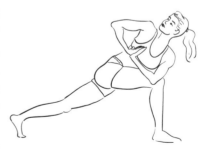

As always, there are lunge modifications for those who are just beginning, or are older and need a bit more support. Try these movements under supervision until you feel comfortable performing them on your own.

Basic standing (not walking) lunge: Keeping hands on hips, step forward a short distance, lunging only slightly. Dip down gently just a few inches. Do not try to achieve a parallel position with the front thigh if you feel any pain or instability.

Supported lunge: If you still feel unstable, try a gentle lunge using the support of your hands and arms. You can either put your hands on a wall in front of you with your forward toes against the wall to provide stability, or you can place two stable chairs at your sides to hold on to while you gently dip down.

Trunk (Core)

There is only one key exercise to review for the core—the plank. Each of the root exercises we just learned utilizes your core muscles. In fact, almost any exercise or activity you do on a daily basis engages your core, whether you realize it or not. As you strengthen your core, try to develop a sense of "core-consciousness" with all your activities, from loading the dishwasher to raking leaves in your backyard. You never have to do sit-ups again if you activate your core throughout the day and practice the suggested exercises regularly.

The Basic Plank

There are different grades within the basic plank depending on your core strength, so let's go from easiest to hardest within the basic level. For each exercise, keep your abdomen, buttocks, and leg muscles contracted and your spine straight.

Level 1: Forearm-knee plank: Assume the plank position illustrated below with your weight resting on your forearms and knees. (Use a mat to make it easier on your knees and elbows.) If you can hold this for two minutes, move to level 2.

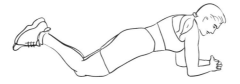

Level 2: Hand-knee plank: Take plank position shifting up off your elbows and centering your weight on your hands and knees. If you can hold this pose for two minutes, move to level 3.

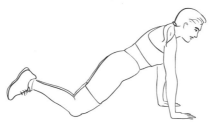

Level 3: Hand plank: This level is basically a push-up position. Weight rests on hands and toes and spine is straight. Don't lift that butt in the air!

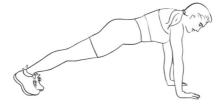

If you can hold hand plank for two minutes, move on to the intermediate, core-building plank exercises below.

Forearm-feet plank: Assume plank position with the weight on your forearms and toes only. Your body should be horizontal; focus on contracting your abs, buttocks, and leg muscles. Hold for 90 seconds to achieve intermediate level goal.

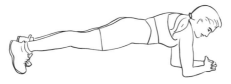

Forearm-side plank: Turn to your side and rest your weight on your forearms with feet stacked on top of each other. Hold for 90 seconds for intermediate level goal.

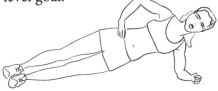

Hand-side plank: Rest your weight on your hand in side plank position. Your top hand can rest on your side or it can reach up straight towards the sky. Hold for 90 seconds for intermediate level goal.

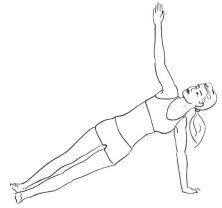

If you can hold the intermediate level exercises for two or more minutes, you have achieved Goddess-Warrior level. You are now ready for some even more challenging variations.

Hand or forearm-side plank with leg lift:
Do a hand or forearm-side plank while lifting your top leg in the air.

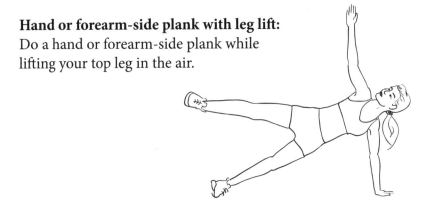

Hand or forearm plank while lifting one arm and opposite leg:
Assume a hand or forearm plank and then lift one of your arms and your opposite leg off the ground. Repeat with the other arm and leg.

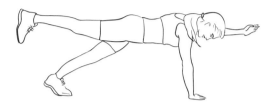

Elevated plank: Once you have perfected your ground level plank, try resting your feet on an elevated surface (bench, chair, etc.) and holding your plank. For an even greater challenge, put your feet on a Swiss ball.

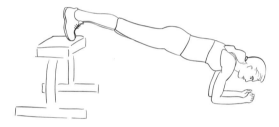

The plank moves discussed above are actual yoga poses. Virtually every major yoga pose will benefit from the core strength and stability you've achieved by perfecting your plank.

The basic plank (level 1) should be appropriate for most seniors and beginners. For additional support, use a cushioned mat to rest points of contact (hands, forearms, knees, etc.).

Tree Applications for Two Key Exercises:
Once you've mastered the basic tree exercises, you can apply them to two key exercises. The first is an invigorating yoga series of poses called Surya Namaskar (sun salutation). The second is an intense total body move known as the burpee. These two very different types of movement provide the balance of a serene, stress-reducing practice and an intense, explosive fitness exercise.

Surya Namaskar (Sun Salutation)

Surya Namaskar is the culmination of the yoga poses mentioned so far. If you are new to yoga, I highly recommend learning the sun salutation. This flow series of poses is energizing in the morning, relaxing in the evening, and provides overall stress relief and improved mental focus throughout the day. Refer to the figure below for the correct sequence of poses, made up of lunges and planks, as well as core movements such as cobra and down dog. Don't depend on the illustration. Yoga is an extremely precise practice that incorporates breath with movement. Take a yoga class, invest in a yoga DVD by an expert like Rodney Yee, watch online yoga videos, or download an app like Yoga Studio by *Modern Lotus*.

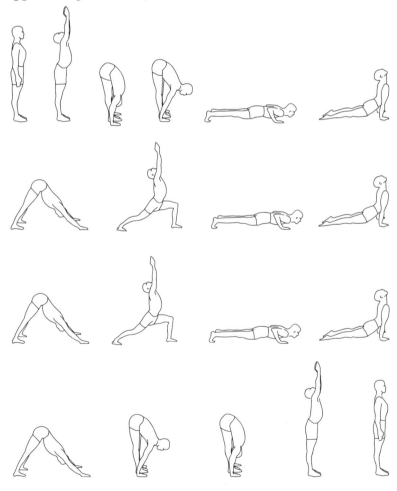

The Burpee

This is the exercise I love to hate. There are not many moves out there that raise your heart rate and fatigue your entire body quicker than burpees. The beauty is that the only piece of equipment you need is your body...nothing else. If you want to run faster, jump higher, or gain that explosive fitness you seek on soccer fields and basketball courts, do burpees! Why not make it a family event and do burpees with your kids? The burpee is really just a quick series of positions that moves through the two core moves, squat and plank, and adds a jump.

How to do a burpee:

1. Start in standing position

2. Drop to a squat with hands on the floor

3. Move immediately to hand plank

4. Walk or jump back to a squat

5. Jump

6. Repeat

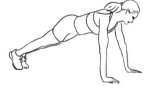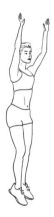

A more advanced version of the basic burpee includes a push-up after assuming plank position. There are many different variations of the burpee to explore with a trainer or like-minded fitness enthusiast.

WALKING FOR HEALTH

Walking should be the basic foundation of your increased activity plan. Walking at a moderate pace will allow you to keep burning the fatty acids you are liberating due to your low-carb, low-insulin eating plan. It will also help lower inflammation, which can flare up due to lifestyle habits and/or intense, endurance exercise. Any exercise program that is so rigorous that you are too tired to walk moderately on intervening days is likely a regimen that needs to be scaled back in intensity.

Regardless of how much exercise you get, be sure you are logging in at least 5,000 steps daily (2.5 miles). The closer you get to 8,000 steps (4 miles) a day, the better. Recall from Chapter 1, that studies showed that South Asians walked fewer steps and were less active than all other ethnic groups. We have a lot of catching up to do!

I urge you to get a pedometer and track your steps daily. Newer generation smartphones have integrated pedometers; so just download one of the many free pedometer apps.

Walking for exercise doesn't mean walking casually. A moderate walking pace has you breathing hard enough that having a conversation requires some effort but is still possible. A vigorous walking pace leaves you breathing primarily through your mouth due to the higher exercise intensity, and carrying on a conversation is nearly impossible. Exercise physiology calls this the "talk test" and researchers from the American College of Sports Medicine determined that it correlates very well with more technical measurements of exercise intensity, such as heart rate and V02 (measure of oxygen consumption).

Here are some variations to add diversity to your walking regimen:

Active walking: For many, the act of walking is fairly passive. We swing our limbs forward and drop each foot on the ground, barely paying attention to the muscles or mechanics involved. When you engage your major muscle groups while walking, you increase your heart rate and get a better workout. Active walking is also an excellent way to practice mindfulness with an awareness of your walking rhythm, rather than letting your mind drift to more stressful matters. With active walking, concentrate on contracting and relaxing your primary walking muscles with each step. As you shift your leg forward, feel and emphasize the contraction of your buttocks, core, and leg muscles. This will soften your foot drop and cushion your heel and forefoot, preventing common conditions like plantar fasciitis, a frequent cause of heel pain. As you swing your arms, contract the biceps of your forward arm and the triceps of your trailing arm.

Resistance walking: If you've got hills in your neighborhood, use them to apply natural resistance to your walks. Otherwise consider wearing ankle weights and/or hand weights while walking to increase workout intensity.

Interval walking: Try alternating fast/slow walking or run/walking. You can also apply the Tabata interval technique (detailed under timesaving workouts).

Timed walks: Most of us have a few set routes we walk. Use a stopwatch to measure your total walk time and try to beat your record as your fitness gradually improves. Better yet, use a motivating phone app like MapMyWalk which automatically tracks distance, walk times, and GPS-enabled location, all while playing your favorite tunes.

Walking corpse: The most restful posture at the end of a yoga practice is savasana, or "corpse pose." One of the reasons this is such a relaxing posture is that the simple act of laying flat on the ground with your palms facing up allows your shoulders to roll back and your chest to open up. Corpse pose is the opposite of the hunched forward position so many of us who live in front of computers have adopted. You can incorporate this same approach to walking. As you walk, face your palms forward, opening up the chest and keeping the shoulders back. Walking like this for even a few minutes after a prolonged sitting session can help relieve compressed tendons and nerves exacerbated by a hunched forward position. Even while you are seated, you can remind yourself throughout the day to roll your forearms out so that your palms face up. When you're ready to type, just roll your palms back towards your keyboard while keeping your shoulders back.

WORKOUT TIPS

I deliberately chose exercises that can be done anywhere to make them time-efficient. No gym or fancy equipment required. Use timesaving, short duration workouts as a back-up plan when you have absolutely no time for longer sessions. I don't recommend completely replacing your one-hour workout with 10-minute, high-intensity sessions. There is a new movement towards what is called the "minimalist workout," with fewer minutes spent performing higher intensity workouts. In my opinion, this modification is another so-called answer to our diminishing attention spans. While exercising too intensely for 45 minutes to an hour accelerates inflammation and is counterproductive to your overall health and wellness goals, cutting each of your workouts down to 10-minute sessions robs you of much needed downtime. Exercise is not just about burning fat and improving endurance. It's also about managing stress, spending personal time away from devices, and dampening the effects of a highly inflammatory lifestyle. You're likely going to use the time you "saved" exercising, to work more or disconnect further from nature. Below are some tips to help you incorporate activity into your busy life.

Working workouts: Truth be told, I wrote the majority of this book while exercising on an elliptical exercise machine. Combining movement with writing helped me stay alert and power through some incredibly productive writing sessions without feeling fatigued or sore from sitting at a computer for hours. Here are five of my favorite tips for performing working workouts:

1. **Working treadmill:** If you own a home treadmill, you can either build or purchase a workstation to place over the console. Alternatively, the *Tread Desk* is the flat floor portion of a treadmill, which can be slipped under any standing desk.

2. **Working elliptical:** I took a $10 resistance band and strapped an old laptop to the display panel of my home elliptical. If

you are thinking of buying exercise equipment for your home, purchase one with a large enough panel so you can convert it to a workstation.

3. **Tablet workouts:** Even if you have a smaller, more portable workout machine, you should still be able to fit your Ipad or similar tablet onto the handlebars. I've skimmed through many e-mails on my tablet while spinning on my stationary bike.

4. **Resistance reading:** You can read headlines and e-mails in front of a monitor while squatting or holding a squat (e.g., yoga chair position). Have you tried plank reading? Slip an Ipad or tablet directly below your eyes while you view your screen. When you're done with a page, switch to side plank, and use your free hand to scroll.

5. **Working meetings:** If you've got a teleconference, strap on your earpiece and take the call while walking. When I'm not an active participant during phone meetings, I'll mute the line and pick up the pace so no one hears me huffing and puffing. Try in-person, outdoor walking meetings with colleagues or clients, instead of the usual sit-down meeting in closed spaces. There's nothing like fresh air, sunlight, and increased blood flow to your brain to breathe some energy and creativity into meetings.

Increase intensity to reduce workout time: Did you know that one minute of high-intensity exercise has the same health benefit as two minutes of moderate intensity exercise? If you are working at high intensity, you should only be able to speak two to three words at a time and should be breathing almost entirely through your mouth. If you've never exercised or are out of shape, start in the low to moderate range and build up your fitness before you start using the techniques below. Again, increase intensity when you're strapped for time, not as a replacement for your overall foundation of increased walking and movement.

Tabata interval workouts: Exercise physiologist Dr. Izumi Tabata developed the Tabata interval protocol, which lasts only four minutes but provides a blistering high-intensity workout for maximum aerobic fitness in the shortest amount of time. Choose an exercise that allows you to perform at full speed/intensity for 20 seconds, followed by a 10-second rest period. Repeat this sequence of intensity and rest eight times for a total of four minutes. The high-intensity, 20-second phase must be done with maximum effort. You should feel exhausted by the end of four minutes. Examples of high-intensity exercises include sprinting, walking as fast as you can (if you can't run or sprint), jumping rope, cycling, doing burpees, etc. Download one of the many Tabata smartphone apps, which beep during your workout to remind you when to alternate between high intensity and rest.

Circuit training: This interval training involves performing a series of exercises in succession with little to no rest period in between. Now that you've learned the tree exercises, you have multiple options for developing your very own circuit or home fitness boot camp. Completing a circuit allows you to efficiently work on strength and cardio simultaneously as you maintain an elevated heart rate during your workout. If you are a beginner, conduct a circuit based on time; for instance, start with 30-second exercises followed by 60-second interval rest periods as follows:

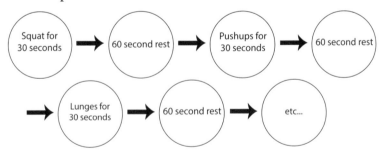

Adjust the intervals based on your fitness level (e.g., shorter rest periods as you get fitter) and add new exercises whenever you can to keep your circuits challenging. I often like jumping rope between sets to keep my heart rate elevated, rather than resting for a full minute between.

Interval setting on cardio machines: If you prefer to use your favorite piece of cardio equipment, use the pre-programmed interval settings and monitor your heart rate to make sure your workout intensity is sufficient. If exercising with friends, use the talk test.

Choose total body exercises: If you don't have the time to select workouts that isolate individual muscle groups, choose ones that engage as many muscle groups as possible. Not only do these types of exercises save time, but they also get your heart rate into your target zone almost immediately. Here's a list of total body workouts to choose from:

- Burpees

- Lunges with upper body exercises (bicep curl, lateral raise, etc.)

- Active walking with weights or up hills

- Faster paced sun salutation

- Jump rope with a weighted rope

- Kettlebell exercises (kettlebell squats, pulls, swings, etc.)

Kettlebell exercises provide some of the most intense, full body, fat-burning exercises you could possibly do. The American College of Sports Medicine reported that the only other exercise that comes close to burning as many calories during a given time is cross-country skiing. Give these bells a try, but be sure you start slow with light weights until you master your form.

Make exercise a habit: One of the most effective ways to incorporate regular movement is to attach it to an existing habit or routine, as opposed to looking for an elusive 30- to 60-minute window to add to your already busy day. Start off with short sessions. Gradually incorporating movement into your daily life helps to rewire your brain and ingrain this habit as part of your new routine. Here are some habit-forming suggestions:

1. **Lunge out of bed:** Start your morning with standing lunges. I especially like rear foot elevated lunges with my back leg raised on the edge of the bed. You can use some other raised surface in your bedroom or bathroom if you don't want to wake your partner. Start with an easy goal...maybe 10 lunges on each leg to start. As you get stronger, do more repetitions and also keep some dumbbells under your bed for weighted standing or elevated lunges.

2. **Toothbrush squats:** Do squats before, during, and/or after you brush. If motivation levels are low, start with ten. Think of how many hours you'll be sitting during the day, leaving those leg and butt muscles completely disengaged. A few minutes of squatting is nothing in comparison!

3. **Post-shower exercise:** Some of us are just not morning people and we need a shower to wake us up. If you can't squat or lunge before your shower, fit some exercise in immediately after you towel off. If you have a non-slip floor and a large enough space to allow a wide stance, you can squat safely in the shower. Add in a plank session right before you get dressed.

4. **Plank time:** A one- to two-minute plank hold can be inserted easily into your morning routine. Maybe while you're waiting for your coffee to brew, or while you read some news headlines or that long-winded e-mail you haven't had time to get to.

5. **Habit walks:** Take walks throughout the day...just before you get into the car to go to work; right when you get to work; during your coffee break; just before and/or after lunch; once you return from work; and before you enter the house. Determine your routine events and habits throughout the day and add standing and walking sessions whenever you can.

You get the picture. Get creative and find ways to incorporate and attach movement to your daily routine. A set of bedside lunges, toothbrush squats, a plank reading session, and a quick morning walk can take less than 10 minutes total. That's 10 minutes of total body engagement and a nice boost in energy levels, and you've barely started your day!

Home Exercise Equipment

Frankly, your body is the best piece of exercise equipment, and all the core movements you've learned can be done without any fancy exercise tools. However, sometimes you will want to challenge yourself by using other pieces of equipment to add resistance or further stimulate your balance and coordination. Using weights, resistance bands, and the like also adds variety to your exercise regimen. I've listed some inexpensive pieces of equipment you can consider adding to your home gym. Remember, the key to maintaining fitness is having an arsenal of exercises you can perform anytime, anyplace.

- Set of dumbbells

- Resistance bands (come in different resistance levels)

- Stability ball

- Yoga mat

- Jump rope

- Exercise DVDs—yoga, kettlebell, boot camp, or circuit training type

- Kettlebells

- Cardio equipment—cycle, treadmill, portable stepper (can fit under your bed or couch)

- Smartphone apps

There are endless fitness tools and coaching apps on your smartphone. Use them to learn yoga or kettlebell training. There are boot camp and crossfit apps that offer a variety of bodyweight exercises with suggested regimens.

Tracking Progress

Tracking various health and fitness metrics is a good way to keep tabs on your progress and can be extremely motivating. Below is a summary of some of the goals we've discussed, as well as a few new ones that can be used as benchmarks for fitness.

Goddess/Warrior status: The tree exercise section gave you a laddered approach by which you start with novice and gradually move up to Goddess/Warrior status. You know you've made progress when you've achieved Goddess/Warrior status in all the core tree movements!

Walk and run times: As discussed, measuring your walk and run times using a stopwatch or a walking/running app can be a great tool for motivation. Even if you're not a runner, but are capable of running, I suggest you measure your one-mile run time. The Cooper Institute Study found that the average one-mile run times of people in their forties and fifties correlated strongly with heart attack risk later in life.[3] Fitness levels are broken down based on run times, as detailed in the following chart. All healthy individuals without any significant physical or medical limitations should be able to run a mile within a reasonable time. Those in the highest fitness level only had a 10-percent lifetime risk of developing heart disease, while the lowest fitness group had a 30-percent lifetime risk.

HIGHEST FITNESS LEVEL	
MEN: 8 minutes or less	WOMEN: 9 minutes or less
MODERATE FITNESS LEVEL	
MEN: 9 minutes or less	WOMEN: 10.5 minutes or less
LOW FITNESS LEVEL	
MEN: 10 minutes or less	WOMEN: 12 minutes or less

Monitoring heart rate: Monitoring your pulse can be an effective way to not only measure fitness, but also to measure heart attack risk. To measure pulse at rest, place your index and middle finger over your wrist, just below your thumb or on the side of your neck. Count the total number of beats in one minute, or count the number of beats in 15 seconds and multiply by four. Check out the sidebar for apps and devices that measure heart rate.

HEART RATE MONITORING TOOLS

Measuring your pulse with your fingers is easy to do when you're at rest but impractical when exercising. Below are some high tech tools for measuring your heart rate.

Standard heart rate monitor: A comfortable chest strap and wristwatch accurately monitor your heart rate during exercise. Set a target heart rate zone and most watches will beep if you are below or under your goal heart rate. Most of the cardio equipment machines at your gym will automatically detect your chest strap, so you won't even need your watch. The display monitor will continuously show your heart rate throughout your workout without you having to grasp the handles.

Wristwatch heart rate monitor: A wristwatch monitor without the chest strap is a bit less cumbersome. Although the standard heart rate monitor has traditionally been more accurate than the watch only monitors, the technology for these monitors is catching up.

Smartphone heart rate app: Yes, there is an app for monitoring heart rate! Most smartphones do a remarkably good job of accurately measuring your heart rate using its camera flash to detect your fingertip blood flow pulsations. I've compared the results to those of a standard heart rate monitor and they are dead on. You can download a free app. Just follow the instructions, and make sure you do not press your fingertip too hard against the flash.

The Metabolic 6-pack: I have already discussed the importance of tracking your 6-pack as you make healthy changes to your eating plan. Do the same as you ramp up your exercise and activity program. Notice changes in insulin resistant markers like blood sugar and triglycerides. If you have high blood pressure, pay attention to the direct impact of exercise on your blood pressure.

Pedometers and activity monitors: We are seeing a rapid evolution from the standard pedometer to state-of-the-art activity monitors integrated into phones and watches or packaged into very small wearable devices. A standard pedometer is all I use to keep track of my daily steps to ensure I'm getting enough baseline physical activity. I've had patients successfully use more advanced activity monitors like the Fitbit or Jawbone Up Band devices, which provide data about steps and grade your activity intensity. These tools also have a nice online platform that allows you to track weekly progress, earn badges for achieving specific goals, and compete or collaborate with buddies. My kids actually keep track of their grandfather's weekly steps and send encouraging e-mails, which has been a huge motivation for him. Find whatever tool interests and inspires you.

Aside from the growing list of trackable goals, pay attention to what matters most. Be in tune with your emotions and more subjective measures, such as your overall levels of energy and happiness and your ability to deal with stress. Do you find activities such as yoga, running, and soccer on the weekends more enjoyable as a result of your newfound fitness levels? Do you have the self-confidence and motivation to sign up for that 5K run, or maybe take up a new sport or recreational hobby? Are you a better parent, spouse, and co-worker due to your physical and mental transformation? Do you feel inspired to motivate others whom you know could benefit from making similar changes?

Resting heart rate (RHR): As you become fitter, your resting heart rate will decrease. Keep track of your RHR periodically as a marker for improved fitness and reduced heart attack risk. A 2010 study tracking middle-aged adults for an average of 12 years found that an RHR over 90 beats per minute doubled heart attack death rates in men and tripled them in women.[4]

Exercising heart rate: Your exercising heart rate serves as a barometer of whether you're hitting your fat-burning zone. Calculating exercising heart rate is as simple as subtracting your age from 220. Roughly 60-70 percent of this number is your fat-burning zone. For example, if you're 40, then 220 − 40 = 180. Sixty to seventy percent of 180 puts your fat-burning range between a heart rate of 108 and 126. If you're extremely fit, you may need to move up to 80 percent.

Heart rate recovery (HRR): Healthy, fit people's hearts take less time to recover after exercise. People who are out of shape continue huffing and puffing while their heart rates take longer to recover. HRR is not just a measure of fitness, but is also correlated with the risk of dying from a heart attack. So how do you measure HRR? Exercise at a high intensity so you're breathing mostly through your mouth, or use your heart rate as a measure. See what your heart rate is immediately after you stop exercising and then check it again one minute after exercising. Studies show that if your heart rate drops by fewer than 13 beats after one minute, you have a higher risk of death from heart disease. Let's say I rode my exercise bike at high intensity and then stopped with an immediate post-exercise heart rate of 160. After one minute, my heart rate drops to 150. That's only a drop of 10 beats, meaning my heart rate didn't recover much, indicating an out of shape, higher risk heart. A decrease of 15-25 beats is the normal range. The more beats your heart rate declines after one minute, the greater your fitness level and the lower your heart disease risk.

Summary

- If you've been unmotivated and too tired to exercise, it's likely due to insulin resistance and excess carb intake. Tackle your diet first as outlined in Chapter 6.

- Focus on core body movements that you can perform anywhere.

- Integrate yoga with your core movements so you can enjoy the additional stress-relieving benefits.

- Acknowledge sitting as a serious health risk and find every opportunity to stand and walk.

- Try "working workouts" if you must get work done.

- Attach movement and exercises to existing habits and daily routines. Start with very realistic, achievable goals.

- Pick recreational activities and exercises you enjoy. Activity should not be a burden or a chore.

- Track and monitor your progress using both measurable (Metabolic 6-pack, etc.) and subjective goals (energy, happiness, etc.).

For Professionals

- For patients and clients who have been chronically sedentary, emphasize nutrition first and slowly introduce very easy, achievable movement goals.

- Prescribe very specific movement and walking goals rather than general recommendations (e.g., 150 minutes of exercise a week). Recommend 5,000 steps daily to start, along with 20 squats each morning.

- Give patients and clients specific measures to follow other than body weight (heart rate, energy levels, plank time, etc.).

- Keep them engaged and motivated by scheduling regular follow-up appointments and sending online messages when possible. Very slowly add on additional movement goals and ramp up walking steps.

CHAPTER 8

RECHARGE! AN APPROACH TO ENERGY AND STRESS MANAGEMENT

MOST OF THE CONDITIONS DISCUSSED thus far have no symptoms. You won't feel high cholesterol, high blood pressure, or high blood sugar until a serious event occurs, such as a heart attack, stroke, or kidney failure. Fatigue, however, is a very real and measurable symptom of poor lifestyle decisions. In fact, many of my patients have become so used to feeling tired that they pretty much accept low energy levels as a normal part of hectic modern life. Feeling energetic—perhaps on the rare occasion of an extended vacation—becomes more the exception than the rule. In this chapter, we will discuss the most common reasons patients experience fatigue and how to quickly correct these conditions and enjoy a higher daily baseline energy level. I call these fatigue factors "S-factors," since they all start with the letter "S." You will learn a systematic approach to neutralizing energy-draining S-factors and to reclaiming those precious energy stores that will help you lead a happier and more productive life.

UNDERSTANDING FATIGUE

In order to get a handle on the true nature of fatigue, let's start with a case study of a patient suffering from severe, progressive fatigue.

Case Study: Manish

Manish is a 45-year-old hotel owner who came to see me for progressive fatigue. He told me that he had always been energetic, motivated, and successful at work and home, but completing simple everyday tasks had gradually become more difficult. He reported waking up feeling unrefreshed, with energy levels dipping mid-morning around 10 am and hitting rock bottom between 2 and 4 pm. He would sometimes nod off at the desk or need a quick nap just to get through the afternoon. By the time he came home, he had no energy left to interact with his two young sons. He used to get by with a cup of coffee in the morning, but recently added a second cup, along with a cup of masala tea in the afternoon. He admitted to high stress levels due to the demands of work, two young children, and a diabetic father with ongoing health issues.

Manish is not alone. Fatigue is one of the most common complaints among patients, regardless of ethnicity, but South Asians definitely complain of low energy more than any other group I see. This is partly due to insulin resistance combined with a high-carb diet. Most patients with fatigue feel helpless and accept a low energy state as a normal part of aging and a permanent side effect of an increasingly busy life. We've discussed how lifestyle changes can improve or reverse risk factors such as abnormal cholesterol, high blood sugar, and excess body fat. One of the most rewarding outcomes of these changes is beating fatigue and feeling a renewed sense of energy and vitality that improves productivity at work and quality of life at home and in the community.

One of my major goals is to be able to competitively play basketball against my young boys for as long as I'm able. Oh, I know they will likely pass me by—in both height and skill level—when they reach their mid-teens, but I have every intention of dragging out the inevitable for as long as possible. I refuse to be the overweight father on the sidelines tapping away at his phone while his boys run up and down the court. These types of goals are hard to quantify, but in the long run provide the most personal fulfillment. I've been pushing the Metabolic 6-pack throughout this book, but consider making your energy levels the critical "7th factor." Besides, achieving most or all of the Metabolic 6-pack criteria should significantly improve energy levels.

The Cardinal Law of Fatigue: "What Goes Up Must Come Down"

I didn't learn about fatigue management during medical training, but was overwhelmed by the amount of fatigue I was treating in the clinic on a daily basis. Clearly, I needed a more systematic way of approaching fatigue that made sense to patients. The Cardinal Law of Fatigue is a general concept I've shared to help patients better understand why they are frequently tired.

> Any substance or state of mind that causes an abrupt rise in energy or alertness will eventually cause fatigue of an equal or greater magnitude.

In most cases, the "substance" is usually caffeine, sugar, or excess carbs, and the "state of mind" is stress—technically an elevation of stress hormones caused by the activation of the fight-or-flight response. The higher and faster your energy level or alertness rises, the harder it will inevitably crash. A sensible exercise program might seem like an exception to this law, because exercise can generate a pleasant improvement in mood and energy levels. However, the natural energy boost you experience from physical activity is very different from the jolt you get from a substance or from fight-or-flight stimulation, and therefore not an exception at all. Movement provides a nice pick-me-up in energy and alertness levels, followed by a gradual return to a calm, centered level of functioning, rather than the crash you are bound to experience after a strong cup of coffee or a carb-rich meal.

Energy Management

Energy management refers to monitoring your current energy level and deciding if it is enough to carry you through your tasks at hand. If you wake up with just enough energy to drop your kids off at school and take care of your usual errands, then you don't need to gulp down a strong cup of coffee. According to the Cardinal Rule of Fatigue, a strong cup of coffee will only lead to a crash in energy levels later in the day when your kids come home and need your attention and energy. On the other hand, if you wake up feeling exhausted, then drinking a mild stimulant such as green tea or a measured dose of coffee might be enough to help you accomplish your goals without an abrupt drop in energy levels later.

The first step in successful energy management is learning to become more energy conscious. I suggest using a green-yellow-red traffic light system to rate your energy throughout the day.

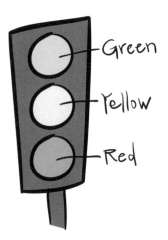

Green means you're ready to go. This is you at your best, firing on all cylinders and ready to tackle just about anything.

Yellow signals you have just enough energy to accomplish your usual daily tasks successfully. Taking on more would require effort.

Red indicates fatigue has stopped you dead in your tracks. Even the simple act of getting out of your chair requires tremendous effort.

Manish's case illustrates an important point. When initially asked to rate his energy levels upon waking in the morning, he indicated yellow. He still went on to consume two cups of coffee by noon. Unfortunately, most people who are leading unhealthy lifestyles have the expectation that energy levels should be green during all waking hours, so they keep consuming stimulants like caffeine to achieve this unrealistic goal, and instead suffer from the caffeine withdrawal crash and disrupted sleep that follow. You cannot expect to have consistently healthy levels of energy if you aren't healthy in the first place. This is like expecting an oversized, gas-guzzling SUV to run like a fuel-efficient sports car. Once you make the shift to a fat burner, you will spend far more time in the green zone with far fewer moments in the yellow zone. Let's explore some of the most important factors that are contributing to your fatigue and keeping you trapped in the yellow and red zones.

The Five S-factors of Fatigue

In my experience, fatigue can be attributed to at least one, and likely more, of the following S-factors more than 90 percent of the time.

- Stress factor

- Sugar/Starch factor

- Sleep factor

- Substances (caffeine, alcohol, medications)

- Sedentary lifestyle

As it happens, Manish fell prey to all five S-factors that cause fatigue. Others may just have one or two factors that bring energy levels down to an unacceptable range. I've developed a systematic approach to fatigue that can significantly improve your energy levels whether you suffer from one or all five energy-depleting factors. Let's work on getting you recharged!

S-FACTOR: STRESS

Stress is one of the most ignored, yet one of the most important S-factors. I see patients who are doing everything right when it comes to nutrition and exercise, but whose excessive stress is wearing them down, making it impossible to reach weight loss goals due to cortisol-driven hunger and fat storage. Stress is not only the underlying cause for nearly every unhealthy lifestyle behavior, but is also a direct proven risk factor for numerous chronic health conditions, from heart disease, memory loss, and cancer to persistent inflammation and accelerated aging. Unfortunately, most of us have a warped perception that a lifestyle of chronic and excessive stress is necessary for success. South Asians impart this belief to their children from an early age, by applying incessant academic pressure that hardwires children's genes and behavior patterns to experience constant stress without appropriate stress-management techniques.

How exactly does stress work? We have small glands sitting on top of our kidneys called the adrenals (Latin for "next to renal," or kidney). They are only about the size of your thumb, but they are extremely powerful battery packs that contain energy-producing chemicals like adrenaline and cortisol. When the pituitary gland in your brain directs the adrenals to release these chemicals into your bloodstream, your heart rate instantly accelerates, causing you to breathe faster and increasing blood sugar levels for a quick energy source for your brain and muscles. The stress response evolved into a complex, high-energy system that provides bursts of emotional and physical activation to help you fight or flee from dangerous situations, also known as the "fight-or-flight" response. If the ground started shaking right now from an earthquake, you would experience a surge in these chemicals that would propel you to move yourself and your loved ones to safety.

Experiencing the continuous stress of modern life is like leaving an electronic device on until the batteries drain, and never recharging it fully.

What happens if you experience modern day, low-level, continuous stress as opposed to the infrequent bursts of intense stress that our primitive ancestors faced? Think of your adrenal glands as your biochemical batteries: chronic stress is like leaving an electronic device on until the batteries drain, without ever recharging it fully. Chronic stress results in a state often referred to as adrenal depletion.

One of the primary stress hormones pulsed out of your adrenals is cortisol. Cortisol contributes to many of the insulin resistant risks we have discussed, such as selective belly fat storage, increased blood sugar, and cravings for high-carbohydrate foods. In addition, elevated cortisol impairs sleep, weakens memory, and suppresses the immune system, making us more susceptible to infections. Take a look at the table below, which compares the stress response that helped our primitive ancestors survive brief, intense, life-threatening stressors to the persistent stressors of modern life that cause rampant disease and disability.

RESPONSE Blood vessels constrict	HUNTER/GATHERER Prevent bleeding	SEDENTARY WORKER High blood pressure
Blood sugar ↑	Provide energy	Diabetes
Belly fat ↑	Calorie storage during famine	Central obesity
Pulse & breathing ↑	Alertness during battle	Palpitations, hyperventilation, anxiety, panic
Muscle tension ↑	Protect internal organs & spinal cord	Muscle spasm, tendonitis, etc

Managing stress is one challenge; the other is measuring stress levels. Many South Asians, especially males, are stress internalizers. They may not look stressed, and may deny being stressed upon questioning, but their behaviors and overall health indicate a different story. Increased irritability, trouble sleeping, and difficulty with memory and concentration are just a few of the more subtle manifestations of stress. Often a spouse, close family member, or co-worker may notice your stress better than you do, since it has become such an ingrained part of your personality over the years. Let's split stress into the more subjective symptoms you can feel and the quantitative signs you can measure.

Stress Symptoms You Can Feel:

1. **Breathing:** Shallow or rapid breathing, a feeling of not being able to take a full breath in, or a suffocating feeling, are all sensations associated with stress and anxiety. Be sure to consult your doctor if you have any issues with your breathing.

2. **Musculoskeletal:** Recurrent pain in any location, especially low back, upper back, and neck pain, can be triggered by muscle tightness and spasm from persistent stress.

3. **Headaches:** Tension headaches are typically caused by muscle spasms and tightness resulting from a combination of stress, prolonged sitting, and poor posture.

4. **Heart:** Palpitations (fast heartbeats) or skipped heartbeats are often caused by an overactive sympathetic nervous system that overstimulates the heart or interrupts its regular, rhythmic beating. See below for how to quantify your stress based on changes in your pulse (heart rate). Consult your doctor if you are experiencing any heart-related symptoms.

5. **Mind and mood:** Excess irritability, anger, impulsiveness, difficulty focusing, memory loss, anxiety, depression, and behavioral changes such as overeating, undereating, oversleeping, or insomnia can all be manifestations of stress.

6. **Digestion:** Did you know your digestive system, often called the "second brain," has more neurons (nerve cells) than your spinal cord does? As a result, excess stress can trigger a wide range of gastrointestinal symptoms like acid reflux, abdominal pain, nausea, bloating, constipation, and/or diarrhea. Those butterflies you feel in your stomach when you're nervous or stressed reflect the powerful mind-gut connection. I have found that the digestive system, especially in the midst of excess carbs, is a major site of stress-induced symptoms.

Stress Symptoms You Can Measure:

1. **Resting heart rate (RHR):** This can be a useful measure of stress for most people. Many people are familiar with their heart rates during exercise, but don't know how real life impacts their pulse. I recommend regularly monitoring your resting heart rate throughout the day, during both relaxing and stressful situations. Once you know what your average RHR runs, checking it periodically can motivate you to slow down and calm down when your numbers run significantly above your normal range. Check your pulse manually by placing your first two fingers lightly over one of the blood vessels on your neck, just to the left or right of your Adam's apple. You can also apply to the spot on your wrist just below the base of your thumb. Count the number of pulses in 10 seconds and multiply by six. You can even use a smartphone app like Instant Heart Rate by *Azumio* that accurately measures your finger pulsations using the flash on your phone. These apps feature an online journal of activities that correspond to your heart rate. Keep in mind that dehydration and stimulants like caffeine can elevate your pulse, as can certain supplements. Likewise, some prescription medications can lower or raise your pulse.

2. **Blood pressure:** As discussed in Chapter 3, some individuals have stress-sensitive blood pressures. In these cases, blood pressure should be monitored periodically. Like heart rate, blood pressure acts as a signal to initiate stress reduction if your numbers run high.

3. **Heart rate variability (HRV):** HRV is the beat-to-beat variations in your heart that are influenced by your breathing. Your sympathetic nervous system causes your heart rate to rise as you take a breath in, and your parasympathetic system causes your heart rate to drop as you breathe out. Exhibiting HRV is actually a good thing because it means your parasympathetic (relaxation) system is active. Low HRV is not only a sign of increased stress, but is also correlated with a higher risk of heart disease.[1] There are portable biofeedback devices

that measure HRV as a stress indicator, such as the EmWave and StressEraser. These devices enable you to directly see the beneficial effects of proper breathing on HRV. There are also smartphone apps like Stress Doctor or Stress Check (both by Azumio) that do a decent job of assessing HRV, while giving you reward points for taking optimal breaths.

4. **Social readjustment rating scale (SRRS or Holmes-Rahe Scale):** This tool is based on a 1967 study conducted by psychiatrists Thomas Holmes and Richard Rahe. SRRS shows that the number of adjustments or life changes, called LCUs (life change units), an individual undergoes is directly correlated to stress and is associated with the risk of developing a medical condition. Individuals that scored highest had the greatest risk of illness. Look up "life change stress test calculator" online and you will find several resources to calculate and interpret your score. For individuals who are stress internalizers and not in touch with their stress symptoms, a high SRRS score reflecting several simultaneous life adjustments should be a flag to manage stress. Even exciting, positive changes produce stress and are accounted for in this assessment. For example, if you just bought a new house, accepted a promotion or a new job, and have a newborn, you will score high. In the midst of such changes, you should consider turning down any new professional or personal responsibilities and instead focus on implementing some suggested stress management techniques. Wouldn't you rather be a calm, focused new parent or new boss than an overstressed, overtired, and irritable one?

Ways to Manage Stress:
It is unfortunate that many of today's South Asians have lost touch with effective stress management techniques like yoga and meditation, which originated from the ancient traditions of their homeland. Thousands of years before scientific evidence confirmed the harmful effects of stress, our ancestors intuitively understood the adverse impact of negative emotions and distressing life circumstances. They developed refined practices to align their bodies and minds

and to connect more directly to their inner selves and higher spirits. In today's high stress, high-tech world, these mind-body healing modalities should be considered modern day necessities.

Yoga: A consistent yoga practice can scale back stress remarkably well. Even 5 to 10 minutes of yoga in the morning and evening can melt away stress and help you energize and relax. Need scientific proof? UCLA researchers studied 45 dementia caregivers, a group known to have high levels of chronic stress, and found that performing 8 weeks of daily 12-minute chants using a yogic technique called Kirtan Kriya Meditation (KKM) significantly reduced the expression of the inflammatory gene NF-kB.[2] Remember, inflammation is the root cause of virtually every chronic, debilitating illness!

Yoga newbies should start with Surya Namaskar (sun salutation), an invigorating flow of 12 different poses that energize every part of your body. (For a description of sun salutation see Chapter 7.) Before attempting to flow through the series, work each individual posture separately until they are all familiar, not perfect. Yoga celebrates gentle progress, not perfection. Yoga requires an open mind; it is a practice that helps you discover and accept your limits. Once you have the basic postures down, work on the flow by smoothly connecting all the postures in sequence, almost like a dance. Once the sequence is mastered, it's time to coordinate breath with movement.

Take a yoga class, hire an instructor, pick up a DVD, watch a YouTube video, or download a yoga app—whatever medium best motivates you. At some point along the way, do get personal instruction in some form (private or group class) since no technology or media can replace a good instructor.

Breath control: Changes in the rate and depth of breathing are one of the earliest indicators of stress. When we are stressed, we take shallow, panting breaths, using only the upper portion of our lungs. This inefficient exchange of oxygen is both an indicator of and a contributor to a stressful state of mind and body. Pay attention to your breath and make a concerted effort to slow down and take deep breaths that activate the entire diaphragm muscle to access the oxygen-rich lower lobes of the lungs. Breathing into the diaphragm requires expanding your stomach upon inhalation—the opposite of what many people routinely do. Don't breathe *up* into the chest, but breathe into the stomach, filling the diaphragm with air. When you regain control of your breathing by taking deep breaths that efficiently exchange oxygen, you literally change your blood chemistry from a stressed to a calm state. I often have patients report what they think is a problem with their lungs, like asthma, but turns out to be a symptom of stress or anxiety. When they manage their stress, their breathing improves.

Most South Asians are familiar with some of the breathing techniques of Pranayama. If not, start off simple with slow inhalations and exhalations. Typically, the exhalation phase is longer than the inhalation phase (for example, a four-second mental count while you breathe in and an eight-second count while you breathe out). Find a pattern that is comfortable for you. You can eventually experiment with a variety of pranayama techniques like kapalabhati, bhastrika, or bellow's breath. Many yoga instructors are familiar with these techniques, but you can also explore online resources, videos, and downloadable apps. The Pranayama app by *Saagara* is an excellent tool I use nearly every morning that allows you to adjust your breathing intervals and provides sound cues for inhalation and exhalation.

Mindfulness meditation: Everyone, no matter how busy, has time to meditate. When patients tell me they have no time to exercise or meditate, I tell them they have the time, but aren't making it a priority. If they were to have a heart attack or some other major medical disaster, then time would magically appear, as regaining health becomes priority number one. Don't wait for a tragic reminder of how important your health is.

Your time is valuable, and mindfulness meditation is a practice that fits seamlessly into the busiest lifestyles. Mindfulness meditation allows you to apply meditation techniques to your daily life, rather than blocking out a specific time for seated meditation (also a worthwhile stress management tool). Mindful eating, mindful walking, mindful driving, and mindful showering all access the vaunted meditative state of total focus and appreciation of whatever is happening in the present moment. When it comes to resetting your high-stress mindset and behavior patterns, simply being mindful during the routine and even mundane elements of your daily life can be even more effective than sitting for a formal meditation session. Jon Kabat-Zinn is a pioneer in the application of mindfulness meditation as a prescribed therapy for stress, anxiety, illness, and chronic pain. There are extensive scientific studies supporting the effectiveness of mindfulness practices in all areas of health. Find a mindfulness center near you, or pick up a book on mindfulness by Jon Kabat-Zinn or other trained practitioners.

Connect with nature: We spend too much time indoors under artificial light, breathing stale recirculated air. Even a few minutes outdoors can have a calming effect that facilitates deep breathing and helps relieve that overwhelming feeling you get when you're staring at an endless inbox of e-mails or whatever other stressors you face daily. Meet with friends and neighbors for outdoor walks or playdates in the park (for your kids and for you grownups too!). Join colleagues for outdoor walking meetings or conduct walking teleconferences with a wireless headset. Basking in the glow of sunlight rather than screen light for even a few minutes can give you a new perspective and make the rest of your day more manageable.

Music meditation: One of the wonders of mobile technology is the access it provides to your favorite music archives anytime, anywhere. I keep an extensive selection of music on my phone, and take advantage of technology to separate my audio files into playlists. I listen to music from my childhood, favorite songs of my late father, Tibetan chants, guided meditations, pop hits, classic rock, instrumental music, and other custom designed sequences depending on my mood and on the activity. Music has the power to instantly put you in a relaxed or positive frame of mind…it can even take you back to a cherished period of your life. Pick some meaningful tracks that you can play in the car or during a walk if your mind is too distracted to enjoy silence or the sounds of nature. There are also dedicated stress-relieving musical apps and downloadable tracks that provide guided meditations and progressive muscle relaxation techniques accompanied by soothing background music. Keep some of these tools handy to help you de-stress when necessary.

Your approach to stress management should be similar to your approach to physical activity. You can't keep looking for that elusive one-hour block of daily time to go to the gym or hit the pavement for a run. Throughout your day, you need to insert physically active moments that involve walking, standing, and lifting. Similarly, when my patients set a goal of 20 minutes of meditation every morning, most of the time they fail. How about getting to work five minutes early, turning on some relaxing music in your car, and then engaging in some mindful breathing? Maybe you do the same when you get home from work, but now you simply take a short walk around the block before you enter the house.

Figure out how you can strategically embed several mindful and stress-relieving moments into your work and home life. Most of us live like pressure cookers, progressively accumulating more and more steam throughout the day. These minutes of mindfulness and quiet reflection release some of that steam before it gets to the point where you snap at your spouse and kids, or reach for that unhealthy snack, or wake up at 3 am unable to fall back asleep, or suffer another panic episode characterized by heart palpitations, rapid breaths, and feelings of overwhelm. Once you experience the subtle benefits of short, intermittent stress relievers, you acquire the motivation and discipline to start incorporating longer, more dedicated sessions of stress reduction. If you're someone who needs numbers or technology to motivate you, then consider investing in a biofeedback device as discussed, or at least downloading the Stress Doctor or Stress Check smartphone app.

S-FACTOR: SUGAR/STARCH

Many of my patients initiate carb reduction for a specific goal like lowering triglycerides, body weight, or blood sugar, and then happen to report an increase in energy levels. This is no coincidence. Almost every individual who removes excess starches from his diet experiences a boost in energy, especially when combined with increased activity. The reason South Asians so frequently complain of fatigue is that they battle the energy-depleting combination of insulin resistance and a very high-starch diet. Manish's breakfast alone consisted of over 150 grams of net carb! Starting his day with already sky-high insulin levels, Manish, of course, fell prey to exhaustion.

Let's use our car analogy to break down how starches and insulin promote fatigue: you are the car, food is your fuel, fat cells that store energy (triglycerides) are your gas tank, and the brain and muscles are your primary engines that power your intellect and move your body. Recall from Chapter 1 how insulin is a storage hormone; meaning it pushes fat and glucose from foods (your fuel) into fat and muscle cells (your gas tank). If your fuel circulated in your bloodstream, it would travel to your primary engines (brain and muscle), keeping you alert and energetic. In the presence of excess insulin, however, fuel is not used as energy but is instead immediately ushered into storage depots as fat. The insulin seals off your gas tank, preventing the fuel from traveling to your engines. The swollen South Asian belly is nothing more than an overinflated gas tank locking away precious potential energy in the form of triglycerides, which never get converted to clean fatty acid fuel...all due to excess insulin from a high-carb diet.

This brings me to my next point: there are actually two types of fuel. Glucose from starches provides your body with a quick-burning form of fuel that rapidly dissipates, leaving you hungry for more glucose sources (sugar and starches). Fatty acid fuel is a much longer lasting, metabolically clean (does not cause inflammation like glucose does), high-octane (lots of nutritional value per calorie in comparison to processed carbohydrates) fuel that is tremendously energizing and does not produce the mood and appetite swings characteristic of glucose fuel.

Recall that dietary fat is converted into two major forms in the body. In the presence of excess insulin, fat is stored in your gas tank as triglycerides. When insulin levels are low, your gas tank (fat cells) converts triglycerides into high-octane fatty acids which are released into your circulation to power your brain, muscles, and other vital organs.

The vast majority of South Asians, especially those with insulin resistance, have untapped fatty acid fuel depots stored as excess triglycerides in fat cells. They run almost exclusively on quick-burning glucose, which leaves them craving starches and sugar every few hours. The thought of skipping a meal or performing intermittent fasting as discussed in Chapter 6 is unthinkable. It's understandable why so many South Asians have high triglycerides, high blood sugar, increased abdominal fat, constant hunger, and low energy levels. As you can see, fatigue and inactivity aren't just a reflection of laziness or lack of motivation. They're byproducts of the amount and type of fuel you are loading into your gas tanks.

Sugar/Starch Assessment

Before his consult, Manish ingested 400 or more grams of net carbs derived primarily from white rice, chapatis, lentils, and abundant Indian crispy snack foods, which he consumed for comfort and to satiate his intense stress-induced cravings. This carb-heavy diet was a key reason for his fatigue. To determine if excess carbohydrates are draining your energy, monitor your Metabolic 6-pack and keep track of your daily net carbs (NC). Your triglycerides, blood sugar, and waist circumference will respond almost immediately to reductions in your net carbs. When these numbers improve, your body is finally making the metabolic switch from burning inefficient glucose fuel to burning long-acting fat fuel.

Sugar/Starch Management

Chapter 6 discusses most of what you need to know to help manage your starch intake and reduce your insulin levels. My most successful patients actually track their quantitative measures against their energy ratings. It helps to make a spreadsheet detailing your net carb intake, lab numbers, and average energy ratings. For example, Manish noticed that lowering his net carbs to below 150 grams dropped his body weight 10 pounds in six weeks, reduced his triglycerides by 100 points, and boosted his mid-morning energy level from yellow to green and his mid-afternoon energy level from red to yellow. All this success without any additional exercise!

Although we tend to think of food as an energy source, mid-morning or mid-afternoon fatigue is often a direct consequence of the amount and type of food you consume at breakfast or lunch. Postprandial somnolence (aka "food coma") is the phenomenon that describes the state of drowsiness following a meal. It is primarily due to over-activation of the parasympathetic (relaxation) component of the nervous system, and is proportional to the amount of food you eat. A small meal may promote relaxation but still keep you in a functional energy zone, while a heavy meal may cause excessive parasympathetic activation, making you feel extremely drowsy and closer to the red zone.

If the meal is also high in carbohydrates, your body succumbs to two additional effects mediated by excess insulin. The first is an abrupt drop in blood glucose, which leaves you feeling wiped out and craving more sugar. The second effect involves the amino acid tryptophan. High insulin levels facilitate the transport of amino acids other than tryptophan into your muscle cells. This leaves more tryptophan available to be taken up by the brain, where it is eventually converted into serotonin and subsequently the sleep-inducing hormone melatonin. It is clear how a heavy lunch, especially one high in carbohydrates (typical for most South Asians), leads to drowsiness through the afternoon.

Really start paying attention to how your body responds to certain meals. We have all been told that eating breakfast is essential, but once your body begins to use fat as fuel, you start to naturally skip breakfast on occasion and may feel more energized in the mornings as a result. Many religious saints and meditation masters practice fasting as a means of increasing alertness and spiritual energy. Their brains are operating on fatty acid fuel. Once you shift into fat-burning gear and can occasionally skip breakfast, you will notice improved focus and concentration during your daily tasks, in addition to improved strength and endurance during workouts.

S-FACTOR: SLEEP

Sleep is an essential part of energy management that inevitably moves down the priority list as we continue to add on more work and screen time. Even before the digital age, South Asians were night owls, often eating dinner close to 10 pm and turning in at midnight or later. Even kids are staying up way past their normal bedtimes for social events or quality time with working parents. A growing number of studies are now showing the deleterious effects of shorter sleep times on chronic health conditions such as obesity, insulin resistance, digestive health, immune function, and general health and well-being. Sleep deficiency is also an S-factor that potentiates the effects of other S-factors. I've included just some of the side effects of insufficient sleep below. This list is by no means comprehensive!

Increased stress: Insufficient sleep reduces your ability to cope with stress and also raises cortisol levels. The REM (rapid eye movement) phase of sleep normally acts to suppress cortisol release; sleeping less removes this inhibition and causes you to produce more cortisol. Think back to how impatient and stressed out you were during a period when sleep may have been persistently disturbed, like when parenting a newborn.

Increased hunger: Reduced sleep increases production of the hunger hormone ghrelin and interferes with leptin signaling to the brain. (Leptin is a hormone that tells the brain when the body is full.) When leptin signaling is blocked, intense hunger and specific cravings for quick energy foods—in particular starches—ensues.

Reduced growth hormone: Growth hormone helps maintain lean muscle tissue and is released primarily during deep phase sleep. When you sacrifice sleep, you lose out on this important, rejuvenating hormone. This is especially true for growing kids. Short changing sleep may reduce their growth potential.

Impaired insulin resistance: Dr. Eve Van Cauter has conducted studies showing that exposing young, healthy, non-insulin resistant individuals to just one week of sleep deprivation can actually make them insulin resistant![3] Imagine what happens to a South Asian who is already insulin resistant and gets insufficient sleep! Sleeping less may result in transitioning from prediabetes to diabetes, or from well-controlled diabetes to uncontrolled diabetes.

Obesity: Weight gain into the realm of obesity is not surprising considering the South Asian battle with insulin resistance. Increased cortisol, increased hunger, reduced growth hormone, and increased insulin resistance (aka excess fat-storing insulin) is a recipe for excess body fat and all associated health conditions.

As you can see, the sleep factor potentiates the stress and starch factors explained above, promotes caffeine cravings, and encourages the sedentary factor since we often feel too tired to move. Even though inadequate sleep may appear to be an isolated problem, it sets off a chain of behaviors and biochemical changes that impact each of the remaining S-factors.

Sleep Assessment

How do you assess something as complex as sleep? You may have a rough idea of how many hours you sleep, but how do you know if it's high quality sleep? Sure, the general recommendation of eight hours of sleep a night sounds sensible, but there is a much bigger picture to address with respect to the quality and effectiveness of your sleep. What's more, world class athletes often get closer to 10 or more hours of sleep to recover from intense training and to allow their body to repair and rebuild lean muscle tissue. Elevated sleep requirements might also be relevant for those under intense stress, such as high-powered executives who travel by jet frequently, or working mothers who have non-stop responsibilities. There are, however, a few ways to assess sleep both quantitatively and qualitatively.

Bedtime/wake time: Calculate the hours from bedtime to wake time. If you sleep mostly uninterrupted through the night, then you'll have a pretty accurate measure. However, if you wake frequently, it is difficult to estimate how many actual hours you spend sleeping.

Sleep motion: You can estimate sleep time based on motion using an instrument called an accelerometer. When attached to your body or placed on your mattress, the accelerometer attempts to detect significant movements, which may correlate with wakefulness. It measures hours slept based on this motion-dependent wakefulness signaling. Many body monitoring devices, including your smartphone (download one of the many different sleep apps), now provide sleep scores based on motion-detection technology. The main inaccuracy of this approach is that you may still be asleep while you are moving around, which would be recorded as wakefulness regardless.

Sometimes you sleep eight hours and wake up feeling unrefreshed; other times you sleep six hours and wake up feeling fine. This discrepancy indicates a difference in sleep quality. Sleep is broken into different stages, all of which are critical for restoration and recovery, both for your brain and your body. The highly restorative, deep phases of sleep in which you are not dreaming are easily compromised when sleep habits are suboptimal. How do you know if you're getting good quality sleep with enough time in deep phase?

Daytime sleepiness, or sleep latency: This is a quick, subjective measure of whether you are getting enough good quality, deep sleep. If you are spending most of your waking hours feeling alert, then you are probably getting the minimum amount of necessary sleep. However, if you find yourself feeling sleepy at different times of the day, especially during tasks that require alertness, such as driving, you may be suffering from either insufficient sleep or possibly an underlying sleep disorder like sleep apnea.

Sleep study: A physician-run, certified sleep lab conducts overnight sleep studies which provide much more detailed information about sleep stages and help to rule out sleep disorders like sleep apnea by measuring apneic (breathless) episodes during the night. A sleep study should be considered if you have excessive daytime somnolence.

Sleep Management

There are a few strategies to help you fix your sleep issues. I'm going to cover some of the most effective behavioral and lifestyle interventions that have helped my patients sleep more soundly. I strongly encourage you to seek out additional resources and professional help if you still have sleep trouble after implementing these suggestions.

Consistent sleep schedule: As you age, your body's circadian rhythm (internal biological clock) becomes increasingly sensitive to abrupt changes in bedtime and wake time. Be sure to keep your sleep schedule as consistent as possible, even on weekends. Don't allow more than 30 minutes variability if possible. Attempts to "sleep in" or go to bed earlier to make up for a poor night's sleep can disrupt your body's internal clock and make sleep disturbances even worse. Sunday night insomnia is a very common phenomenon since many people sleep in on Sunday mornings and then try to go to sleep earlier than usual to start the workweek fresh. This practice will especially backfire if you had a late Saturday night bedtime.

Optimize environment: Your bedroom should be a sanctuary dedicated to sleep and intimacy only. Unfortunately, this sleep sanctuary is now commonly contaminated with digital devices, televisions, and even bedroom home offices. You do not want to associate your bedroom with work or other non-relaxing endeavors. A home temple, which is very common in South Asian bedrooms, is great, and can be incorporated as part of a relaxing bedtime ritual. Light a candle… maybe some incense…and focus on your breathing while performing a session of prayer or meditation.

Whether you have difficulty falling asleep or wake frequently in the middle of the night, do not spend more than 15 minutes in bed awake. The more time you spend tossing and turning, the stronger the association becomes between your bed and wakefulness. Your bed, in effect, is transformed into a place where you "fail" to fall back asleep. Instead, leave your bedroom and engage in a relaxing activity, like a few yoga poses or some fiction or leisure reading. Don't read materials that are related to work or are otherwise of a serious nature that requires concentration. As you strive to optimize your sleep habits, you may have to get out of bed a few times, but gradually you should be able to fall back asleep more quickly and easily in your bed.

Restrict light: There is a growing body of scientific evidence that links screen time with reduced sleep time. The blue light emitted from laptops, tablets, phones, etc. has been scientifically proven to disrupt the natural release of the body's sleep hormone, melatonin. Your brain registers blue light as a mild form of sunlight and triggers your body's wakefulness signals. Not to mention, work performed on these screens is mentally stimulating and requires full concentration. Whether it's work e-mail, social networking, or vacation planning, you are activating your brain with unnatural light and extraneous thoughts, instead of calming your mental faculties with sleep-inducing activities. I've minimized the number of times I wake during the night, simply by restricting my screen time after dark. Patients have shared similar experiences.

Here are some tips that will help you limit nighttime light and preserve your natural bedtime melatonin release:

1. **Dim your lights after sunset:** Shut down unnecessary lights and screens in your home as it gets dark. Dim your lights as much as possible to sync your indoor environment with Earth's circadian rhythm and to optimize your natural internal rhythms that are strongly influenced by the planet's light and dark cycles. Investing in some electric candles is a safe (and romantic) way to welcome the evening.

2. **Use orange light:** If you must be on a screen, then consider purchasing a pair of orange or yellow lens sunglasses, which filter out the melatonin-disrupting blue light spectrum emitted by regular light bulbs and digital screens. Some of my patients have switched out white bulbs for orange bulbs in their bedrooms and home offices to mellow things out after dark. Orange bulbs are available at large home supply stores like Home Depot and Lowes.

3. **Install f.lux software:** This free software program synchronizes your computer display with the time of day by recalibrating the "color temperature" of your screen after it gets dark. You can download this software at stereopsis.com/flux/.

4. **Stay active:** Your goal is not just to get more hours of sleep, but to optimize cycling through all the necessary phases of sleep, from the dreamy REM sleep that sorts through and organizes information processed during waking hours, to the slow-wave deep sleep that restores and rejuvenates mind and

body for the day ahead. The best way to prepare your body for a successful night of sleep is to increase your physical activity levels. If you've ever done a full day of yard work or a long hike that leaves your entire body aching, you've probably noticed that you slept like a baby that night. That's because your body innately understands that you require more deep sleep to recover from exertion. Stress, or mental exertion, normally has the opposite effect.

"The more mental activity (i.e. stress) outweighs physical activity, the worse you sleep"

Ideally, you want to crawl into bed feeling moderate physical fatigue, the perfect parameter to counterbalance the day's mental and emotional stress. The more physical fatigue outweighs mental activity, the deeper you will sleep. I think back to childhood trips to India where I saw rickshaw pullers and other laborers sleeping soundly on slender ledges and stairwell steps in the middle of loud, congested streets and train stations. And here, so many of us struggle to sleep in dark, quiet, temperature-controlled rooms on expensive mattresses! No mattress or sleep device compares to physical exertion when it comes to facilitating a goodnight's rest.

Don't take these suggestions to the extreme, however. A significant amount of exercise right before bedtime is not advised because the elevation of body temperature and increased blood flow can lock you in an activated state for a while afterward, interfering with attempts to fall asleep. However, a little bit of exercise can administer a nice sedative effect when its time for bed. Personally, a few sets of squats with a kettlebell before bedtime, especially on my most inactive days, tend to impart a nice sedative effect.

Nap when necessary: Even when you are doing everything right, your body will occasionally experience significant fatigue and sleepiness during the day. A short nap lasting as little as 10 minutes can be refreshing and is preferable to a coffee break, which may interfere with sleep. I've taken naps in my car before giving a lecture, and frequently put my head down on my desk for a few minutes during my lunch break. I'm amazed at how those few minutes of refreshment power me through the rest of the day. On a chemical level, when you can close your eyes and settle into a relaxed state of mind you rebalance the easily depleted sodium/potassium levels in your brain. When you return to an active state, your synapses are literally refreshed and reenergized for peak cognitive function in the hours ahead.

The best time for and duration of a nap are highly personal and can vary based on your overnight sleep patterns and levels of activity and stress. Some individuals require shorter naps (15-20 minutes or less) in the early afternoon to prevent disrupted sleep during the night. Others can take long, late afternoon naps and still sleep fine during the night. Generally, a 20-minute nap between the hours of 1 and 3 pm, when sleep-inducing melatonin levels tend to rise and you consequently might experience high levels of what scientists call sleep pressure, is ideal for most people. To learn more about the science behind and best strategies for napping, check out Dr. Sara Mednick's book, *Take a Nap, Change Your Life.*

Sleep restriction therapy and CBT (cognitive behavioral therapy): I have seen many patients struggle with insomnia and other disorders despite making honest efforts to implement the aforementioned suggestions. If you still struggle, consider seeing a therapist that specializes in CBT for insomnia. There are some powerful behavioral modifications that can be taught in a structured manner to help you sleep. There are also books and online CBT resources available.

Sleep restriction therapy is a specific protocol that attempts to dramatically improve sleep efficiency (amount of time you stay asleep) by initiating the minimum amount of sleep necessary, and then gradually moving your bedtime earlier in set time intervals. Check out online resources and protocols for sleep restriction therapy.

S-FACTOR: SUBSTANCES

The most problematic substances for sleep are caffeine-containing products and alcohol. These substances leach hours of quality, deep sleep from your life, and have a cumulative toxic effect on your health. Enjoy these two tempting substances in moderation.

The Caffeine Craze

A few words first about caffeine, since it is gaining continued prominence in many forms, from traditional coffee and tea drinks, often supersized, to high-energy sweetened beverages that are consumed by kids and adults alike. Caffeine is a prime example of the Cardinal Law of Fatigue. I am not recommending that everyone stop consuming all products containing caffeine, but I'd rather you view caffeine as a prescription medication instead of an automatic component of your daily routine. Would you chew on a blood pressure pill just because of its savory taste even if you had normal blood pressure? I hope not, because the side effect could be a drop in your blood pressure low enough to cause you to pass out. Similarly, if you use our traffic light system and rate your morning energy level an acceptable yellow, do you really need to drink a strong cup of coffee that will potentially drop your energy levels to the red zone by early afternoon and possibly ruin a good night's sleep? To avoid caffeine pitfalls, take a look at the quick guidelines below.

Caffeine sensitivity: Each person metabolizes caffeine differently. For some, even a small amount of caffeine amps them up and makes them feel jittery. For those with a high tolerance for caffeine, an espresso shot at bedtime won't impede sound sleep. To determine your level of sensitivity, first cut back completely and then gradually add the lowest caffeine dose necessary for you to achieve a reasonable, not hyperactive, energy level. In order to monitor caffeine intake, you'll need to know the level of caffeine contained in various foods and drinks. There are many helpful Internet resources. I've started you off with a chart that reveals the caffeine content of popular items.[4]

Item	Caffeine mg
Venti Starbucks coffee (20 oz)	415
Grande Starbucks coffee (16 oz)	330
Jolt Energy drink (12 oz)	280
Tall Starbucks coffee (12 oz)	260
5-hour Energy (2 oz)	208
Monster, Rockstar, Venom, NOS energy drinks	160

Item	Caffeine mg
Starbucks espresso (2 oz)	150
Folgers Classic Roast instant coffee (12 oz)	148
McDonalds coffee (16 oz)	133
Black tea (8 oz)	30-80
Red Bull (8.4 oz)	80
Snapple lemon tea (16 oz)	62
Green tea (8 oz)	35-60
Mountain Dew (12 oz)	54
Diet Coke (12 oz)	47
Coca-cola, Coke Zero, Diet Pepsi (12 oz)	35
Arizona Iced tea (16 oz)	15

Think before you drink: If you believe you are sensitive to caffeine, then step back and ask yourself if you really need that cup of coffee. If your energy level falls in the acceptable yellow zone, then it may be worth passing up a dose of caffeine, or only drinking the smallest amount and strength possible, to avoid side effects later in the day and at night.

Earlier is better: Do not underestimate the sustained effects of caffeine on your sleep. The term "half-life" refers to the amount of time it takes for half of a substance to be eliminated from your body, and is a common measurement to track the effects of drugs on your metabolism. The average half-life for caffeine is about four hours. This means if you have 100 milligrams of caffeine in your bloodstream at 12 noon, you'll have 50 milligrams in your blood by 4 pm, 25 milligrams by 8 pm, and 12.5 milligrams still hanging around at midnight, etc. The half-life of caffeine varies greatly among individuals and can be influenced by medications, alcohol, and smoking. For example, birth control pills can increase caffeine's half-life to 10 hours. If you absolutely need to drink caffeine, drink it as early in the day as possible. No caffeine after noon is a good rule of thumb, but for very caffeine-sensitive individuals, even morning caffeine can disrupt a good night's sleep.

Less is more: If your energy level is not acceptable, then drink the least amount of caffeine necessary to accomplish the task at hand.

This may require some experimentation on your part. When my energy level is low, one cup of green tea is usually all I need for a slight boost. On more challenging days, I may increase my caffeine intake with a cup of black tea or coffee. In a world where caffeine is now served in supersized designer coffee drinks and energy beverages, portion control is critical to minimize the potential side effects of caffeine and sugar overload.

Watch your carbs: Hopefully by now you are carb-savvy enough to avoid high-carb caffeine beverages like frappuccinos, sodas, and sweetened energy drinks, and to resist the cumulative effects of adding sugar to several cups of coffee and/or tea daily. In addition, many South Asians love to eat biscuits or some other crispy sweet with coffee or tea, a dangerous combination you want to avoid when at all possible. Otherwise you may give yourself a double S-factor dose of a Substance (caffeine) plus a Sugar.

Alcohol: Nightcap or Sleep Disrupter?

Alcohol is often consumed in the evening after work or later at night as a "nightcap." Some people even use alcohol as a sleep aid. While that glass of wine or serving of scotch does deliver a sedative effect, alcohol actually interferes with the optimal cycling through all phases of sleep. Falling asleep under the influence of alcohol interferes with the critical deep phase sleep and makes you more susceptible to nighttime awakenings. Alcohol-induced sleep often results in waking unrefreshed and feeling slightly groggy throughout the day. In addition, just like your morning or afternoon tea triggers cravings for sweet and crispy snacks, alcohol often triggers urges for crispy, salty treats like chips. If you drink alcohol regularly at night, or have a sense that alcohol might be interfering with your sleep, conduct a similar elimination experiment as you did with caffeine to see if alcohol is indeed the culprit.

In addition to caffeine and alcohol, be aware of the following sleep-inhibiting substances:

Prescription drugs: Medications, such as beta-blockers for high blood pressure, can cause fatigue.

OTCs: Over-the-counter medications often contain stimulants, such as caffeine, or sedating ingredients. Cough and cold preparations traditionally feature stimulants like dextromethorphan (cough suppressant) and pseudoephedrine (decongestant).

Diet pills, herbals, and Ayurvedic medicines: Herbs and tinctures, no matter how natural, often contain stimulants or sedating ingredients that can cause withdrawal fatigue. For example, even though the stimulant ephedra has been banned in diet pills, it is still an occasional ingredient in some herbal remedies and Chinese medications.

If you are experiencing persistent fatigue after cutting back on caffeine, digital stimulation, and inconsistent bed and wake times, stop taking your supplements (herbals, Ayurvedics, etc.) for a while, and talk to your pharmacist or physician about possible fatigue side effects from any prescription medications you might be taking.

S-FACTOR: SEDENTARY LIFESTYLE

It has been my experience that individuals who sit in front of a computer all day (like our case study Manish) complain about fatigue far more than those whose jobs require more walking and physical activity. The human body was not designed to remain in a seated position for hours on end, which might explain why fatigue has become an epidemic in our modern, high-tech society. Even though cutting your starch intake and improving your sleep can be energizing, improving activity levels and adding exercise can enhance and sustain energy long term. In addition, increasing activity levels has a positive influence on your other S-factors. It helps manage stress, improve sleep, metabolize starches, and reduce the need for substances like excess caffeine and alcohol.

Shifting your body's fuel source from short-acting carbs to longer-acting, energizing fat is one milestone; benefiting from this fuel by delivering it to your brain and muscles is another. Remaining sedentary is as useless as converting an oversized mini-van into a sports car and then leaving it parked in the garage. The fuel just sits in the gas tank! In order to deliver energy through your circulation (fuel lines) to your engine, you have to get your heart pumping faster and your muscles working harder so they can use the fuel for energy. Stagnant fatty acid fuel from inactivity is less likely to be used by your brain and muscles and more likely to be taken back up by fat cells for storage. Your brain gets the signal that you don't need energy because you're sitting for hours, and so stores it in your gas tank (fat cells). Remember that even the simple act of standing burns three times as many calories as sitting. Get the fat out by eating fewer carbs and lowering your insulin levels, and then deliver it to your brain and muscles by standing (i.e., set up your standing work desk) and moving as much as you can.

HOW TO RECHARGE YOURSELF ONCE AND FOR ALL

You may have noticed that the five S-factors are not independent entities, but are intimately connected in various ways.

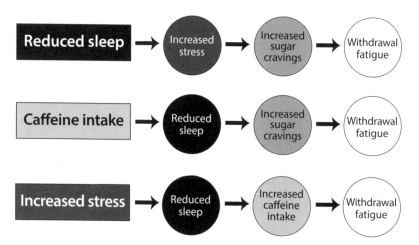

You get the picture. Tackling all five S-factors may seem over-whelming, but focusing on one or two factors at a time may be all you need to break the rest of the chain. Manish cut the excess sugar/ starch factor, which helped him shed body fat and gave him the energy to exercise, which in turn enabled him to better manage his stress and sleep more peacefully.

Look Back to Find the Culprit

Any time you feel unduly fatigued, you can almost always look back over the past 12 hours and notice some strong contributing factors. For example, if you feel exhausted at 3 pm, it could be due to the white rice, pasta, or chapatis you had for lunch, the poor night's sleep, and/or the caffeine withdrawal from your morning cup of coffee. How could this fatigue have been minimized? If you slept poorly and know you can't survive without your morning coffee, choose the least amount of caffeine possible to get you through the morning. Next, make sure you eat a lighter lunch that is high in protein and healthy fats with minimal carbs. Recall that even if you eat the ideal nutrient composition for lunch, the volume of food itself can overactivate your parasympathetic system, causing excess grogginess in the afternoon. You may still feel tired in the afternoon from the lack of sleep, but making these simple changes can be the difference between your energy levels being in the functional yellow zone versus the paralyzing red zone. Whenever you feel fatigued, look back to find the cause, and then work to prevent history from repeating itself. Keeping a fatigue journal to document your energy levels (red, yellow, or green) and S-factors at different times of the day is a helpful way to identify the causes. Eventually, you will intuitively make the necessary adjustments to maximize your energy levels given various circumstances.

Planning Ahead for Peak Performance

Once you become more energy aware and familiar with the effects of the different S-factors, you will be able to tailor your energy levels to maximize performance in every area of your life. Let's look at this practice at work in one of my patients.

Case Study: Vikram

Vikram is a 48-year-old sales executive who complained of intermittent bouts of fatigue that were reducing his productivity at work. He visited me on a Monday and told me he was giving the "presentation of a lifetime" on Friday at lunch and needed to be at his best. He came to me asking for a sleeping pill so he would be alert for his big day. I advised Vikram that since he was not used to taking sleeping pills, this might backfire and leave him feeling even groggier during his presentation. Instead, I told him that it was critical to prepare for this important event at least two days in advance. I recommended he eliminate caffeine after 12 pm on Wednesday and Thursday to help him get two nights of good sleep. I also suggested a Friday morning workout followed by a healthy, high-protein breakfast only if he felt hungry. I explained how fasting or having a light, low-carb or no-carb breakfast can improve focus and alertness. If he slept poorly on Thursday night because of anxiety about his big day, then it would be acceptable to have a small cup of coffee about two hours before his presentation. Drinking caffeine too early in the morning might lead to a crash by 12 pm, and drinking it too close to his presentation could make him more jittery and nervous. Vikram was happy to report that his presentation went without a hitch.

Athletes train for events with similar preparation. They don't just randomly go from hour to hour, letting their hunger and emotions dictate eating and behavior. Take some control of your life and prepare your mind and body for peak performance! Also keep in mind that the weekend before a big event is an opportunity to energize, rather than overwork. I often prepare for big presentations by spending a full Saturday with the kids on a long hike, or playing soccer or basketball at the park. Physical activities spent with my loved ones charge my batteries so that I am energetic and fully engaged for work the next week. Making weekends an extension of the workweek, without adequate time for rest and play, will only impair performance and diminish your overall sense of well-being. Incorporate some advanced preparation with the principles in this chapter and you will conserve and replenish those precious energy stores for the moments in your life that matter most.

MEDICAL CONDITIONS THAT CAUSE FATIGUE

If you have tried your best to correct the S-factors in your life but still suffer from persistent fatigue, then see your doctor for a thorough evaluation. Don't sweep fatigue under the rug and treat it as a normal part of life. There are some common medical conditions that cause fatigue, including…

- Thyroid disorders

- Depression and anxiety

- Anemia

- Diabetes

- Common medication side effects

- Sleep disorders: sleep apnea and restless legs syndrome

Thyroid Disorders

The thyroid gland controls your metabolism. An underactive thyroid (hypothyroidism) is the more common cause of fatigue, but an overactive thyroid (hyperthyroidism) can also lead to tiredness. A simple blood test called the TSH (thyroid stimulating hormone) is used to screen for thyroid disease. Some common signs of thyroid diseases are listed below.

Hypothyroidism:
Intolerance to cold weather
Unexpected weight gain
Constipation
Hair loss
Leg swelling
Fatigue

Hyperthyroidism:

Intolerance to heat
Unexpected weight loss
Diarrhea
Hair loss
Palpitations
Anxiety
Fatigue

Depression and Anxiety

Constant fatigue may be a symptom of depression or anxiety. An imbalance in the brain chemical serotonin can cause a drop in energy levels. Be on the lookout for the following symptoms:

Depression:

Persistent feelings of sadness or hopelessness
Loss of interest in normal daily activities
Frequent crying spells
Fatigue
Trouble sleeping
Lack of motivation
Irritability
Restlessness
Feelings of worthlessness
Difficulty focusing
Difficulty making decisions
Suicidal thoughts or behavior

Anxiety:

Restlessness
Feeling keyed up or on edge
Fatigue
Difficulty concentrating
Irritability and impatience
Easy distractibility
Excess sweating
Shortness of breath

Heart racing
Stomachache or diarrhea
Headaches

Anemia

Anemia occurs when your red blood cells drop below a normal level. Red blood cells carry oxygen to your muscles and vital organs, so a reduction in these cells can produce fatigue. Anemia can be caused by blood loss, poor nutrition, chronic exercise, chronic disease, and a number of other conditions. A simple blood test called a complete blood cell count (CBC) is used to diagnose anemia. In many of my menstruating female patients, iron deficiency with or without anemia causes fatigue. A blood test for iron levels can be done if indicated, and if iron deficiency is present, then taking an iron supplement can boost energy levels within a few months. Vegetarians are at risk for anemia due to nutritional deficiencies such as iron and vitamin B12.

Diabetes

Fatigue is a common symptom of diabetes and is tied to insulin resistance as we've already discussed. Other symptoms of diabetes include:

Excessive thirst
Frequent urination
Unexpected weight loss
Blurry vision
Extreme hunger
Irritability

Sleep Disorders

Sleep apnea results from abnormal breathing during sleep, while restless legs syndrome is a discomfort in the legs that disrupts sleep. The unpleasant sensation of restless legs syndrome has been described in various ways, including creeping, crawling, jittery, tingling, aching, or burning. Either condition can reduce the amount of good quality sleep, producing daytime fatigue. Symptoms for each are listed on the following page.

Sleep apnea:
  Loud snoring
  Disrupted breathing during sleep (usually noticed by bed partner)
  Excessive daytime sleepiness and fatigue
  Morning headaches

Restless legs syndrome:
  Leg symptoms are worse at rest, especially when lying or sitting
  Leg symptoms improve with movement
  Leg symptoms get worse at night
  Symptoms cause daytime sleepiness and fatigue

There are other types of sleep disorders best determined by a sleep study and consultation with a specialist who can help identify the cause.

Chronic Fatigue Syndrome (CFS)

If fatigue is present for at least six months and there is no identifiable cause or medical condition, then CFS needs to be considered. The eight major symptoms of CFS are:

  Impaired memory or concentration
  Exhaustion following physical or mental exercise
  Unrefreshing sleep
  Joint pain (without redness or swelling)
  Persistent muscle pain
  Headaches of a new type or severity
  Tender neck or axillary (underarm) lymph nodes
  Sore throat

Serious Disorders

Heart disease, lung disease, infection, autoimmune conditions, and cancer are some of the serious medical diseases that can cause fatigue, but usually other symptoms are present. It is imperative to have a thorough medical evaluation for persistent fatigue in order to rule out these chronic conditions. Sudden onset of fatigue without an identifiable cause warrants immediate medical attention.

Summary

- Become more energy aware by using the traffic light system to grade your energy throughout the day.

- Identify which S-factors are contributing to your fatigue.

- Focus on one or two S-factors first. Don't set goals that are unrealistic or unsustainable.

- Make stress reduction a high priority. Chronic stress should not be considered a normal part of life.

- Fatigue is tied closely to insulin resistance and excess carbs in the diet. Follow the CARBS plan in Chapter 6 while monitoring your Metabolic 6-pack.

- Be sure to see your physician for persistent or abrupt onset of fatigue.

For Professionals

- Encourage individuals with fatigue to keep an energy journal, using the traffic light system.

- Ask questions regarding the S-factors when doing a fatigue evaluation.

- Recognize fatigue as a common symptom of insulin resistance and a high-carb diet.

- Be sure to ask about stress and provide appropriate support and resources as needed.

- Use the Metabolic 6-pack as a biometric guide to energy levels. As numbers improve, so should energy levels.

- Keep on the lookout for medical disorders that cause fatigue, like nutritional anemia in vegetarians.

CHAPTER 9

OPTIMAL HEALTH FOR
SOUTH ASIAN WOMEN

SOUTH ASIAN WOMEN FACE many challenges in the quest for optimal physical and emotional health. The traditional South Asian female of generations past served as head of household, managing several children and extended family members. Despite the tremendous responsibilities involved, a broad family support system helped to prevent feelings of isolation, enhance self-worth, and share in many of the tasks. Prior generations of South Asian women enjoyed better health and life satisfaction due in large part to this familial network. Many modern South Asian women, however, have migrated away from their native lands, leaving behind many of these health-promoting cultural traditions. Consequently, they face a new set of challenges. In the Western world, family units are typically much smaller, and the supportive extended family and cultural ecosystem is often lost as a result.

Today, a vast number of South Asian women have entered the workforce, balancing tremendous professional pressures while still managing the majority of domestic responsibilities. The modern day lifestyle stressors I've discussed throughout this book, such as inactivity, a toxic food environment, limited sunlight exposure, and digital stress, significantly impact a woman's body composition and metabolism. This is especially true following a typical South Asian pregnancy fueled by an unhealthy diet and prolonged inactivity, often perpetuated by false myths and traditions that aggravate insulin resistance and promote obesity after delivery.

In this chapter, I highlight the modern lifestyle challenges that have a particularly detrimental impact on South Asian women, and end with a special section on healthy pregnancy considerations. Let's start with a case of an insulin resistant mother and daughter.

Case Study: Anita

Anita is a 45-year-old woman who came to see me for diabetes prevention advice. She had a history of PCOS (polycystic ovarian syndrome) as a teenager, a condition that went undiagnosed at the time. She recounted battling with weight issues, irregular periods, terrible acne, and excessive facial hair—factors that led to mild depression. Unfortunately, both she and her family knew nothing about PCOS at the time. She was able to diagnose her affliction only after noting similar symptoms in her 16-year-old daughter.

The birth of her daughter was complicated by gestational diabetes. Anita has remained prediabetic since her pregnancy, with her fasting blood sugars inching closer towards diabetes each year. She has had difficulty with weight loss, despite trying multiple different diets. A detailed history revealed a daily carbohydrate intake above 300 grams, mostly obtained through whole wheat chapatis, lentils, some rice, and abundant amounts of fruit. Her physical activity was limited to 20-minute walks, three times a week.

I told Anita that she needed to break the female tradition of insulin resistance in her family. I put Anita on a lower carbohydrate-eating plan and recommended the same eating plan for her daughter, who had a high likelihood of developing diabetes given her PCOS and obesity. They also took part in joint personal training sessions twice a week and walked every evening. Anita eventually shed 25 pounds and normalized her blood sugars. Anita's daughter lost 10 pounds and experienced improvement in her PCOS symptoms.

THE PCOS EPIDEMIC

Every South Asian woman needs to know about polycystic ovarian syndrome, which is the most common endocrine disorder in females. The overall global incidence of this condition is between 20 to 30 percent. One study showed that the highest reported incidence in an ethnic group was among South Asian immigrants in Britain—just over half of South Asian women (52 percent) had PCOS![1] Researchers also found that the degree of insulin resistance uncovered in these non-diabetic women with PCOS was similar to that of a type 2 diabetic. Compared to Caucasians, South Asians develop PCOS at an earlier age and have more severe symptoms, greater associated insulin resistance and excess insulin levels, and a higher incidence of infertility.[2]

What exactly is PCOS and how is it related to insulin resistance? The extra insulin resulting from insulin resistance triggers the formation of cysts in the ovaries, the production of excess male hormones called androgens, and the accumulation of excess body fat. Over half of women with PCOS are obese due to insulin-driven body fat storage. The extra fat tissue makes the problem worse because fat produces male hormones that contribute to the hormone imbalance characteristic of PCOS. This hormone imbalance disrupts normal menstrual cycles and may cause infertility. Blood testing and diagnostic imaging are confirmatory, but the diagnosis of PCOS is made primarily from observing one or more of the following symptoms:

- Irregular menstrual cycles

- Evidence of excess male hormones (androgens), which produce symptoms like acne, excess facial and body hair, and hair loss over the scalp (alopecia)

- Obesity, especially insulin resistant central obesity

- *Acanthosis Nigricans*—a rash consisting of dark brown/ black-colored velvety or thick textured skin lesions found in body skin folds (back or side of neck, armpits, groin, etc.)

It is critical for South Asian women, and particularly parents of teenagers, to recognize the symptoms of PCOS early on and seek medical attention as soon as possible.

Besides the physical harm incurred, PCOS can be psychologically devastating to teenagers and young women. Obesity, acne, and facial hair adversely impact body image, particularly during adolescent years. The fertility difficulties can be disastrous to those wishing to start a family. Furthermore, the following downstream risks of PCOS caused by insulin resistance are an even greater threat to health:

- Risk of diabetes is over seven times greater than it is for someone without PCOS

- Increased risk of heart disease with more extensive atherosclerosis of blood vessels

- High blood pressure

- Increased risk of metabolic syndrome

In fact, all of the insulin resistant conditions discussed thus far are more prevalent and often more severe in women with PCOS. It is critical for South Asian women, and particularly parents of teenagers, to recognize the symptoms of PCOS early on and seek medical attention as soon as possible. Lifestyle changes to reduce body fat and medical treatment for PCOS symptoms can help control this condition, neutralize dangerous long-term risk factors, and dramatically improve psychological health and overall quality of life. To summarize:

- Women and family members should be aware of PCOS symptoms

- Seek medical attention early on if you suspect PCOS

- Exercise, a healthy eating plan to reduce body fat, and emotional support are critical

- Women with PCOS should be screened regularly for signs of insulin resistance, in particular the Metabolic 6-pack

- If lifestyle changes do not manage symptoms effectively, medical treatment is available

Remember, excess fat can make PCOS significantly worse; I have seen patients with PCOS do very well merely by losing fat through carb reduction. Teenagers may not have to undergo strict carb reduction to reduce body fat. Anita's daughter simply had to eliminate sodas, sweets, and processed foods, particularly those containing high fructose corn syrup (HFCS), to alleviate her PCOS symptoms.

INSULIN RESISTANCE AND HEART DISEASE

While heart disease rates are higher in males, females are certainly not immune to the heart disease and insulin resistance epidemic. Unfortunately, many South Asians still view heart disease as a man's disease and as a result, women are not being adequately screened for insulin resistance and cardiovascular risk factors. A California study conducted between the years 1990 and 2000 looked at ethnic variations in heart disease risk among whites, African Americans, Chinese, Japanese, and Asian Indian women. All groups exhibited a reduction in heart disease mortality (death from heart disease) over the 10-year period, except Asian Indian women, who actually experienced increased heart disease mortality.[3] Many South Asian women limit physician visits to obstetrics care during pregnancy and pediatric visits for their children. Routine annual health exams are usually lacking. This trend needs to be overturned. South Asian women must be screened regularly for the Metabolic 6-pack criteria discussed in Chapter 1.

FEMALE DIFFICULTIES REDUCING EXCESS BODY FAT

I frequently see couples in my office for a joint health and medical consultation, and often end up putting them both on the CARBS eating plan. Wives usually complain that husbands lose considerably more weight, even though the women frequently make more disciplined efforts to eat right and exercise. Indeed, when it comes to fat loss, most men do have an advantage over women. The primary reason is baseline body composition. Recall how a high fat-to-muscle ratio is a major driver of insulin resistance and insulin overproduction. The average female, not only South Asian but all ethnicities, has a higher ratio than the average male, making her much more susceptible to fat gain and much more resistant to fat loss. The high prevalence of PCOS in women, combined with this high-insulin state is a contributor to the excess body fat in South Asian women. For a typical sedentary, high-carbohydrate-eating South Asian woman, the tendency to accumulate body fat can become precipitously worse after pregnancy, because hormonal changes can stimulate even further fat storage.

There are numerous examples of elite female track and field athletes not just competing after having children but winning Olympic medals and setting national and world records!

Interestingly, pregnancy does not automatically program a woman to be overweight and out of shape for the rest of her life. There are numerous examples of elite female track and field athletes not just competing after having children but winning Olympic medals and setting national and world records! Russian high jumper Anna Chicherova took a leave from athletics in 2010 to have a child, and then went on to win the World Championships in 2011 and the Olympic gold in 2012. There may be physiologic changes—such as an increase in blood volume and the effects of the hormone estrogen—that enhance endurance and reduce injuries, thereby promoting such athletic accomplishment. Other experts speculate that the benefits are mainly psychological—women become more resilient all around for having endured pregnancy and childbirth. For those of you who are not quite looking to break world records, do understand that there are major health benefits to staying fit through pregnancy and, of course, after childbirth. One study found that women who maintain their fitness during pregnancy continue to exercise at a higher level after they have children than those who stop exercising when they become pregnant.[4]

South Asian women often hit a weight loss plateau due to lack of strength training. Walking seems to be the almost exclusive form of exercise among most South Asian women. Once I convince South Asian women to add more intense resistance and weight training, they break through plateaus and notice more significant changes in body composition. Adding brief, intense workouts to one's routine improves the fat-to-muscle ratio. This helps reduce insulin resistance, and is also critical for bone and musculoskeletal health. Fears about getting too "bulky" from weight training are based on complete myth. Unlike men, women do not naturally have the levels of testosterone required to support the building of bulky muscles.

The type of drastic cyclical dieting that many South Asian women periodically engage in—which often involves periods of severe caloric deprivation from exclusive juicing and Ayurvedic techniques—leads to a loss of not only fat but also precious lean muscle tissue. Consequently, the ratio of fat to muscle doesn't change, so the level of insulin resistance remains the same and body fat is easily piled back on once these unsustainable interventions are completed.

Here are some key tips to help South Asian women break through weight loss plateaus:

1. **Reduce carbs further:** South Asian females may need to initially reduce net carb intake to 50 grams a day or less in order to drive down fat-storing insulin. Removing staple South Asian grains and dropping to a net carb intake of less than 50 grams jumpstarted Anita's fat loss!

2. **Eliminate wheat:** Don't underestimate the appetite-stimulating and fat-storage-promoting effects of modern wheat, as detailed in Dr. William Davis's book, *Wheat Belly*. Try going wheat-free for three to four weeks using the substitutes discussed in Chapter 6.

3. **Add resistance training:** Focus on exercises that involve large muscle groups like your legs. If you are hesitant to join a gym, you can gain considerable strength and muscle with simple body weight exercises done in the privacy of your own home. As these get easier, you can add weights.

4. **Add sprinting:** Try high-intensity sprint training, where maximum effort bursts are interspersed with rest intervals. This type of training, often called "interval training," can help unlock stubborn fat cells in less time.

5. **Get some sun exposure:** Be sure vitamin D levels are normal by obtaining adequate sun exposure on large skin surface areas of your body during the months of peak solar intensity at your latitude. Chapter 11 highlights vitamin D recommendations.

6. **Get calcium:** Consider adding more dietary calcium (including high-fat dairy products) which has been shown to support weight loss in women.

7. **Control stress:** Chronically elevated levels of the primary stress hormone cortisol act as major fat loss obstacles for many modern citizens immersed in hectic lifestyles. Stress-induced cortisol release not only increases fat storage, but also contributes to emotional eating. Moderating life stress restores a more natural appetite based on real hunger, rather than cortisol cues.

8. **Optimize sleep:** Lack of adequate sleep increases insulin resistance and promotes fat storage. Like stress, insufficient sleep also causes hormonal changes that drive hunger and fat storage.

9. **Eat more fat:** Yes, adding more fat to your diet can assist with weight loss! Emphasize monounsaturated fats, omega-3s, and healthier saturated fats like coconut oil and ghee. Be sure to restrict your carb intake. Totally avoid trans fats and vegetable oils. Remember that fat doesn't increase insulin and can help improve mood and energy, reduce hunger, and optimize hormonal balance.

10. **Try intermittent fasting:** If you experience mild hunger while fasting, indulge in sparkling water, coffee, or tea with coconut oil and a handful of nuts. If you develop unbearable hunger, end your fast and eat a *South Asian Health Solution*-approved meal. Fasted morning workouts can be effective in promoting fat loss, but be sure to stay well hydrated.

11. **Eat more vegetables:** Be sure you are getting adequate micronutrients in your diet through abundant servings of vegetables and sensible consumption of seasonal fruits. High-nutrient-value plants are lacking in most South Asian diets, a deficiency that can impair fat burning.

12. **Check your thyroid:** If you are still having trouble, talk to your doctor about screening for thyroid disorders and anemia. An underactive thyroid can promote easy weight gain, and anemia can often cause fatigue and difficulty initiating or increasing exercise levels.

BONE AND MUSCULOSKELETAL HEALTH

Let's shift our attention to bones and tendons. I see a tremendous amount of early arthritis, tendonitis, and osteoporosis (reduced bone density increasing fracture risk) in South Asian women. Many of these conditions are related to the risks and lifestyle factors that predispose South Asian women to fat gain. A high ratio of fat to muscle not only promotes more fat gain and insulin resistance, but it also leaves joints and tendons unprotected and exposed to premature arthritis and musculoskeletal injuries. Muscles, unlike fat, not only provide a sturdy protective layer to joints, but they also take up the brunt of our daily repetitive and impact-related activities, sparing the joints from early wear and tear. Arthritis is even further advanced by excess blood glucose from insulin resistance, which triggers the production of advanced glycated end products that promote increased inflammation and cartilage degeneration. Add significant vitamin D deficiency to the mix (vitamin D is essential for building strong bones), and now you have thin, fragile bones connected by worn out joint cartilage and surrounded by overstressed tendons and ligaments due to lack of muscle. Many of the South Asian females I see in my practice have developed significant ankle sprains and injuries while doing minor household chores or activities—all due to inadequate muscular support! The overall musculoskeletal frame of an average South Asian patient is not upright and sturdy. It's hunched forward and unstable, especially in South Asian women. So how do we prevent these musculoskeletal issues and rebuild a sturdier frame?

1. **Adequate weight-bearing exercises:** "Weight bearing" means staying upright so your body works against gravity. Such exercises include walking, hiking, jogging, racquet sports, yoga, and dancing. Swimming is a great exercise, but not considered weight bearing.

2. **Additional weight training:** Adding weights will further strengthen and protect bones.

3. **Ensure optimal vitamin D levels and dietary calcium intake:** Vitamin D allows your body to absorb dietary calcium, necessary for strong bone building.

4. **Screening for osteoporosis:** Age-appropriate screening for osteoporosis with a DEXA scan (imaging test measuring bone density) usually starts at age 65, but may be indicated sooner if you carry risk factors. Discuss screening with your doctor.

5. **Anti-inflammatory eating plan:** An anti-inflammatory diet consists of abundant plant-based foods and healthy fats. Cut back excess sugar and carbohydrates to reduce arthritis risk.

PREGNANCY PEARLS

Pregnancy is a very broad topic, but I'd like to highlight a few important points. Arm yourself with knowledge, work with an experienced nutritionist, and stay connected to your obstetrician and physician throughout the entire process. It is proven beyond a doubt that the health and nutritional status of the mother before and during pregnancy are critical factors that influence the immediate health of the child and his or her adult health as well. Treat pregnancy like an Olympic sporting event. Actually, it's far more important than an Olympic event! If you want to ensure optimal health for your baby during childhood and beyond, you need to enter pregnancy in the best shape of your life. What you put into your body will have a direct impact on your baby's genetic blueprint.

> *The health and nutritional status of the mother before and during pregnancy are critical factors that influence the immediate health of the child, as well as his or her adult health.*

From Low-birth-weight (LBW) Babies to High-risk Adults

Fetal programming explains how the nutritional environment of the developing fetus influences its genetic code. The placenta is the lifeline between mom and fetus through which nutrient-rich blood is delivered to allow growth and development. Both maternal overnutrition and undernutrition contribute to reductions in placental blood flow, leading to intrauterine growth restriction (IUGR). IUGR has several immediate complications for the baby such as hypoglycemia (low blood sugar), pneumonia due to a condition called meconium aspiration, and motor and neurological complications. Most parents are less familiar with the future repercussions of IUGR, especially when these complications arise due to overfeeding.

Researcher David Barker conducted pioneering studies that showed how LBW babies had a higher risk of insulin resistance and heart disease later in life. Recall from Chapter 1 that insulin resistance developed as an evolutionary adaptation that allowed humans to conserve energy during times of famine. Placental malnutrition basically produces a state of fetal famine, which in turn exerts intense pressure on fetal genes, making them express a state of insulin resistance that endures into adulthood. This translates to a higher risk of developing conditions such as diabetes, high blood pressure, and heart disease—all programmed from birth! Many South Asians start off as thin babies and children, and end up as insulin resistant and overweight adults. Sound familiar?

The WHO/UNICEF report indicates that South Asia has the highest incidence of LBW babies in the world. Although the majority of these LBW babies are due to severe malnutrition, LBW babies are all too common at every socioeconomic level. Below is a list of some of the important factors and lifestyle modifications South Asian women need to be aware of to reduce their chances of delivering a LBW baby. Keep in mind that even South Asian women that do everything right may still have an innate predisposition to deliver LBW babies, and this should not be viewed as a form of personal failure. I encourage all family members to be aware of the factors listed below, since often it is familial influence that drives the behaviors of pregnant women. The impact of secondhand smoke exposure from a spouse or unhealthy foods prepared by a family member can have direct effects on the health of the fetus.

1. **Quit tobacco and nicotine:** If you smoke, quit. If you are around someone who smokes, insist that they quit or smoke outside, far away from you and your unborn child.

2. **Improve nutrition:** Severe maternal malnutrition is an obvious cause of IUGR. However, poor nutrition does not always

mean undernutrition. You can be taking in more than enough calories and still be malnourished due to a lack of adequate macro and micronutrients. A diet filled with empty carbohydrates, which for Anita was the repetitive pattern of dal, rice, and chapati with very little vegetables, can result in an overweight mother who provides inadequate nutrition to the developing fetus.

3. **Supplement with folate:** A deficiency in folate, also known as folic acid, is associated with premature babies, neural tube defects (birth defect of brain and spinal cord), and LBW babies. Folate is included in prenatal vitamins to reduce the risk of these complications. Foods such as leafy green vegetables and beans are rich sources of folate.

4. **Protect against insulin resistance and diabetes:** These conditions can cause LBW or oversized babies, both of which are associated with risk later in life. I strongly encourage all women planning to become pregnant to have their Metabolic 6-pack monitored in order to pick up on insulin resistance as early as possible, even before blood sugar starts to rise.

5. **Lower blood pressure:** Be sure to get your blood pressure screened regularly before pregnancy since hypertension is associated with IUGR.

6. **Give up the alcohol:** Given the high risk of IUGR in South Asians, a complete abstinence from alcohol during pregnancy is mandatory.

7. **Load up with vitamin B12:** A study done on women in urban Bangalore showed an association between maternal vitamin B12 deficiency and IUGR.[5] Vitamin B12 deficiency is especially common in vegetarians. I recommend being screened and, if low, incorporating more vitamin B12 in the diet and discussing supplementation with your doctor.

8. **Ensure vitamin D intake:** One study showed an association between low vitamin D levels and LBW babies.[6] It is hypothesized that low vitamin D reduces available calcium for fetal bone growth and decreases hormones necessary for glucose and fatty acid production to fuel fetal growth and development.

9. **Monitor iron intake:** A meta-analysis of 48 randomized trials made up of 18,000 pregnant women showed that daily iron supplementation was associated with an almost 20-percent reduction in risk of delivering a LBW baby.[7] For every 10 mg increase in dose up to 66 mg per day, there was a four-percent risk reduction.

10. **Be cautious of caffeine:** There is a slight association between caffeine and LBW babies, but the effects are not nearly as strong as those linked to tobacco smoke and malnutrition. During pregnancy, do not consume more than 200 mg of caffeine daily. The less the better. Caffeine doses vary greatly depending on the drink. An average 6 oz cup of home brewed coffee contains about 100 mg of caffeine. A large cup of coffee at your favorite coffee house may be loaded with over 400 mg of caffeine! Masala tea and green tea have much lower caffeine doses. See the chart on page 213 for caffeine levels in popular beverages.

11. **Screen for infection:** The TORCH test, which stands for Toxoplasmosis, Rubella, CMV, Herpes, and HIV, screens for infections associated with IUGR and other fetal complications. Syphilis is another infection associated with IUGR.

12. **Beware of other associated conditions:** Chronic kidney disease, heart disease, respiratory disease, anemia, and autoimmune disorders like lupus can increase the risk of delivering a LBW baby.

A combination of several factors increases the risk of delivering a LBW baby. Major factors include the health and nutritional status of the mother, in addition to significant toxins like tobacco smoke. However, an accumulation of more subtle, yet common factors such as vitamin D and B12 deficiencies, coupled with excessive caffeine intake may also have a marked impact on the birth weight of the baby. Maintaining a balanced exercise program is also important in preventing IUGR-related conditions such as insulin resistance and hypertension.

Detecting Gestational Diabetes Risk Before Pregnancy

Gestational diabetes—diabetes that occurs in conjunction with pregnancy—has become an epidemic among South Asian women. Often women with underlying insulin resistance but no prior history of blood sugar abnormalities become diabetic as a result of pregnancy. This was the case with Anita, who had completely normal blood sugars until her pregnancy. It's not that the pregnancy alone caused the diabetes. The insulin resistance was already there, but the physiological state of pregnancy accelerated it into a state of diabetes. You will be routinely screened for gestational diabetes at the time of pregnancy, but it is critical to detect insulin resistance as early as possible using the Metabolic 6-pack.

Recall how measures of abdominal fat, high triglycerides, and low HDL cholesterol can signal insulin resistance long before changes in blood sugar occur. Detect these markers before becoming pregnant, and you can implement the lifestyle changes necessary to dramatically reduce your risk of gestational diabetes, and all of its associated complications. Risk factors for gestational diabetes include…

- Any of the Metabolic 6-pack factors discussed in Chapter 1
- Being of Asian descent (South Asian or East Asian)
- A family history of diabetes
- Being overweight before pregnancy
- Previously giving birth to a baby weighing more than 9 pounds
- Prior history of gestational diabetes
- Prior history of giving birth to a stillborn baby

Risks of Gestational Diabetes for Mother and Baby

Gestational diabetes elevates blood sugar, which is then transferred to the fetus. We've learned how glucose promotes obesity through the fattening effects of the hormone insulin. Excess glucose fed to the fetus via maternal circulation also produces a supersized baby who is prone to complications at the time of birth, and to obesity and diabetes throughout his or her life. Following is a summary of the risks to mother and baby caused by gestational diabetes:

Risks to baby:

1. High-birth-weight baby, which increases the risk of birth injuries and the chance of a C-section.

2. Low-birth-weight baby due to a higher risk of premature delivery (babies delivered early are lower birth weight).

3. Respiratory distress syndrome due to immature lung development in premature babies.

4. Low blood sugar (hypoglycemia) due to excess insulin.

5. Jaundice due to an immature liver that can't break down a pigment called bilirubin, causing yellowing of the skin and eyes.

6. Type 2 diabetes later in life.

Risks to mother:

1. High blood pressure, which damages your arteries, heart, brain, and kidneys if left unchecked.

2. Preeclampsia and eclampsia, which pose a serious threat to both mother and baby. Preeclampsia occurs when the mother develops high blood pressure and protein in her urine. Eclampsia is a more serious form of preeclampsia that induces seizures.

3. Higher future risk of diabetes and heart disease after pregnancy. Studies generally report a 30-percent conversion rate to diabetes after pregnancy.

Your health and that of your future child depend on your nutritional status. <u>Stop</u> procrastinating and <u>start</u> shedding that extra body fat, adding muscle, and eating a nutrient-dense diet.

Management of Gestational Diabetes

A comprehensive discussion of the management of gestational diabetes is beyond the scope of this book. If you have been diagnosed with gestational diabetes, you will need the close supervision of a multidisciplinary team consisting of your obstetrician, nutritionist (preferably diabetes certified), and endocrinologist. You will also need to monitor your blood sugars directly using a glucose meter. You will most likely be asked to track your carb intake daily; I encourage you to use Chapter 6 as a resource for exploring your low-carbohydrate dietary options. Since your goal is not to lose weight during your pregnancy, be sure to stick to your medical team's recommendations for caloric intake and weight gain. Your focus during pregnancy is going to be strict blood sugar control while maintaining a healthy increase in weight.

Nutrition Before and During Pregnancy

If you are not yet pregnant but are planning to become pregnant in the future, you should follow the eating principles outlined in Chapter 6, especially if you are overweight and have any of the Metabolic 6-pack risk factors. Your goal is to shed that extra body fat, add muscle, eat a nutrient-dense diet, and improve your overall fitness. If you've been procrastinating making these changes and plan to have children in the near, or even the not-so-near future, then the moment to make a change is now. Your health, your future child's health…even your grandchild's health depend on it. Your nutritional status directly affects your child's genes, which he or she will then pass on to future generations. Remember, you are training for one of the most important events in your life, and the earlier you start, the better your chances of avoiding gestational diabetes and its associated complications.

What are the appropriate nutritional guidelines for women who are already pregnant, and is it safe to eat a lower carbohydrate diet? Excess carbohydrate consumption plays into the extremely high incidence of gestational diabetes among South Asian females. During pregnancy, your goal is to cut back on the junk and empty carbohydrates that provide little to no nutritional value, while being careful not to severely restrict carbohydrates in an effort to lose weight. A healthy amount of weight gain during pregnancy is essential, and should be tracked by your obstetrician and possibly a nutritionist. Drastic carbohydrate reduction during pregnancy can complicate healthy weight gain and act as an additional metabolic stressor. Avoid more aggressive fat-burning techniques like fasting during pregnancy. If your body is not adapted to the lower carbohydrate eating lifestyle, pregnancy is not the time to start experimenting with drastic carb reduction.

Here are some basic nutrition guidelines for pregnancy:

1. **Remove junk carbohydrates:** Cut sugar, sweets, sodas, and processed foods with high fructose corn syrup (HFCS).

2. **Ban all trans fats:** Trans fats cross the placenta to the fetus and have been shown to have adverse effects. Trans fats, otherwise known as hydrogenated or partially hydrogenated fats, are abundant in Indian baked goods, crispy snacks, sweets, and packaged and processed foods. Vanaspati is a partially or fully hydrogenated vegetable oil that is a cheap, dangerous substitute for ghee, used widely in Indian cooking and packaged foods. Stay away from it. Have zero tolerance for these fats, especially during pregnancy.

3. **Add plants:** Consume at least six to eight servings of fresh vegetables and fruits per day. Eat a variety of different colors and enjoy dark, green, leafy vegetables like spinach, kale, and Swiss chard, which are loaded with vitamins A, C, K, and folate.

4. **Eat a balanced macronutrient profile:** Carbs are usually more than prominent in a South Asian diet, so focus on increasing protein and healthy fat intake (especially omega-3s). A carb-predominant diet will increase the risk of elevated blood sugars, insulin resistance, and gestational diabetes. Consider eliminating or limiting rice intake, or switching to small portions of brown rice, especially if you show signs of insulin resistance.

5. **Don't forget eggs:** Eggs are a near-perfect pregnancy food with high quality protein, vitamin B12, and another B vitamin called choline, which is an excellent nutrient for fetal brain development.

6. **Get your healthy dairy:** Greek yogurt in particular is recommended since it has twice the protein and fewer carbohydrates than regular yogurt does. Dairy is an excellent source of calcium and vitamin D, two essential nutrients that help build strong bones for mother and baby.

7. **Eat your beans:** I know beans are on the restricted list for the CARBS eating plan, but when you are pregnant beans are allowed, especially if you are vegetarian. They are a good source of protein, fiber, and vitamins, including folate. The FDA does recommend avoiding raw, sprouted beans such as mung bean sprouts due to a higher risk of bacterial contamination. Well-cooked bean sprouts are safe for consumption.

Fish and Omega-3s

Studies have shown that consuming abundant amounts of fish rich in omega-3 fatty acids during pregnancy can improve your child's overall brain function, visual acuity, attention, and behavior. DHA, the most important omega-3 related to fetal brain development, is absorbed into the brain most efficiently during the third trimester and first two years of life. In fact, DHA represents 97 percent of the omega-3 fats in the brain and 93 percent of all omega-3s in the retina. Mothers should boost their DHA intake during the pre- and post-natal periods so that the fetus receives DHA during pregnancy and the baby receives DHA-rich breast milk. A general recommendation is 300 mg of DHA taken daily. An additional advantage of adequate DHA during pregnancy is a lower risk of postpartum depression.

Oily, coldwater fish like salmon are excellent sources of brain-boosting DHA omega-3s. The FDA has set a limit of 12 oz a week for fish due to concerns regarding mercury toxicity from excess consumption. This limit, however, is controversial. Several studies are now showing that the risk of limiting fish intake and its brain-healthy DHA may exceed the potential risks of mercury toxicity.

Consuming any 12-ounce fish won't do. There are better fish than others to eat when it comes to maximizing DHA intake and minimizing mercury contamination. For example, salmon provides over 10 times more DHA than catfish or tilapia does. Choose wild salmon whenever possible; farmed salmon is rife with contaminants. Keep in mind that the majority of Atlantic salmon is farmed. I've listed DHA levels in parentheses per 100 grams of fish consumed:

- Wild salmon (1500 mg)

- Rainbow trout (677 mg)

- White tuna canned in water (629 mg); Light tuna canned in water (223 mg)

- Atlantic sardines, canned in oil (509 mg)

- Atlantic cod (154 mg)

- Shrimp (144 mg)

- Catfish (128 mg)

- Alaskan king crab (118 mg DHA)

- Tilapia (110 mg)

All the data, except for that of tilapia, comes from the USDA website. Limit your intake of big, predatory fish—like shark, swordfish, tilefish, albacore tuna (canned tuna is ok), and raw fish—which have more mercury. The website, www.gotmercury.org, calculates the amount of mercury consumed based on your body weight, the type of fish, and the serving size.

Many of my vegetarian patients eat plenty of plant sources rich in omega-3 ALA, such as leafy greens, flaxseeds, chia seeds, and walnuts. When it comes to your baby's eye and brain health, ALA is safe, but is an ineffective substitute for DHA. It is very inefficiently converted to DHA by the body. There are some studies showing that algal DHA (DHA from algae) may be a more effective vegetarian alternative to boost DHA in babies.

The Organic vs. Conventional Debate

I realize buying organic foods and produce puts a definite strain on the food budget, but if you can make the stretch during pregnancy, it's worth it. A developing fetus is extremely susceptible to all the potential pesticides, contaminants, and hormones present in inorganic foods. Consider the additional money spent going organic as an investment towards a potentially healthier, happier, and even smarter baby. The following foods should be high priority for buying organic during pregnancy.

Meat: Buying grass-fed, organic meat not only ensures fewer contaminants, but also guarantees significantly more brain-boosting omega-3s. This is especially true for fattier meats like beef.

Milk: Milk that is organic and grass-fed has no hormones, pesticides, or contaminants and, like meat, contains greater amounts of omega-3s.

Butter and ghee: Many of the chemicals and hormones you want to avoid are highly concentrated in butter, so choosing organic butter is a smart move, especially during pregnancy. You can make your own ghee out of organic butter, or purchase organic ghee.

Eggs: Eggs with yolk are a pregnancy-healthy food. However, fat-soluble pesticides can seep into the yolk, so try to buy your eggs organic.

Leafy greens: Spinach, kale, and lettuce have greater surface area and so absorb more pesticides. Buy these organic.

Apples: Never buy conventional apples, which are one of the most heavily contaminated fruits. Studies also show a greater amount of healthy antioxidants in organic apples.

Fish: Wild caught fish is preferred over farmed.

The Environmental Working Group's (EWG) annual "Dirty Dozen" list ranks produce with the highest levels of pesticide residue. As mentioned above, apples usually top this list with 98% doused with pesticides. Check out this list, along with the recommended "Clean Fifteen," at www.ewg.org/foodnews. If buying organic meats is too expensive or they are not accessible, then buy the leanest cuts possible. Most pesticides and contaminants hang out in the fat, so trim the fat when you prepare the meat. Buy staple foods you eat on a daily basis organic if possible, since pesticides and contaminants have a larger impact given your frequency of consumption.

Vegetarian vs. Non-vegetarian Considerations

If you have a choice, I absolutely recommend you choose to be non-vegetarian during your pregnancy. Incorporating foods like fish, meat, eggs, and dairy provides both macro and micronutrients, such as B vitamins, vitamin D, omega-3s, choline, and iron, that are essential for an optimal pregnancy. If you are a strict vegetarian for religious or personal reasons, then you still have many options for eating a nutritious, optimal protein diet, in addition to consuming fats and healthy carbohydrates. However, it will be important for you to take supplements to fill some of the nutrient deficiencies in your pregnancy eating plan. If you are unable to gain sufficient weight during your pregnancy, work with your nutritionist to discuss adding healthier, calorie-dense foods to your diet.

Important Pregnancy Supplements

Your goal is to try to get the majority of your key pregnancy nutrients from natural foods, but I realize this can be challenging. Below is a list of supplements that may help bridge some of these gaps. Confirm dosages with your physician since recommendations are constantly being updated. If you have any questions about the safety of a particular supplement or brand, discuss with your doctor.

Folic acid: The general recommendation is to take between 0.4 to 0.8 mg daily of folic acid to prevent neural tube defects. Start supplementing at least one month before and for two to three months after delivery. Since a large percentage of pregnancies are unplanned, it is reasonable to take this dose throughout a woman's childbearing years.

Iron: For women who do not have anemia (low red blood cell counts), the World Health Organization recommends taking 60 mg of iron daily. This appears to be a more optimal dose than the CDC recommended 30 mg per day, especially for reducing the risk of delivering a LBW baby. Many physicians, however, recommend 30 mg of iron based on CDC recommendations, and most prenatal vitamins contain around 30 mg of iron, so supplement accordingly. Adequate iron consumption is especially critical for vegetarians who are susceptible to iron deficiency. I recommend vegetarians screen for anemia with a blood count before they become pregnant.

Calcium: The general daily recommendation for calcium is 1,000 mg daily for pregnant and lactating women 19 to 50 years of age, and 1,300 mg for women between 14 and 18 years of age.

Prenatal vitamins (PNVs): These typically contain a combination of folic acid, iron, and calcium. Your doctor may recommend a specific type. Be sure to add up all your daily nutrient amounts from multivitamins and additional supplements to make sure you are not undershooting or overshooting the recommended doses.

Vitamin D: There is no standard recommendation for vitamin D supplementation during pregnancy. Vitamin D deficiency has been associated with conditions such as gestational diabetes, low birth weight, and preterm labor, but it has not been proven that supplementation reduces these complications. Given that many South Asian women are severely vitamin D deficient, and given the frequency of conditions like LBW babies and gestational diabetes, I recommend screening and treatment to raise vitamin D levels to a normal range. Vitamin D levels are stabilized primarily through sun exposure and secondarily through supplementation, with diet contributing only minimally to your vitamin D requirements.

Vitamin B12: Vegetarians are at high risk for B12 deficiency, especially strict vegetarians who avoid dairy and eggs. The general recommendation is to consume 2.4 micrograms of vitamin B12 daily. I think it is reasonable for vegetarian South Asian women to be screened for B12 deficiency with blood testing. You can be treated with injectable or oral vitamin B-12 depending on your levels.

Omega-3s: It is preferred that you get your omega-3s, especially DHA, from fish. There are no good studies showing that taking a supplement, rather than consuming fish, has significant benefit. If you cannot eat fish, then it is reasonable to take an omega-3 that supplies the daily target of 300 mg of DHA. If you are a strict vegetarian who will not use fish oil capsules, algal DHA supplements may be worth looking into since they are superior to flaxseed and other plant-based DHA sources; there are also studies showing some benefits of this form of DHA in pregnant women.

I strongly recommend discontinuing any herbal or Ayurvedic medications during your pregnancy. Studies have detected unacceptable levels of lead, mercury, arsenic, and in some cases prescription drugs in some Ayurvedic products labeled "Indian" or "South Asian," sold in stores and online. If you feel strongly about taking any of these, discuss the specific product with your doctor. Healthy growth of the fetus is a very delicate process that can be impaired by these potentially toxic substances.

Exercise During Pregnancy

Many South Asian women become excessively sedentary during pregnancy, and family members often encourage extended periods of rest. The worry of having a LBW baby often motivates South Asian mothers to avoid exercise for fear of burning too many calories. This is definitely not the case, unless you are doing highly intense, exhaustion-level exercises almost daily. Pregnancy is a nine-month marathon that can be emotionally and physically exhausting. It is an event you need to get in shape for and stay in shape during! Here are some of the many benefits of being physically fit during pregnancy:

- Aerobic fitness reduces pregnancy-related fatigue and improves mood

- Staying active prevents and treats insulin resistance and gestational diabetes

- Strength and flexibility training (like modified yoga) can reduce pregnancy-related low back pain

- Exercising helps manage stress and improves sleep, which is frequently interrupted during pregnancy

- Physical activity reduces pregnancy-related constipation by keeping bowel movements more regular

- Exercising reduces recovery time after pregnancy and helps you lose that extra baby fat quicker

- Working out may make labor more tolerable

At least 30 minutes of daily moderate level exercise is recommended during pregnancy. Talk to your doctor about any specific activity restrictions your pregnancy may dictate. A high-risk pregnancy may call for more limited activity or, in rare cases, complete bed rest. Most studies show that moderate level exercise does not increase the risk of delivering a LBW baby. In fact, many studies suggest that both mother and baby share the heart healthy benefits of exercise. Babies born to fit mothers tend to have healthier hearts, and, given the rates of heart disease in South Asians, exercise is something every woman should prioritize throughout her pregnancy.

Postpartum Depression (PPD)

The birth of a newborn is often anticipated as the most thrilling and joyful event a mother can experience. There is a flipside, however. Postpartum depression (PPD) is a condition that can cause extreme feelings of sadness after delivery, resulting even in anger and apathy towards the child. Since South Asian women are often expected to internalize and endure domestic hardships, many women suffer silently from PPD. South Asians who migrate to other countries are especially susceptible given that they are often isolated and lonely, trying to adjust to a new culture, with limited support from spouses who work long hours.

The general rates of PPD in American women are 1 in 10, but the incidence in immigrant South Asian women appears to be considerably higher. A 2007 study published by Deepika Goyal in the *Journal of Obstetrics and Gynecology* reported that 28 percent of Indian American women suffered mild symptoms of PPD, and 24 percent suffered major symptoms. Unfortunately, only half of women are properly diagnosed, and the resulting stress can significantly interfere with the mother-child relationship, the relationship with the spouse and other family members, and the overall development of the child.

PPD manifests as the following symptoms:

- Overwhelming feelings of sadness

- Lack of bonding or attachment to the baby

- Extreme impatience, irritability, and anger

- Complete lack of emotion

- Overeating or undereating

- Oversleeping or undersleeping

- Difficulty concentrating

- Significant memory loss

- Physical symptoms (headaches, constant back pain, nausea, upset stomach)

- Thoughts of hurting yourself or that life is not worth living

Husbands, wives, and close family members need to be aware of the symptoms of PPD early on. A prior history of anxiety or depression significantly increases the risk. If you suspect PPD at any point, it is important to seek help from a professional immediately. This is a treatable condition. Family or caretaker support for the baby and related chores can help ease some of the stress while the mother tries to manage her PPD. To prevent and treat PPD, consider the following:

Delegate: Delegate some responsibilities to your spouse and/or family members, especially during the first weeks of pregnancy when the adjustment is most intense. Family members should contribute to baby care to give mothers personal time for exercise and other non-baby activities.

Seek professional help: Connect with a lactation consultant during pregnancy to increase your knowledge and reduce the stress related to infant feeding.

Take your vitamins: Omega-3s may help prevent and manage PPD symptoms, and B-vitamins may help balance your mood.

Exercise daily: Exercise releases mood-enhancing chemicals called endorphins.

Pamper yourself: Massages, even for 15 minutes, can help ease PPD symptoms.

Sunbathe: For sufficient vitamin D, expose large skin surface areas to sunlight during the peak times of day and year depending on your location.

Socialize: Connect with other mothers who share similar challenges. Resist the impulse to completely disconnect from others.

Prioritize sleep: Even short naps throughout the day can be energizing and improve mood. Spouses and family should help mothers set aside adequate time for rest.

Get help: Mother-infant bonding is critical to the baby's healthy emotional and physical development. Do not internalize your feelings. Reach out to family, friends, your medical team, a mental health specialist, or support groups. Postpartum support international (http://postpartum.net/Default.aspx) provides comprehensive online resources and a list of support centers.

A positive mood, nutritious food, and regular physical activity are the cornerstones for a successful pregnancy outcome. South Asian women have several simultaneous issues which may warrant special attention, such as high rates of insulin resistance and gestational diabetes, significant rates of LBW babies, severe vitamin D deficiency, and a vegetarian diet deficient in B vitamins. It is important for South Asian women and their healthcare team to be aware of these issues and implement any necessary early screening tests. Monitor the Metabolic 6-pack for insulin resistance and screen for vitamin deficiencies as early as possible to correct and prevent health issues.

Finally, beware of advice from well-intentioned family members. Opinionated mothers and mother-in-laws may enforce their own rules about avoiding exercise and encouraging the intake of high-sugar, high-carb foods during pregnancy. If any of their advice seems contradictory to what you've learned in this chapter or to what your healthcare professional has told you, don't follow it. Our longstanding tradition of insulin resistance is aligned with many cultural myths and conventions regarding what constitutes a healthy pregnancy. Remember, this is your pregnancy and your future child's health, so make sure you remain in charge.

> *Beware of advice from well-intentioned family members, who may promote poor eating habits or discourage healthy exercise.*

Summary

- South Asian women are at high risk for insulin resistance and heart disease.

- Recognize PCOS early on.

- South Asian women need a primary care doctor and annual physicals and labs, in addition to routine gynecological exams.

- Resistance training can help with fat loss and bone health.

- Maternal health and nutrition during pregnancy influence childhood and adult-onset diseases.

- Gestational diabetes and LBW babies are common in South Asian women.

- Healthy eating, supplements, and exercise improve pregnancy outcomes.

- DHA, an omega-3, is critical for optimal brain and eye development in children.

- Vegetarians must increase protein and healthy fats and consider taking supplements to fill nutrition gaps. If you have a choice, choose to be non-vegetarian during pregnancy.

- Be aware of postpartum depression and seek help if you have symptoms.

For Professionals

- Encourage women to get annual general physical exams. Gynecologists should advise women to establish routine primary care in addition to gynecological care.

- Screen for PCOS early by asking about symptoms.

- Metabolic 6-pack screening should be conducted annually in most women to detect early insulin resistance.

- Have a low threshold for screening for vitamin D, vitamin B12, and overall anemia, especially in vegetarians.

- Encourage resistance training in South Asian women and recommend home-based exercises for those uncomfortable with public gyms.

- Counsel women of childbearing age early on about common pregnancy issues like gestational diabetes, LBW babies, and PPD.

- PPD should be screened for and discussed by multiple providers, including the gynecologist, pediatrician, and primary care doctor. Support resources should be provided.

CHAPTER 10

BUILDING A HEALTHIER FUTURE
FOR THE SOUTH ASIAN CHILD

THE SOUTH ASIAN COMMUNITY must take a family approach, not an individual approach, to living healthier. We are facing a pediatric obesity crisis in America, and the crisis is particularly severe among South Asian children of all socioeconomic levels and in all geographic locations. The scientific evidence is mounting: the way we raise our children today affects their healthy tomorrows. Quite simply, we are rearing unhealthy children who, if they do manage to escape adolescence without any significant health crises, will pay the price as they step into adulthood. It's up to us to monitor the health choices of our young ones and to model appropriate nutrition, exercise, and lifestyle decisions along the way. Even if your kids are grown, I encourage you to read this entire chapter because some day you may be a grandparent, an aunt, or some other family member who plays an important role in the growth of a child at all stages.

I am not a pediatric physician, but my wife, Dr. Shally Sinha, practices in Fremont, California where the vast majority of her patients are of South Asian descent and range in age from newborns to teenagers. She's seen countless cases of obesity, adult onset diabetes (in children!), and high cholesterol. Dr. Shally's pediatric training never covered cholesterol disorders; why should it have? Cholesterol problems don't rear their ugly heads until adulthood! Or so we thought…

Unfortunately, cholesterol issues (and their associated risks) are becoming all too common in our children. So much so that expert groups are currently hard at work establishing guidelines for screening and treating heart disease risk factors in youth. Type 2 diabetes used to be called "adult onset diabetes," but we're now seeing it manifest in kids as early as age 11. The future is not very bright for an 11-year-old with diabetes, no matter how highly he or she ranks academically. The natural course of diabetes predicts a high risk of complications, including eye disease, kidney disease, and high blood pressure as early as the late teens. If you think it's already stressful shuttling your child between school, sports, and other extracurricular activities, be prepared to add regular doctor visits, nutritionist visits, pharmacy visits, etc. to help manage his diabetes. In addition, that dangerous plaque we discussed in Chapter 2 can start forming in childhood, especially in kids who have conditions like pediatric diabetes, high cholesterol, and obesity. A plaque that forms in early childhood is the precursor for a serious event such as a heart attack or stroke in a young adult.

The way we raise our children today affects their healthy tomorrows.

Beyond Dr. Shally's pediatric practice, we are seeing a general trend of South Asians developing diabetes and heart disease about 10 years earlier than other ethnic groups. The root of the crisis lies in the combination of insulin resistant genes, highly sedentary lifestyles, and unhealthy Indian and Western foods. It's not uncommon to hear of a thirty-or forty-something South Asian having a heart attack. What will happen to the new generation of even more sedentary, obese South Asians who are consuming even unhealthier diets? Are they going to develop heart disease in their twenties? By all indications, this seemingly far-fetched scenario is entirely possible, unless we take drastic action immediately.

A SOUTH ASIAN PARENT'S TOP 10 CONCERNS ABOUT HEALTH

Visits to the pediatrician are key in understanding crucial information that can help guide the healthy growth of your child. Let's start with a typical case study.

Case Study: Suneel

Suneel is an eight-year-old boy whom my wife, Dr. Shally, has been following since age three. He was born as a low-birth-weight baby and like most babies his size was overfed early on to help him "catch up" to what his parents deemed a normal percentile range on his growth chart. As a toddler he was a "fussy eater" with no regular feeding times, and preferred drinking milk as his primary source of calories. As he grew older, parents and family members fed Suneel the foods he craved and demanded, such as fast foods, sugary desserts, and crispy snack foods. Even though Suneel ate normal quantities of food on his own (which were appropriate for his size), his family continued to heap on extra meal servings and to supplement with junk foods in order to meet their inflated expectations. They found it much easier to feed him junk foods he enjoyed, than to face the challenge of getting him to eat nutritious meals and snacks. As long as he took in calories and gained weight, they felt he was making healthy progress. As a result, Suneel went from being a low-birth-weight baby to being an overweight eight-year-old with high triglycerides on his cholesterol panel.

Suneel's parents, with list in hand, came to see Dr. Shally for their son's routine checkup. It is a rare occasion that my wife does not see a list pulled out when treating a South Asian child. The topics on these lists seem to be pretty much the same, give or take a few, so she's put together the 10 most common concerns South Asian parents have about their kids' health.

1. *Suneel's too skinny and isn't gaining weight.*

2. *Suneel won't eat any fruits or veggies. He hardly eats and only wants to drink milk.*

3. *Suneel won't eat unless I force feed him or sit him in front of the TV. He doesn't eat anything at school.*

4. *Suneel won't sleep unless we go to sleep with him at the same time. His bedtime is the same as ours.*

5. *Suneel has a hard time waking up in the morning and often ends up skipping breakfast or eating very little.*

6. *Suneel spends hours on the Ipad, watching TV, or playing video games.*

7. *There's no time for Suneel to exercise during the weekdays due to schoolwork, piano practice, and his academic enrichment homework.*

8. *Suneel's too short. What can we do to make Suneel taller?*

9. *Suneel's not eating enough. What kind of supplements should we give him?*

10. *How do I make Suneel smarter?*

We'll use each of these concerns as a trigger to delve deeper into common health issues faced by South Asian kids and teens. Each of these concerns played an active part in Suneel's transformation from an underweight baby to an overweight eight-year-old with a cholesterol disorder that primes him for cardiovascular disease and diabetes.

Growth
1. *"Suneel's too skinny and isn't gaining weight."*

This is a common complaint from South Asian parents, and it is almost always unwarranted. It's important to understand that when a parent treats a child as though he/she were growth deficient it creates emotional stress for both parents and children and leads to inappropriate feeding habits for the child; not to mention the long-term effects it has on a child's relationship to food and the body. Unhealthy dietary habits can escalate into eating disorders such as binge eating, anorexia, and bulimia.

> *The guilt you may temporarily feel when not fulfilling the expectations or heeding the advice of well-intentioned family members pales in comparison to the permanent pain you will feel when watching your obese child develop chronic health issues you could have easily prevented.*

Suneel's family was anxious about his low birth weight and made an aggressive effort to put some meat on his bones. This anxiousness stems from a prevalent misconception among South Asians that having some extra visible body fat (or looking more rotund) speaks of good health and affluence. Extended family members often aggressively perpetuate this myth by making parents feel inadequate if their child appears too "scrawny," when in fact the child may be at an ideal body habitus for preventing chronic disease. When parents leave for work, determined live-in family members may take matters into their own hands by rolling up their sleeves and preparing fattening meals and snacks to quickly increase body weight. Be prepared to confront family members—do what's healthy for your child and not what you think will please your parents or in-laws. The guilt you may temporarily feel when not fulfilling their expectations or heeding their advice pales in comparison to the permanent pain you will feel when watching your obese child develop chronic health issues you could have easily prevented.

Distorted perceptions of what a healthy child looks like are reinforced when parents misinterpret government-published growth curves. In order to alleviate much of this anxiety and hopefully convince you and others to nourish your children appropriately, let's first understand how to correctly interpret growth charts. The two most commonly used growth charts in the US are the CDC (Centers for Disease Control) and the WHO (World Health Organization) curves.

CDC growth charts: These charts from the United States Government's Centers for Disease Control and Prevention (CDC) have been used since 1977 to track the growth of infants, children, and adolescents in the US. The charts show age-appropriate percentile curves representing typical body measurements in mostly Caucasian children who were either formula or breastfed.

WHO growth charts: Data from the World Health Organization (WHO) was derived from a more racially diverse population than was data from the CDC. The WHO looked at the growth and development of 8500 infants and children in Brazil, Ghana, India, Norway, Oman, and the US between 1997 and 2003. The goal was to establish a single international standard, representing children worldwide who were mostly breastfed for at least 4 months, and still breastfeeding at 12 months, under normal environmental conditions.

Currently, US guidelines recommend pediatricians use the WHO curve for ages 0-2 years, and the CDC curve for ages 2-18 yrs. The reason is that breastfeeding, reflected by the WHO curves, is the recommended standard for feeding up to age one. The WHO curve is also based on a higher quality study designed to track normal physiologic infant growth. The CDC charts are based on smaller sample sizes for the first six months of life, with no weight data between birth and three months. The CDC charts reflect how children in the US *did* grow during a specific time period, which is not necessarily indicative of ideal growth. As a result, the CDC charts are inferior to the WHO charts for children under age two and do not serve as ideal benchmarks for growth. The WHO growth charts set standards and show how children *should* grow under optimal conditions. Despite being less accurate under age two, the CDC growth charts are used for children two years and up since they use similar methods as the WHO curves.

Reading and accurately interpreting these curves is a challenge in and of itself. There are separate charts for weight, height, and body mass index (BMI), which are plotted on the vertical axis, while age is plotted on the horizontal axis. Boys and girls have separate charts for each of these measures. The growth curve is a distribution of measurements on a bell curve that shows several different percentiles (5th, 10th, 25th, 50th, 75th, 90th, 95th), with most children clustering around the middle of the curve. For instance, if a child has an average weight or height for his age, he will have a point on the 50th percentile curve of the corresponding weight or height chart.

Keep in mind that these are not academic curves to be met with the goal of achieving the highest percentile possible. Many parents don't understand this concept and worry if their child is not plotting on the 90-95th percentile for height and/or weight. If your child plots at the 95th percentile for weight on the weight chart, that means he is heavier than 95 percent of children his age. Some South Asians may rejoice at this number since they think this means he is well fed, while others may panic that their child is too heavy. Neither interpretation is accurate. Looking at a single percentile number at any given time provides no useful information. You need to look at your child's personal growth trend over time. A child's growth pattern is the result of many complex factors working together simultaneously, such as genetics, gender, hormones, nutrition, and physical activity. As long as your child is growing in a consistent pattern and following a trajectory on any of the percentiles, he or she is doing fine.

To illustrate a real world example, let's refer to the WHO weight chart below for boys, from birth to two years of age. The age is plotted on the horizontal axis and weight on the vertical axis. Whether a child grows consistently along the 15th percentile curve (2nd curve from the bottom) or along the 50th percentile curve (middle curve), he is developing normally. One percentile is not superior to the other. If a child drops percentiles or climbs percentiles too quickly, it may signal that the child is either underfed or overfed. In order to assess whether a jump in percentiles is indeed cause for alarm, you'd need to analyze your child's BMI and length curves.

Weight-for-age BOYS
Birth to 2 years (percentiles)

World Health Organization

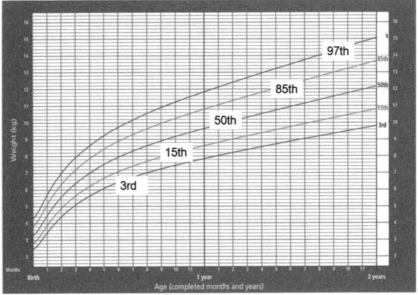

WHO Child Growth Standards

Genetic predisposition has a lot of influence on whether your child plots below or above average, especially for height. Dr. Shally commonly sees South Asian babies plotting at a lower percentile for weight compared to height. Let's return to Suneel to illustrate this point. As an infant, Suneel plotted at the 20th percentile for weight and 70th percentile for height. Pushing Suneel to the highest percentile for weight may mean he's gaining weight too fast, propelling him closer to obesity, diabetes, and heart disease later in life due to accelerated weight gain as a child. Unfortunately, this is exactly what Suneel's family did. They panicked at his low-infant-weight percentiles and were determined to get him abruptly to a higher percentile.

Pushing Suneel to the highest percentile for weight may mean he's gaining weight too fast, propelling him closer to obesity, diabetes, and heart disease later in life due to accelerated weight gain as a child.

By the time Dr. Shally saw Suneel for his eight-year-old checkup, his weight was 73 pounds, which put him at the 90th percentile on the weight chart, while his height was 50 inches, which put him at the 44th percentile on the height chart. The BMI curve, based on his height and weight, was abnormal. Recall from Chapter 3 that BMI= weight (kg)/ height^2.

The BMI curve reflects the calculations by age and is shown as a bell curve with percentiles. The range is as follows:

<u>Underweight:</u>   5th percentile or lower
<u>Normal:</u>   Between the 10th and 85th percentile
<u>Overweight:</u>   Between the 85th and 95th percentile
<u>Obese:</u>   95th percentile or over

Suneel's BMI was 20.6, which put him at the 94th percentile. He went from being what his parents and family thought was an underweight baby to a borderline obese eight year old. His growth results at age eight are summarized below:

Suneel at Age 8	Results	Percentiles on Growth Chart
Height	50 inches	44th percentile
Weight	73 pounds	90th percentile
BMI	20.6	94th percentile

The BMI chart below illustrates how Suneel has landed just below the top curve, representing the 95th percentile cutoff for obesity.

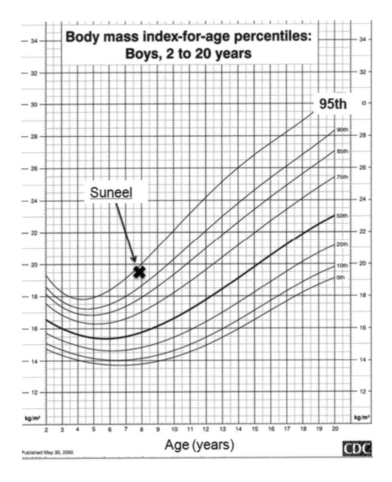

Body mass index-for-age percentiles:
Boys, 2 to 20 years

95th

Suneel

Age (years)

Published May 30, 2000.

CDC

What if Suneel's weight percentile started at the 25th, but then dropped with each visit...from the 25th to the 10th and then to the 5th percentile? That's a red flag that he's not gaining sufficient weight, and your pediatrician would then assess if this decrease were due to low caloric intake or some other medical problem.

Another way to gauge your child's growth is to look at the growth trends children usually follow at various stages of development. These may vary if your baby was born premature or with a very low birth weight. The growth trends are listed on the next page.

Weight Trends:

AGE	EXPECTED WEIGHT GAIN
2 weeks old	Regain birth weight, then gain 1.5 to 2 pounds per month
3 months old	Gain 1 pound per month
1 year old	Triple birth weight
1-6 years old	Gain 4-5 pounds per year
6-10 years old	Gain 5-7 pounds per year

Depending on when puberty starts, girls can gain a total of 15 pounds during their peak growth spurt (usually ages 11-13) and boys can gain a total of 30 pounds (usually ages 13-15).[1]

Height Trends:

AGE	HEIGHT
0-12 months age	10 inches gain
1-2 years age	4-5 inches gain
2-6 years age	2-2.5 inches per year
6-10 years age	2-3 inches per year

Notice from the table above how the initial rapid growth in the first year of life slows down in subsequent years. This is reflected on the growth curves by the steep slope in the first year and the shallower slope during childhood. Many parents get anxious when they see their toddler not growing as fast as he did during infancy. Please note that between ages one and two, only a four to five pound weight gain is expected.

Additional growth spurts occur in puberty, which occurs between ages 8 and 14 for girls and 9 and 14 for boys. Adult height is attained four to five years after the peak growth spurt.

Recall that Suneel plotted along the 25th percentile on the weight chart as an infant. This was his normal, genetically pre-programmed weight range. As he aged, we would have expected some fluctuations according to normal nutritional intake, but overzealous feeding led to an abrupt jump in percentiles, landing him in the overweight category based on BMI. The metabolic consequence of these unnatural shifts is that he is now programmed for insulin resistance and all its complications (obesity, diabetes, heart disease, etc.) later in life, unless his parents intervene and reverse this early damage. There is, of course, always room for exceptions. Some babies who are undernourished during pregnancy will be born at a low birth weight and may need to cross percentiles for catch-up growth. Interpreting growth curves throughout a child's life is a complex process, and you'll need to work closely with your pediatrician to determine the healthiest course.

Summary of age-appropriate growth:

- Treating a child as though he/she were growth deficient is emotionally stressful for everyone.

- The misconception that your child is too skinny may be fueled by a misinterpretation of government published growth curves, reinforced by incorrect cultural perceptions of a healthy body weight.

- Doctors usually use the WHO curve for children less than 2 years of age and the CDC curve for kids ages 2-18.

- Don't expect your child to be in the 90-95th percentile for height, weight, or BMI. She can be on any percentile trajectory as long as the percentiles for each category are within the same range.

- If your child's weight drastically jumps percentiles, it's a sign he is gaining too much weight too fast and may be headed for obesity, diabetes, and heart disease.

- If your child's weight consistently jumps down percentiles, then there's cause for concern that he might be losing too much weight.

- You can gauge your child's growth by analyzing documented growth trends for weight and height, but due to multiple complex variables, you'll need to work with your pediatrician in interpreting these values.

Nutrition and Feeding Behavior

2. *"Suneel won't eat any fruits or veggies. He hardly eats and only wants to drink milk."*

3. *"Suneel won't eat unless I force feed him or sit him in front of the TV. He doesn't eat anything at school."*

Suneel is the child. It is his parent's responsibility to make sure he is eating a nutritious diet. How can a child who has absolutely no knowledge of nutrition and health and who naturally acts through impulse rather than reason be expected to choose to eat fruits and veggies? Even grown, rational adults have a hard time sticking to good eating habits. Just like you control his bedtime (hopefully!) and monitor the programs he watches on TV, you also need to influence and enforce his eating choices. It can be challenging to work with our finicky little ones. Here are some clever tricks to get kids to eat veggies and fruits:

Mix them into the foods they love already. For example, add assorted vegetables to their favorite pasta dishes, or top off their pizzas with vegetables rather than just meat or cheese. Set rules/negotiate: "You can't eat pizza unless you eat the veggie toppings." If they only like cheese pizza, then they must eat a small salad before, or eat the toppings separately. Don't give in to pressure and manipulation...you are the boss of what your kids eat!

Blend them into lentils, sauces, curries, soups, and smoothies. If you don't have one already, invest in a high-powered blender or food processor. Blending your own soups, smoothies, sauces, and baby foods is an excellent way to provide extra servings of vegetables and fruits. Our kids love making fresh smoothies after school or on the weekends. We'll leave a variety of fruits and vegetables out and they chop, load, push the buttons, and pour.

Dip them into dips and spreads such as hummus, guacamole, or nut butters (peanut, almond butter). Tasty spreads and dips make raw vegetables more appetizing for kids.

Combine them into different shapes and colors. Baby carrots, mini-peppers, edamame, cherry tomatoes, sugar snap peas—kids love variety and color!

Train them by not giving in to a pouty "no." Babies need to be offered a food at least 10 to 15 times before it belongs in the rejection pile. Your influence over your child's taste buds is greatest early on so don't wait to introduce a wide variety of vegetables, fruits, and other healthy foods to his/her developing palate. Veggies should be introduced between four and six months of age. Once they've taken in a variety of vegetables, introduce their palates to fruit. Children should also be repeatedly reintroduced to healthy foods cooked in a variety of ways. Shaking up your preparation methods increases the probability that your kids will accept the nutritious goodies you're offering.

Involve them in the process of preparing and serving vegetables and fruits, and you increase the odds they will eat them. Give them a cutting board and a kid-safe knife and have them cut their own salad, or they can mix their own blend of pre-packaged fresh vegetables. Have them grow their own vegetables in the family vegetable garden. Let them create their own smoothies and soups. Make it a game and ask them to give their creations names, such as "Suneel's Super Smoothie!"

Present them as artistic creations just waiting to be gobbled up. Dinosaur chicken nuggets surrounded by broccoli floret trees and fruit skewers…or fruits and vegetables carved into fun shapes. Don't worry if you're not a natural culinary artist. Even presenting foods in separate compartments in a lunch container, such as a bento box, makes eating far more appealing.

Remember, don't give up or give in to your child's demands for quick, easy non-nutritious foods. It's your job to help them develop their tastes for healthy foods, which will benefit them throughout their life.

An important rule of thumb to apply is that kids decide *how much* they eat, while parents decide *what* they eat. If a child says they're full or shows signs they're full, you stop the feed. If a child refuses to eat the healthy snack or meal you prepared for them and insists on eating junk, they don't get fed. You must remain in control of their food choices since young kids usually lack the maturity and knowledge to know which foods will help their bodies grow and develop in a healthy fashion. Too often parents complain that "my child only wants to eat pizza" or some unhealthy fast food option. This is a sign that your child has assumed control of what he or she eats, which is only acceptable if your child makes healthy food choices.

Now that we've got the basics covered, let's discuss some age-specific recommendations that focus on feeding behavior and nutrition essentials for toddlers, school-aged kids, and teenagers.

Toddlers (ages 1-3): Inappropriate feeding behavior is a common predicament for South Asian kids. Toddlers lack set feeding times, and eat at 1 pm one day and 3 pm the next with dinner anytime between 7 and 9 pm. Not only that, parents often feel their child isn't eating enough at these meals, and try to compensate with unhealthy, unsatisfying, and nutrient-devoid snacks throughout the day. Beware of crispy Indian snacks, cookies, plain chapati, and other carbohydrate-loaded and insulin-spiking foods. Toddlers quickly develop an affinity for these types of foods over healthier options.

Many toddlers dislike feeding time and prefer to just drink milk to satisfy hunger. Parents often succumb to this pressure since milk is a quick and easy source of calories, and giving in to a toddler's demands avoids confrontation. This isn't a healthful tactic, however, as kids ages one to three only require 16 ounces of milk per day and no nighttime feeds. Replacing precious, nutritious snacks with extra portions of milk deprives them of the opportunity to eat other forms of protein, in addition to healthy fats, fruits, and vegetables. Heavy milk consumption commonly results in constipation due to a lack of dietary fiber, and iron deficiency due to a lack of iron-rich foods in the diet.

The first step in establishing good feeding habits is to set consistent feeding times for breakfast, mid-morning snack, lunch, mid-afternoon snack, and dinner. Sit your toddler down in a booster seat or high chair and do not allow him to roam around while eating. The goal is to get him to self-feed as much as possible. Don't offer any milk, juice, or snacks in between scheduled feeding times. If they're thirsty, give them water, and let your toddler feel hungry for the next feed. Developing an early awareness of hunger and satiety (fullness) cues your toddler to feed based on natural impulses and prevents mindless overeating later in life. Toddlers eat every two to three hours, and they only eat very small portions at a time. A meal can be just four to five tablespoons (composed of 1-2 tablespoons of a whole grain, 1-2 table-spoons of a protein source, and 1-2 tablespoons of a fruit or vegetable). These blends can be made with healthy fats such as olive oil, coconut oil, coconut milk, ghee, and butter (preferably organic, grass-fed).

To help reinforce the feeding schedule, make sure meals and snacks don't last more than 20 minutes. If your toddler refuses to eat what you have put out or begins to throw the food down, end the feed right then. Do not force feed. Once your toddler averts his head from the spoon or stops eating on his own, the meal is over. Eating should be a pleasant experience. Don't turn meals into power struggles between toddler and parent by trying to sneak in some extra bites of food using force or tricks. Even when your child rejects his food, avoid feeding anything until the next scheduled feeding time. If your toddler rejects two to three meals in a row or eats very little, don't succumb—stick to this plan for a few days to allow him time to adjust. During this time, he will need to stay hydrated with fluids, which can be monitored by making sure he continues to produce the usual wet diapers. He will be okay if he doesn't eat many solids for a few days.

Another common habit is to feed kids in front of the TV. Avoid using TV as a distraction that allows you to sneak food into your toddler's mouth. Such a habit prevents toddlers from learning to self-regulate and often results in overfeeding. Children become con-ditioned to eat beyond fullness, ignoring their satiety signals. Such behavior eventually leads to overeating and excess weight gain. Let your child self-feed until he or she feels full, not until you feel satis-fied that he's eaten enough.

Let's summarize these principles:

- Schedule feeding times and stick to them.

- Encourage toddlers to sit and self-feed. Don't chase kids with spoons and bite-sized chapati pieces!

- Set limits—20 minutes and the meal or snack is over regardless of how much food has been eaten.

- Don't force feed. Feeding time should be pleasant, not a battle between parent and toddler.

- Avoid TV and other digital distractions during feeds.

Elementary school-aged kids: Elementary school-aged kids also eat irregularly. They are often rushed off to school in the morning with no or very little breakfast. Lunch typically consists of either unhealthy cafeteria options or an unbalanced serving of excess carbohydrates, processed quick foods, and sugar. For example, a typical Indian packed lunch may consist of just a chapati, rice, and vegetable curry. Kids often return home famished since a lunch like this provides virtually no protein or healthy fats. They are then loaded up with high-sugar snacks followed by a dinner that is usually their best, and only, complete meal of the day.

How can kids sustain adequate focus and attention during long school days if their brains are not supplied with healthy, consistent fuel sources? It is imperative that children start the day off right with a healthy, unhurried breakfast made up of an appropriate balance of protein, healthy carbohydrates, and fat. A quick bowl of sugary cereal or a waffle is not acceptable. A carbohydrate-dominant breakfast deprives children of the healthy protein, fat, and nutrients necessary to fuel their brains and muscles throughout a day of learning and play. Instead, try options like eggs (as an omelet or scrambled with veggies and cheese), fruits with nut butter (apple with almond butter spread), and low-fat or full-fat Greek yogurt. Avoid juices and other concentrated sources of sugar. Offer fruit servings in raw form to maximize fiber and nutrient intake and minimize sugar overload.

I realize school cafeteria lunches are convenient for busy parents, but really scrutinize the monthly menu and try to pack healthy home lunches on days when the school offering is unhealthy. Keep in mind that many younger school-aged kids do not eat much while at school. They may be too distracted by friends and classmates, leaving little time to eat lunch. Don't worry. Just make sure you provide a good breakfast in the morning, and give a meal or heavy snack right after school.

Older school-aged kids who have money and access to vending machines on campus may fill up on junk foods like candy, cookies, and crispy snacks. The simplest solution is to not provide any money for access to unhealthy vending machine foods and to instead pack healthy snacks as their only option. If you have latchkey children who come home from school to no parents, be sure your fridge and pantry shelves have healthy options only so they don't gorge on junk foods. A nutritive-stocked pantry will benefit all family members, young and old.

One way to get kids to eat healthier is to educate them about nutrition and have them participate with mealtime preparation. This could be as simple as setting the table or cutting veggies for a salad with a kid-safe knife. Meal preparation should be a family responsibility, not just one parent's. In addition, aim for at least four dinners per week when the entire family sits at a table and eats together. Putting into practice regular family meals has not only been associated with decreased obesity, but has also been shown to promote family bonding and better communication between children, teens, and parents.

In an attempt to "fatten the child up," grandparents who live at home can thwart your efforts to maximize your children's nutrition and health by feeding them extra sweets, junk foods, and empty carbs. This can completely disrupt the child's eating schedule and push them towards obesity and a higher risk of chronic health conditions like diabetes. It's a common cultural misconception that chubby kids are healthier kids. Relatives expect the child to keep their cute baby fat even as toddlers and preschoolers. As long as your child is gaining weight adequately from year to year, he is growing on target and is healthy, no matter how skinny he looks to you. Remember that the BMI curve naturally dips between the ages of two and five. I realize it's hard for many parents to let go of their child's baby fat, but do understand that kids are not meant to be chubby during the toddler/preschool years and beyond.

To summarize:

- Don't let your child skip or skimp on breakfast.

- Pack a healthy lunch, especially on days when the cafeteria options are unhealthy (this might be every day!).

- Substitute fruit juices with fresh fruit.

- Have children participate with meal prep.

- Aim for at least four family dinners per week.

- Be aware of what other family members are feeding your kids. Take charge of what your child eats and put your foot down!

Teens: Most of the nutrition principles discussed so far apply to teens as well. Teenagers are susceptible to irregular eating patterns and poor food choices due to late bedtimes and early school hours. They are sent off to learn with no breakfast (or a high-sugar breakfast) and limited fuel, which is further drained by the consumption of excessive fast food meals and junk food. Teens need to eat meals and snacks that are a proper balance of healthy fiber, protein, and fat just as younger kids do.

Teens, however, need to be particularly vigilant about moderating their intake of high-calorie, sugar-sweetened beverages. According to Dr. Harold Goldstein, executive director of the California Center for Public Health Advocacy in Davis, CA, sweetened beverages are considered one of the primary factors in accelerated childhood obesity rates in recent decades. Today's average teenage boy (and we are talking across the globe, not just in America) consumes over a quart of sugar-sweetened beverages daily. A typical 12-ounce can of a sugar-sweetened beverage contains 10-12 teaspoons of sugar. Sugar-sweetened beverages include sodas, juices, sports drinks, iced teas, and iced coffee drinks. The metabolic consequences are dire and the link between these beverages and conditions like obesity and diabetes has been repeatedly confirmed. Do not keep these beverages in your house. More important, act as a role model and do not consume any of these beverages. Also remember that your neighborhood coffee house, a common congregation hub for teens, serves up all types of sugar-sweetened, caffeinated beverages, contributing as much to teenage obesity as nearby fast food restaurants do.

The other side effect of excess sugary beverage intake is the overconsumption of caffeine. Sodas, energy drinks, iced tea, and coffee beverages are the major caffeine culprits. Consuming over 100 mg per day of caffeine is associated with symptoms like heart palpitations, high blood pressure, anxiety, headaches, and disrupted sleep. Caffeine may seem to provide an academic advantage by allowing teens to stay up later to cram in more schoolwork, however, the benefits are overshadowed by sleep disturbances and attention and focus problems due to hyperactivity and severe fatigue from caffeine withdrawal crashes.

What are some healthier beverage options for teens and their families? Water reigns supreme as the beverage of choice. You can also create your own flavored waters (aka "spa water") by filling a pitcher of water and adding citrus wedges, crushed mint and herbs, ginger, etc. If you miss the sensation of carbonation, use sparkling water. If you want a sweeter taste, blend ice, sparkling water, a handful of berries, and some mint for a refreshing, naturally sweetened beverage.

Apart from sweetened beverages, the intake of fast foods and junk foods continues to escalate in teenagers. From the vending machines at school to the mini-market and chain fast food restaurants, teens are the target of most unhealthy foods because teens tend to make more impulsive food choices. Even popular coffee house chains where teens meet for study groups and social gatherings offer up plenty of sugar-laden pastries, muffins, and cookies to accompany their signature sugar-sweetened, caffeinated beverages. It is essential to instill healthy eating habits in children from the earliest age possible, so that they make the healthy choice when you are no longer there to make it for them. Instilling healthy habits early on helps to avoid the inevitable confrontations parents face when trying to convince a teenager with a long history of poor eating habits to abruptly start eating healthier foods.

If you are struggling to convince your teen to make healthier food choices, try to play a role in preparing, or even better, having them prepare as many meals and snacks at home as possible. Most teens should at least be eating their breakfast and dinner at home, and getting teens to prepare their own school lunch ensures that most of their meals are homemade. When teens play an active role with food preparation, they are more likely to enjoy eating healthy. Have them join you on trips to the grocery store or local farmer's market and teach them the essential lifelong skill of cooking as early as possible. Remember, your teenager will be in complete control of their food choices when they ship off to college (and be tempted to gain that notorious freshmen 15+ lbs), so you want to make sure they have a solid foundation of healthy nutrition and eating habits to take with them. This is more valuable than anything they can learn in school. Finally, make an effort to have the family sit together for meals as often as possible. Results from a Canadian study of over 26,000 adolescents ages 11 to 15 showed that each additional family dinner during the week led to fewer emotional and behavioral problems and greater emotional well-being and life satisfaction, regardless of gender, age, or family economics.[2]

Specific tips for teens:

- Moderate, or ideally eliminate, all liquid sugar sources (sodas, juices, energy drinks, designer coffee drinks, etc.).

- Limit caffeine intake (coffee, tea, energy drinks, sodas, etc).

- Moderate or eliminate consumption of junk foods and fast foods. Forbid junk food inside the home!

- Teach teens to cook and involve them in meal preparations.

- Eat together as a family as often as you can.

Sleep

4. *"Suneel won't sleep unless we go to sleep with him at the same time. His bedtime is the same as ours."*
5. *"Suneel has a hard time waking up in the morning and often ends up skipping breakfast or eating very little."*

South Asian children typically have very late bedtimes. Researcher Jodi Mindell conducted a study of over 28,000 infants and toddlers from around the world; results showed that Indian and Asian kids slept significantly fewer hours than their Caucasian counterparts.[3] Common reasons cited included late dinners (8-9 pm), overworked parents who come home late and keep their children up in order to spend time with them, and extra academic work assigned by parents. Sacrificing your child's sleep for the sake of extra academic knowledge harms, rather than helps not only their health, but also their ability to learn. Keeping your kids up later to get their homework done means they will be less able to pay attention to and absorb information the following day during school.

Late bedtimes translate to difficulty waking up and remaining alert at school, and skipped or inadequate breakfasts certainly contribute to focusing difficulties. The child starts the day both tired and hungry, leading to poor attention span, irritability, and restlessness during school hours. Adults know what it feels like to be sleep deprived. Our mood changes, we are less energetic, less productive, and unhappy. These effects are even more pronounced in children whose growing bodies and developing brains depend on sufficient rest. Kids, unlike adults, don't have the emotional maturity to suppress feelings of exhaustion and fatigue, so they instead become irritable, have tantrums, and act defiant.

Many parents claim that their kids start homework later because they come home tired and need to take a nap first. You can break this cycle by encouraging an earlier bedtime. Lack of sleep is not a situation to be taken lightly. Sleep is not only essential for proper emotional and brain function, but is also essential for growth. Avoid overscheduling and prioritize your child's activities to allow for an earlier bedtime. Keep bedtime and wake times as consistent as possible on weekdays and weekends. If your child or teen likes to sleep in on weekends, let them do so, as their bodies may be craving much-needed rest and recovery from the long school week. However, excessive sleep on weekends is a likely sign that your child is not getting enough sleep during the week.

In order to establish healthful sleep patterns sign up for social events and activities that protect your child's sleep time. Make sleep a priority, especially on Sundays and school nights so that they have proper rest for the school day. For example, plan Sunday morning hikes or other outdoor activities. Plan a lunch get together rather than the more common dinner event which often extends into late nights and prolonged bedtimes.

Consistency is key, so be strict about enforcing bedtime. Bedtimes should be set based on the required hours of sleep and optimal wake-up time. Elementary school and middle school-aged kids need about 10 to 11 hours of sleep, while teens require at least 9 hours of sleep. So if Suneel, an eight year old, needs to wake up at 7 am to allow enough time for a healthy breakfast before school, he should be going to bed between 8 and 9 pm to ensure the essential 10-11 hours of sleep. You'll know based on his level of tiredness whether 8 pm or 9 pm is best. Unfortunately, it's not uncommon for South Asian kids like Suneel to go to bed between 10 and 11 pm, short-changing their sleep time significantly.

Don't give in to pleas for a half hour more of TV watching or video game playing. Speaking of which, stimulating activities such as watching TV, playing video games, or chatting with friends on the computer should be avoided at least two hours before bedtime. Likewise, tone down the artificial light in the home once evening commences (this includes bright lights from a computer screen). Use study lamps for bedtime reading. Soft lighting allows your child to wind down by increasing the body's release of the sleep-inducing hormone melatonin.

Replace your child's TV and computer time with a relaxing bedtime ritual, such as a shower or bath followed by a bedtime story read by a parent or older sibling. These will evolve into healthful habits as your child grows older. A relaxing bath and some light reading in bed will help sleep come easily for your child as an adolescent, teen, and adult.

Many parents of young children make the mistake of overstaying their welcome. Say goodnight to your child and leave the bedroom, avoiding the temptation, or request of your child, to stay until she has fallen asleep. This is a natural, and important, part of the weaning process. You don't want your child to depend on your presence in order to fall asleep. There will be many nights in the future when you will be unable to be at her bedside, and you need to prepare her for these circumstances by teaching her to sleep independently. This includes escorting your child back to her room when she comes to your bedroom in the middle of the night. Reassure her if she's had a nightmare and is scared, or if she's convinced a monster is underneath the bed, but don't allow her to curl into bed with you. If you're having a particularly difficult time getting your child to master sleep, consider implementing a reward system. Positive reinforcement can come in the form of praise, or as a token reward system for the nights your child stays in bed without any interruptions.

Summary of sleep guidelines:

- Staying up late hinders your child's ability to learn and adversely affects their health.

- Insufficient rest can lead to irritability, tantrums, defiance, and attention problems.

- Enforce an earlier bedtime and keep bedtime consistent.

- Don't overbook your kids with activities. Prioritize their sleep!

- Elementary/middle school-aged kids need approximately 11 hours of sleep, while teens require at least 9 hours of shuteye.

- Avoid digital activities at least two hours before bed.

- Implement relaxing bedtime rituals.

- Darken the lights once evening falls.

- Don't stay with your child until he has fallen asleep. Encourage independence.

- Don't allow your child to sleep in your bed, no matter how scary the nightmare.

- Promote good sleep habits with positive reinforcement.

Digital Parenting

6. *"Suneel spends hours on the Ipad, watching TV, or playing video games."*

Screen time has become a significant issue for children and parents. Parents are becoming increasingly reliant on an extended family of digital devices to help raise their kids. When a child misbehaves, many parents simply hand their child a smartphone or tablet so they can watch a cartoon or play a video game, rather than explaining why the behavior is inappropriate. It's an easy way to transmute squeals and tears into laughter, but it's ineffective in the long run.

> *Parents are becoming increasingly reliant on an extended family of digital devices to help raise their kids.*

Distracted moms and dads routinely answer questions and converse with their kids from the side, without eye contact, while answering e-mails and texts. Face-to-face conversations and interactions, and intimate parent-child relationships are being gradually diluted by our obsession with digital devices. New mothers are now trending toward using devices while nursing, disrupting one of the most intimate human connections.

What are the consequences of digital parenting? Research now shows that infants and toddlers need direct interaction with parents and other caretakers for healthy brain growth and proper language development.[4] Handing your child a smartphone or tablet with an educational app is not a replacement for direct parent-child inter-action and learning. In fact, that educational app or game may be backfiring since screen time may be linked to behavioral problems in children. A study published in the journal *Pediatrics* suggests a significant association between early exposure to television and sub-sequent attention-related problems.[5] Based on this correlation, con-sider setting the following house rules.

Rule #1: Limit total screen time: Total screen time includes time spent in front of a computer, television, tablet, smartphone, or simi-lar electronic device. Screen time should be no more than two hours a day for children over the age of two. Children under two years old should not be subjected to any screen time. According to the afore-mentioned study, children are most susceptible to screen-related attention problems in the early years of development. Track screen time with a timer, app, or other computer software program. Avoid estimating time, as both kids and parents usually don't realize how much total daily time is spent with a digital companion.

Rule #2: Enjoy a digitally-free dinner: Turn off all devices and screens at dinner and allow for conversation between family mem-bers. Don't underestimate the beneficial effects of family dinners, such as a lower risk of obesity, a lower risk of teenage smoking and alcohol abuse, better school grades, and improved communication between parents and kids.

Rule #3: Keep electronics out of the bedroom: Do not keep a computer or TV in the child's bedroom. A permanent desktop in a bedroom is an ongoing invitation to spend more time on the com-puter. Instead, keep it in a room where other family members come and go often so you can track online time and monitor content. For older children who need computers for schoolwork, opt for a laptop instead so you have better control over digital-free time.

It's imperative that parents take an active role in monitoring the content of the TV programs, video games, and Internet surfing their child is exposed to. Passwords can be set for streaming entertainment. Even with parental controls in place, it's easy for a child to stumble upon inappropriate materials. Two hours of fast-paced, highly stimulating, potentially inappropriate content can cause adverse behavior changes, whereas age-appropriate content will help stimulate fitting behavioral changes. For example, exposure to media violence has been associated with more aggressive behavior in certain susceptible kids and teens.

> *Recovery time improves behavior and facilitates learning. If your computer and digital devices need to hibernate and recharge, so do your kids.*

Rule #4: Stimulate your child with non-digital hobbies: Be sure to provide your child with enough non-digital hobbies, such as outdoor/indoor play consisting of athletic activities, art or science projects, music, reading, and essential down time. That's right, daydreaming and idle time foster a strong sense of creativity and imagination. Habitually sticking your child in front of a screen leads to idle minds, because the device provides the imagination and content! An imaginative child grows into an innovative, successful adult. Idle time also gives your child's brain a chance to rest and recover. Recovery time improves behavior and facilitates learning. If your computer and digital devices need to hibernate and recharge, so do your kids.

Take a minimalist approach when entertaining your kids. A backyard, a ball, and a stick can provide plenty of entertainment when kids are left to their own devices. Don't give in to their initial whining and complaining. In other words, don't let your own shortened attention span as a parent perpetuate the same problem in your child by immediately handing him a digital device. This may curtail the whining, but it also silences imagination and spontaneous creativity. Give your child a chance to explore the wild outside, and they will surprise you and themselves with the many games and activities they creatively concoct.

Rule #5: Monitor your own online addiction: Parents who suffer from their own form of online addiction are often the ones who don't participate in or create non-digital activities for their children. If you're inundated with work that requires you to be on the computer, handing a child a screen is sometimes the easiest way to stay on track and get your job done. This is fine to do every now and again as long as it's not exceeding your child's daily screen time quota. If you can't pull yourself away, take your laptop outdoors into the backyard or a local park so that your child can play and burn off some energy. Another option is to take your child to the local library so they can read or explore while you get some work done. If you continue to struggle and your finances allow for it, perhaps it is a good idea to hire an afternoon babysitter a few times a week to keep your kids outdoors and physically active while you take care of your work and daily errands.

Summary of digital parenting tips:

- Set strict screen time limits. Two hours per day maximum!

- Screen-free mealtimes.

- Screen-free bedrooms.

- Monitor content carefully and use passwords for streaming entertainment.

- Facilitate non-digital hobbies.

- Minimalist entertainment policy: turn them loose in the backyard!

Activity and Exercise

7. *"There's no time for Suneel to exercise during the weekdays due to schoolwork, piano practice, and his academic enrichment homework."*

Childhood should be synonymous with generous amounts of activity and play, indoors and outdoors, but unfortunately sedentary behavior is a modern day misfortune. Play is an essential part of growth that is now being short-changed. Many South Asian parents seem to be in a hurry to accelerate young kids into advanced academics and more mature behavior. Play is often viewed as a waste of productive time, and most forms of physical play have now been replaced by sedentary video games played on TV screens and portable devices. Some parents have the misperception that digital play is somehow superior to physical play in terms of intellectual stimulation and strategy building. As a consequence of this sedentary behavior, children are putting on extra weight and even developing vitamin D deficiency from limited sunlight exposure.

A study conducted by the British Heart Foundation showed that British South Asian kids were the least active of all ethnic groups.[6] Intense academic pressure and role modeling after inactive family members who don't exercise were cited as common reasons for childhood sedentary behavior. Recall from Chapter 1 that studies done in Canada and the UK showed South Asians to be the least active of all ethnic groups. British researchers took this one step further and measured heart rate variability (HRV) in South Asian kids between seven to nine years of age and compared the results to age-matched white European kids.[7] (Low HRV indicates a higher risk for future heart disease.) This study found that South Asian kids had lower HRV; as early as seven years of age they exhibited signs of aerobic deconditioning and greater cardiovascular risk!

How can you incorporate more activity into your child's life? The trick is to discover what makes your child tick. Encourage participation in activities she enjoys, rather than forcing her to perform in a sport she doesn't like. Perhaps you were a former soccer star who has envisioned passing on your fancy footwork to your child, or perhaps you wish to live vicariously through their tremendous athletic accomplishments, imagining a room full of trophies and medals. Unfortunately, these fantasies usually don't come true, and if your child repeatedly rejects a chosen sport, you need to get creative and find an activity *she* enjoys rather than one *you* enjoy. Otherwise your child may develop low confidence and a negative association with all forms of sports and physical activities. If organized team sports are not working, transition to individual sports (tennis, golf, gymnastics, dance, martial arts, etc.) or more unstructured activities (biking, climbing, running, skateboarding, etc.). Check your local community college class list for great ideas. Our kids, who are Star Wars fanatics, even took classes in the art of the light saber. They would come out of every class soaked in sweat, with huge smiles on their faces!

Even if your child participates in group or individual sports, it's important to encourage unstructured physical activities and hobbies that will last a lifetime, such as running, hiking, dance, jumping rope, and practicing yoga. Many of my adult patients who are now overweight and suffering from chronic health issues were former high school athletes, but they had no other exercise skills or habits. Unfortunately, when their competitive sports careers ended, they became sedentary. Having a few lifelong activity hobbies at hand, allows your kids to continue exercising long after they've outgrown their sports.

Physical activity becomes habitual when it's incorporated into your child's daily schedule and into your family's routine recreational activities. For example, schedule some form of outdoor play immediately after school. This may be at the school playground right after pick up or in your backyard before they enter the house. After-school exercise will improve their mood, help them focus on their homework, and allow them to sleep better. Add physical activities to family recreation as well. Two of the most popular family pastimes are eating out and going to the movies. Add active options to your weekend or weekly traditions: hiking, cycling, picnics with playground play, etc. Even an after-dinner neighborhood walk a few times a week is a great opportunity to get in some physical activity and quality family time.

All of us spend enough time seated indoors at school and work, so avoid duplicating this sedentary behavior during recreational time. Fun competitions can also get the entire family motivated. My kids live to beat me in basketball. Play sports with your kids, such as tag or ultimate Frisbee. If you're not yet physically fit enough to keep up with the young ones, make walking a friendly, competitive game. Purchase pedometers for everyone in the family and see who can log in the most steps daily or weekly.

Finally, be an active role model. Inactive parents lack credibility when they try to push their kids to be more active. Yelling at your kids from the sidelines to run faster during their soccer games when you hardly get out of your chair is not setting a good example. Exercise and play with your kids. Have them watch you while you exercise at home, in the yard, or at the local park. Educate them about why you exercise: "Exercise makes me healthier, charges my batteries, gives me more superpowers…" Let them know you're going for a run or heading to the gym, so it sinks into their subconscious that their parents are making activity a priority.

Hopefully by now you realize that insulin resistance and chronic disease are not individual issues for South Asians, but family problems that require a family solution. A child who watches his parents make healthy choices is much more likely to become an adult who does the same.

Summary of activity and exercise tips:

- Discover the best activity for your child: team sports, individual sports, or unstructured activities.

- Incorporate physical activity periods into your child's daily schedule.

- Create active family outings to balance out the inactive ones.

- Be an activity role model.

Vertical Height

8. *"Suneel's too short. What can we do to make Suneel taller?"*

Most scientists agree that the potential range of outcomes of your adult height is mostly hardwired into your genes, but that environment and lifestyle can exert some influence. Peter M. Visscher of the Queensland Institute of Medical Research in Australia studied 3,375 pairs of Australian twins and found that genetics accounted for 80 percent of reported height, also known as height heritability. However, raising your child with good food, sleep, and exercise habits may allow him to reach his maximum height within his genetically constrained range of outcomes. For instance, let's say your child's maximum height range is five foot ten inches. Feed him right and make sure he gets enough rest and exercise and chances are high that he will reach his maximum. However, if the same kid grows up on junk food, insufficient sleep, and limited exercise, he may only reach five foot seven inches, short of his full genetic potential. No matter what superfoods you feed him he won't grow to be six feet tall, as this is outside his genetic potential.

The mid-parental height formula has been a standard since the 1970s to estimate a child's adult height based on the height of both parents.[8] The formula is as follows:

Girl's height prediction:	**Mom + Dad's height (inches) - 5** <hr> **2** (with a standard deviation of +/- 2)
Boy's height prediction:	**Mom + Dad's height (inches) + 5** <hr> **2** (with a standard deviation of +/- 2)

Let's say Suneel's mom is 62 inches tall and his dad is 67 inches tall. Based on the formula for boys, Suneel's estimated adult height would be:

$$\frac{62 + 67 + 5}{2} = 67 \text{ inches, or 5' 7" (+/- 2 inches)}$$

While this calculation holds true for most children, remember that it's just an estimate. Respect the hardwired aspects of your child's genetic recipe and focus on raising him or her to be as healthy as possible. Do not let children feel inadequate if they are smaller than average in stature. Parents should not view this as a parenting failure, especially if they are making sincere attempts to improve all major lifestyle factors. Appreciating genetic boundaries also prevents overzealous family members from overfeeding kids, which can lead to an unhealthy increase in width instead of height. Your goal is to maximize your child's genetic potential for growth by optimizing the lifestyle factors below.

> *Respect the hardwired aspects of your child's genetic recipe and focus on raising him or her to be as healthy as possible.*

Diet: A healthy, balanced diet is crucial to fuel normal growth and development. Empty calories in the form of sugars, processed foods, and excessive carbohydrates, need to be replaced with nutritious proteins, fats, and vitamins from vegetables and fruits. Even excess amounts of so-called healthy foods like wheat in the form of chapatis may impair bone development due to an ingredient called phytic acid, which impairs absorption of minerals such as calcium. A study made up of South Indians documented the link between low dietary calcium and high-phytate consumption and low levels of vitamin D.[9] Fuel your kids with lower net carb, nutrient-dense meals and snacks as discussed in detail in Chapter 6.

Exercise: Leading an active lifestyle plays an important role in growth. One cultural myth is that stretching or even hanging from a bar will increase height. Despite advice from family members or information you've found on the web, neither has been shown to have any impact on height. Stretching is, however, a healthy component of exercise.

Sleep: Optimal sleep habits and duration is not only essential for proper emotional regulation and brain function, but also necessary for spurring growth. The majority of growth hormone is actually produced during sleep. One study showed that sleep is significantly related to growth as early as the first few months of life.[10]

Vitamin D: Maternal vitamin D levels are an important contributor to proper fetal skeletal growth and development. One small study in Ireland found that babies born to mothers with low vitamin D levels (due largely to the fact that most of their pregnancy occurred in the fall/winter months) had shorter thigh bones than babies born to mothers pregnant mostly in the spring and summer months.[11] Shorter thigh bones in babies may correlate with reduced height in adult life. In addition, studies link low vitamin D in girls to increased body fat and decreased height[12], as well as premature puberty.[13] Obesity also promotes lower vitamin D levels since vitamin D is absorbed by fat cells.

Obesity: In addition to these lifestyle factors, the pediatric obesity crisis is causing hormonal changes that may adversely affect growth and development. For instance, excess body fat triggers early puberty. A study conducted by pediatric endocrinologist Dr. Louise Greenspan of Kaiser Permanente San Francisco Medical Center, found that young girls with increased body fat and higher BMIs experienced an earlier onset of puberty than did those with normal bodyweight.[14] While puberty timelines vary greatly among individuals, lifestyle factors that influence premature puberty for your child can cause an early closure of bone growth plates, potentially leading to stunted growth. Premature puberty in girls is also associated with an increased risk of future breast and uterine cancers.

Dr. Robert Lustig, professor of pediatrics at UCSF, explains that obese girls have higher levels of the hormone leptin, which leads to early puberty, higher estrogen levels, greater insulin resistance, and further fat accumulation.[15] Since you still have nearly total-control of your young daughter's diet, be diligent about keeping her at a healthy weight as she approaches puberty.

Summary of maximizing your child's height:

- Your child's height is determined 80% by genetics and 20% by environmental and lifestyle factors.

- You can maximize your child's potential for growth with healthy lifestyle choices.

- A healthy diet made up of protein, fats, veggies, and fruits fuels growth.

- Physical activity plays an important role in your child's growth.

- Sufficient sleep helps spur growth.

- Adequate vitamin D during pregnancy helps proper fetal skeletal growth and development.

- Encourage sun exposure (low levels of vitamin D have been shown to stunt growth and promote obesity).

- Obesity leads to early onset puberty, which hinders growth and increases your daughter's future risk for breast and uterine cancers.

Supplements

9. *"Suneel's not eating enough. What kind of supplements should we give him?"*

When parents request supplements for their kids, it's usually a sign that they are not feeding their children healthy foods or perhaps not being creative enough in their presentation of nutritious foods.

A healthy diet provides most of the essential nutrients your child needs, and will always be nutritionally superior to a capsule. On the other hand, a diet full of excess sugars, processed foods, and predominant carbohydrates (rice, Indian flatbreads, lentils)—especially in the absence of abundant vegetables, fruit, healthy proteins, and fat— will deplete existing nutrients from your child's diet.

Most children who eat a well-rounded diet and have no dietary restrictions do not require supplements by the time they reach middle childhood. An exception is breastfed infants who require a daily vitamin D supplement until they switch to cow's milk at or after age one. If, despite your best efforts, your child is a picky eater, has a poor appetite, or eats a restricted diet (e.g., vegetarian and/or no dairy products), then a supplement such as an iron-containing multivitamin or vitamin D should be considered. Talk to your pediatrician before starting your child on any supplement and always strive to meet most or all nutrient requirements through natural, healthy foods first. Supplement requirements are constantly changing based on updated studies, so confirm dosages with your pediatrician and refer to a reputed website like healthychildren.org for guidance.

Grand academic, musical, and artistic ambitions of youth can truly go to waste if your child doesn't achieve a bare minimum of daily activity.

Intelligence
10. "How do I make Suneel smarter?"

The question of intelligence is a running diatribe among South Asian parents. The smart factor seems to be the attribute parents obsess over the most. It also happens to be what often drives many unhealthy behavior changes and future health challenges for our children.

Is the answer to sign your children up for more enrichment courses, to push their bedtimes even later so you can cram more information into their little brains, to add on another structured "activity" so they can keep up with their peers? Even summer vacation, which used to be a time for kids to rest, enjoy plenty of play time, and join fun recreational activities like summer camp, has been replaced by intense summer school sessions in an effort to push kids ahead academically. Although some of these activities may be beneficial by some linear measurement, if they are compromising any of the bigger principles (sleep, nutrition, unstructured play, etc.) then these academic enrichment activities are doing more harm than good to your child's intellectual and emotional development. We've already touched on some of the consequences, but I'd like to delve deeper into how fitness, sleep, nutrition, and stress are related to your child's intellectual development.

It is clear that a fit human is a smarter human. The famous Indian saint, Swami Vivekananda said:

"The brain and muscles must develop simultaneously. Iron nerves with an intelligent brain—and the whole world is at your feet."

Iron nerves don't mean a super-athlete, but someone who makes a point to achieve at least the bare minimum of activity and physical fitness competency. This is especially relevant for children, who in this digital age have become couch potatoes for the first time in recorded history.

As a health practitioner in the affluent, ultra high-tech Silicon Valley, I am well aware of the competitive academic environments, busy schedules, and safety fears that get in the way of your children enjoying the long hours of unstructured, outdoor play that you were lucky enough to have experienced in your childhood. However, it should be noted that any grand academic, musical, or artistic ambitions of youth might truly go to waste if your child doesn't achieve a bare minimum of daily activity. Aside from the long-term health consequences and elevated disease risk correlated with childhood obesity, it has been proven that fitter kids do better in school. Don't believe me? Here's the proof:

EXERCISE FOR SMARTS

→A 2002 California Department of Education study of 954,000 California students matched performance on the standardized Stanford Achievement Test with performance on the state-mandated Fitnessgram, a comprehensive physical fitness test. The result: "Statistical analysis indicating a distinct and linear correlation between students' academic achievement and fitness scores."

→A Swedish study done at Sahlgrenska University Hospital and made up of more than one million 18-year-old males showed that better fitness consistently correlated with higher IQs. This finding also applied to genetically identical twins. The fitter twin had a higher IQ than the less fit sibling, despite sharing the same genes! Proof that IQ is not purely genetic but also depends on external factors like fitness.

→Studies from the University of Illinois found that just 20 minutes of walking before a test raised scores, even if the child was otherwise unfit or overweight.

We now know that there are brain-boosting chemicals like brain derived neurotropic factor (BDNF) that increase after just a single exercise session, which is why those pre-test walkers scored higher. There are a number of other beneficial hormonal, metabolic, and circulatory changes that are enhanced by increased fitness levels. There are no two ways about it: the fitter you are, the smarter you are. Understand the spirit of the message here and try to look at activity as a lifestyle benefit, not just a short-term brain booster to try with your kid before a big test. There are no shortcuts, and the benefits extend far beyond scientific quantification.

Sleep: There are a large number of studies supporting the fact that sleeping less leads to academic underachievement. All of the brain faculties needed to maximize your child's intellectual potential—such as attention, memory, and creativity—can be compromised with as little as 20 minutes of sleep deficiency. A child's brain is much more sensitive to even small amounts of sleep deprivation, and children lack the maturity to be able to deliberately increase focus and concentration when they feel tired or sleepy. One study showed that children who sleep less scored lower on neurocognitive testing, which measures mental tasks related to learning. In particular, tasks involving visual and spatial skills were most severely compromised.[16]

High school students who sacrificed sleep did worse on tests and had difficulty learning information in classes, regardless of how much they studied. This particular study involved 9th, 10th, and 12th graders who completed daily diaries for 14 days. Results showed that regardless of how much a student studied each day, sacrificing sleep time for study time resulted in more trouble understanding material in class the following day. Staying up late to cram in more information actually backfired.[17]

Sleep disorders can sometimes be misdiagnosed as attention disorders such as ADHD. A misdiagnosis can have disastrous effects on your child's cognitive development. ADHD medications have been proven to worsen sleeplessness. If ADHD is the right diagnosis, insufficient sleep can exacerbate symptoms. Snoring is a sleep disorder that has also been linked to academic underdevelopment. Studies have shown that children who snore, especially if overweight, have significantly lower IQ scores and poorer academic performance. Even snoring medical students were found to be at a higher risk of failing their exams.

Many of you may be thinking, " but my child goes to bed and still gets straight As because of all the extra work he does at night!" All-star academic performance may be an indication of good health, but not necessarily. Let's examine a bigger picture. Beyond the grades, do teachers report that your child has a good attention span and participates and behaves well in class? Is your child energetic and happy overall? Does your child easily fall asleep at night and wake up easily in the morning in a decent mood? If you have observed all these positive factors, then your child is likely getting enough sleep. Don't let good grades or high gymnastic scores serve as an excuse to fall short on basic healthy lifestyle habits such as adequate sleep. If your child is inattentive, hyperactive, emotionally unstable, irritable, and so forth, insufficient sleep may be a key factor.

Nutrition: Healthy food is a critical part of brain development. Cut back foods that have a negative impact on mood, behavior, and learning. This includes foods with sugar and fructose, and most packaged, processed foods, which contain a growing list of chemicals and preservatives that are being linked to all types of learning disorders. A child's developing brain is particularly susceptible to these artificial additives, so keeping home meals and school lunches and snacks fresh and naturally prepared is preferred. We've discussed many of these points already, so here's a summary of key nutrition points that can help with learning and academic performance:

- Provide kids with a healthy breakfast every morning.

- Try to make each meal and snack as fresh, natural, and nutritionally dense as possible by incorporating a fruit or vegetable.

- Provide brain-boosting omega-3s found in salmon, walnuts, spinach, kale, Brussels sprouts, and flaxseed.

- Don't forget nuts, nut butters, nut milks, seeds and seed butters (which are protein), fiber, and healthy fat-containing options that can be incorporated into meals, snacks, and recipes.

- Remember that a cranky child who can't focus on her academic work is often a hungry or tired child. Stop the work, feed your child, add on a few minutes of play, and then try hitting the books again.

Reduce stress: Today's child is exposed to unprecedented amounts of stress imposed by overdriven parents. Academic pressures are tremendous, and even organized sports come with their own set of tensions. Playing a sport used to be a carefree activity among friends conducted in neighborhoods and parks. Now it's more often a structured, costly endeavor that increases stress in children because parents instill intense competitiveness from an early age. A healthy dose of competition is fine, but playing a sport often becomes another rigid, extracurricular activity for overscheduled kids. Let them enjoy the sport with positive encouragement, rather than harsh criticisms or comparisons to others who may excel. Sports are a form of play and should build self-esteem and confidence, not add stress and negative emotions. If that's not the observed effect, you need to change your approach and expectations as a parent, or change to a different sport or activity.

> *A young, delicate, developing brain is often unprepared to take on the intense academic and athletic activities common today. Rather, it craves freedom, openness, and spontaneous exploration.*

A young, delicate, developing brain is often unprepared to take on so many intense activities. Rather, it craves freedom, openness, and spontaneous exploration. You need to schedule free play time and "quiet time" into your child's schedule as eagerly as you schedule music, sports, and academic enrichment. Stress is the modern day equivalent to the threat our primitive ancestors faced from predators. Exposing a child to intense levels of stress without giving them the time, space, and emotional tools to manage stress is like sending a young child into the harsh wild without any training or preparation.

Not only does stress cause physical symptoms like headaches, musculoskeletal aches and pains, and digestive disorders in kids, but also it can adversely affect academic performance. Stress disengages the intellectual region of the brain known as the prefrontal cortex, and stimulates the areas of emotion and even aggression. This makes learning a struggle and holding attention nearly impossible. Exercise is a common and very effective way to manage stress, but meditation is also turning out to be an excellent stress management tool for kids.

Visitacion Valley Middle School in San Francisco was plagued by low test scores, high dropout rates, and tremendous socioeconomic pressures with 20 percent of students having one or both parents incarcerated during the 2009-2010 school year. In lieu of this desperate situation, school principal Jim Dierke decided to conduct a novel experiment and adopt filmmaker David Lynch's *Quiet Time* transcendental meditation program. The program at Visitacion incorporated 12-minute meditation sessions before and after school for all students. Academic scores and school attendance soared, and children reported reduced anger and better focus during school hours.[18] Students learned to control their emotional and aggressive brains in the midst of personal stressors, and to engage their intellectual brain in the classroom.

Now that you have a handle on some of the major lifestyle factors that affect your child's intelligence, let's look at a typical daily schedule for a South Asian child and how it progressively sabotages these crucial elements.

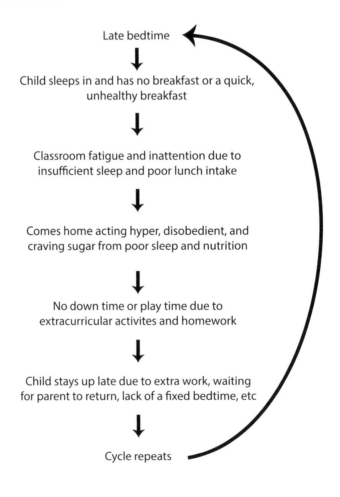

Late bedtime

↓

Child sleeps in and has no breakfast or a quick, unhealthy breakfast

↓

Classroom fatigue and inattention due to insufficient sleep and poor lunch intake

↓

Comes home acting hyper, disobedient, and craving sugar from poor sleep and nutrition

↓

No down time or play time due to extracurricular activites and homework

↓

Child stays up late due to extra work, waiting for parent to return, lack of a fixed bedtime, etc

↓

Cycle repeats

In my generation, as in the current generation, there is a push from parents for children to become physicians or other highly trained professionals. Although these physicians are professionally successful, a large percentage of them are obese and have the same insulin resistant conditions they are treating in their patients. I see a growing number of physicians as patients in my South Asian consult practice. Ask yourself: do you want to raise a fit and healthy physician, lawyer, engineer, writer, musician, etc., or do you want your son or daughter burdened by chronic health issues that you may have been able to prevent as a parent? The lifestyle choices you make on a daily basis (bedtime, snack and meal choices, etc.) may seem inconsequential and routine, but can make the difference between a healthy future and a life cut short.

Summary of how to enrich your child's academic performance:

- Help your kids reach their fitness goals. Fitter kids do better in school!

- Even small amounts of sleep deficiency can damage academic performance.

- Cut back on sugary, processed foods, which negatively impact mood, behavior, and learning.

- Minimize stress and encourage relaxing activities such as meditation.

Preventing Ravi's Death: A Lifespan Approach to Disease Prevention

In Chapter 1, I introduced the tragic death of Ravi. A combination of insulin resistance and a highly inflammatory lifestyle led to the rupture of an atherosclerotic plaque, which blocked off his coronary (heart) arteries and produced a fatal heart attack. Armed with what we learned from this chapter, let's now take a total lifespan approach to heart disease risk by rewinding to Ravi's early childhood and tracing the origins of his insulin resistance and heart disease.

Ravi was considered underweight, as are most South Asian babies. Although he appeared too skinny, he was in fact skinny-fat, since his body had high fat levels relative to very little muscle mass. This tendency towards a "thin-fat" South Asian infant body habitus was validated by a study conducted in Pune, India. The study directly compared body measurements of South Asian babies in Pune to those of Caucasian babies born in Southampton, UK. Although the South Asian babies had a lower body weight, they had higher amounts of preserved body fat and less lean muscle compared to the UK Caucasian babies, thus earning them the label of "thin-fat."[19]

With good intentions, Ravi's parents and extended family were determined to get him looking "healthy" again by overfeeding to achieve "catch-up growth." Bombarding a "seemingly" underweight baby with excess calories initially programmed Ravi for a lifetime of insulin resistance. Granted, Ravi was a child who needed some extra calories for growth, but the amount he was fed as an infant far outstripped his growth needs. How can you prevent this fate for your child? Follow the growth curves and allow your child to track along their percentile, rather than jump up to higher percentiles.

Today's modern lifestyle layered upon insulin resistant genes is a recipe for early onset heart disease and other chronic illnesses.

Even though Ravi's body was set up for insulin resistance early on, he still had the ability to eliminate or significantly reduce his chances of developing diabetes and heart disease later in life. The key is instilling healthy lifestyle changes as early as possible. Unfortunately, Ravi's early childhood and adult life were marked by excessively sedentary behavior due to intense academic and professional pressures, in addition to poor eating habits which further strengthened and reinforced the insulin resistant predisposition he acquired at birth. This eventually led to metabolic syndrome at a young age, complicated by his first heart attack, which mirrored his father's history. By the time Ravi implemented healthy lifestyle changes, it was already too late. His existing insulin resistance, inflammation, and high-stress lifestyle culminated in a second, and this time fatal, heart attack. What about the two children Ravi left behind? I would argue that they face an even greater risk of earlier heart disease than any generation before them. They are exposed to...

- a more toxic, unnatural food environment

- significantly less physical activity

- vitamin D deficiency due to minimal sun exposure

- higher stress levels and overstimulation from digital devices

Today's modern lifestyle layered upon insulin resistant genes is a recipe for early onset heart disease and other chronic illnesses. It is time for us to reset priorities, traditions, and outdated belief systems, and focus on helping future generations become healthier and happier.

For Professionals

- Educate parents as early as possible about common South Asian growth patterns, so they know what to expect.

- Emphasize the short-term and long-term risks (insulin resistance, obesity, etc.) of pushing infants and children out of their normal growth percentiles through overfeeding.

- Be aware of the impact of extended family members who overfeed infants and children at home.

- Promote physical activity and free play time at every visit.

- Encourage more consistent sleep schedules and earlier bedtimes.

- Counsel families against overscheduling children with too many activities that compromise sleep, exercise, and free play, while adding stress. Emphasize that adequate sleep, fitness, and free play are strongly correlated with intelligence.

CHAPTER 11

ANTI-AGING AND IMPROVING
THE HEALTH OF THE ELDERLY

OUR MODERN LIFESTYLES have turned chronological age into a virtually insignificant number when it comes to examining the big picture of aging. Aging is not just the number of years you've inhabited planet Earth, but rather the degree of wear and tear your body, brain, and vital organs are expressing at a given point in time. Let's take a look at a case study to see accelerated aging at work.

Case Study: Suresh

Suresh is a 34-year-old computer programmer who came to see me for a new patient physical exam prompted by a recent car accident that had landed him in the local urgent care clinic. Suresh complained of neck pain and tingling in his left arm, so the physician on duty took x-rays of his cervical spine. The x-rays showed some chronic degenerative changes, but no fractures from the accident, and Suresh was diagnosed with "whiplash syndrome." Suresh's x-ray showed severe degenerative arthritis typical of that found in someone above the age of 70! The natural curvature of Suresh's cervical spine was absent (normal cervical spines have a slight curvature), and his head was markedly shifted forward about two inches into a turtle-like posture. The physician asked that he follow up with a primary care doctor. As part of his physical exam, I ordered Metabolic 6-pack lab tests. His results showed metabolic syndrome with a high hs-CRP level indicative of inflammation.

Skeletal misalignment and related arthritis are the physical signs of the times for today's sedentary, screen-facing workforce. I can look at a person and predict how many hours they sit in front of a computer based on their deviated head position. The human spine's natural curve in the cervical region allows the head, which weighs between 8-10 pounds (about the weight of a bowling ball) to sit above the body's center of gravity. Every inch your head moves forward from this natural position exerts about 10 additional pounds of stress on the neck. Shifting his head forward two inches means Suresh is carrying about twenty extra pounds on top of his already 10-pound head weight—that's 30 pounds of neck stress! Our recent ancestors would never have fallen prey to such an extreme degree of arthritis by the third decade of life; they moved too frequently, ate natural foods, and obtained plenty of bone-building vitamin D through outdoor sunlight exposure.

Suresh became susceptible to degenerative arthritis at such a young age because he led a highly inflammatory lifestyle, as evidenced by his insulin resistance and elevated hs-CRP test. Suresh was also victimized by something called advanced glycated end products (AGEs), which are the byproducts of insulin resistance and a high-carb diet. AGEs permit the immune system to eat away at your protective joint cartilage and accelerate aging. Suresh's chronic neck pain stems from a combination of the adverse mechanical effects of poor posture on his spine, and the tendency of insulin resistance to increase the body's inflammatory response to pain.

Suresh's forward head posture didn't just develop during his adult life, but likely started shifting when he was a child. The progression of poor posture and movement mechanics at a young age is becoming an epidemic. Infants are placed in unnatural seated props and kids are constantly protruding their heads towards all sorts of screens and loading oversized backpacks onto inactive, poorly conditioned spines. Such practices are turning arthritis, which used to be a condition seen almost exclusively in the elderly, into a disease for all ages.

ACCELERATED AGING

Before moving to the Bay Area to take care of a large group of South Asian patients, I began my practice in Southern California where I treated a predominantly non-South Asian population. Many of these patients worked jobs involving hard labor, often outdoors. I could easily predict the age of these patients. I completely lost that predictive ability when I started seeing South Asians, especially my mostly sedentary, high-tech employees. Many were thirty-something men who looked like they were pushing fifty. They carried protuberant pot bellies and hunched forward postures reminiscent of those of old men with curved spines. Were my South Asian patients actually aging at an accelerated rate? In addition to all the health risks we've discussed thus far, let's add one more: *premature aging*, which unfortunately targets South Asians at an accelerated rate.

Biological Markers of Aging

Let's first discuss some biological markers of aging, and then discuss the impact of selected lifestyle factors on these markers. There is a great degree of overlap between the process of aging and inflammation. Lifestyle practices that promote ongoing systemic inflammation will make you age faster. Lifestyle practices that reduce excess inflammation in the body will help delay the aging process.

Telomeres: Our genes are encoded onto twisted, double-stranded DNA molecules called chromosomes. The tips of our chromosomes are protected by critical DNA end pieces called telomeres. These telomeres can be compared to the plastic caps that protect the end of shoelaces from fraying. Telomeres determine the health of our genetic material and allow cells to divide. Each time a cell divides, that cell ages and the telomeres get shorter. When telomeres become too short, the cell can no longer divide and the cell dies. Keeping our telomeres long and healthy slows down the process of cellular aging, and thus human aging. An enzyme called telomerase replenishes telomeres after cell division. As we age, the amount of available telomerase is depleted and telomeres consequently grow shorter. Having keyed in to the link between telomeres and cellular aging, scientists are now studying the effects of various lifestyle factors on telomere health.

AGEs (advanced glycation end products): Proteins are the building blocks for muscles, blood vessels, and organs, as well as the collagen that maintains your cartilage, bone, and skin. When proteins begin to break down, you start to look older: your skin starts to wrinkle and your body feels less flexible as joint cartilage wears away and arthritis follows. Much of this damage to proteins can be attributed to the accumulation of substances called AGEs. AGEs form when sticky glucose (sugar) molecules in the blood bind to proteins, making them dysfunctional and highly inflammatory. Vital organs like your brain, heart, liver, and kidneys can be adversely affected by the physical accumulation of inflammatory AGEs at these sites. Recall that AGEs bind to receptors on immune cells called RAGEs (receptors for advanced glycation end products); this process stimulates the production of a chemical called NF-kB that, when activated, leads to rampant inflammation and blood vessel changes that are key triggers for atherosclerosis.

Glycohemoglobin (HbA1C): Although AGEs cannot be easily measured with a blood test, glycohemoglobin (HbA1C)—the blood test routinely used to diagnose and monitor diabetes—measures the amount of glycated hemoglobin (sugar bound to the protein hemoglobin) and can serve as a rough marker for excess AGEs. Even a gradual rise in your glycohemoglobin levels can indicate accelerated aging. Fortunately, modifying your diet by reducing excess carbohydrates typically improves your glycohemoglobin level within a few months. See Chapter 1 for details on the glycohemoglobin test.

Four Major Age Accelerators

Let's summarize four key age-accelerating factors that speed the shortening of our telomeres and increase the production of AGEs.

1. **Poor nutrition:** Excess carbohydrates in the South Asian diet, especially in conjunction with insulin resistance, translate to

higher levels of circulating blood glucose. Higher circulating blood sugar leads to the excess production of AGEs, and AGEs are associated with virtually every major age-related medical condition, including:

- Heart disease

- Arthritis

- Alzheimer's disease

- Cancer

- Diabetes

- Eye disease

- Nerve damage

- Kidney disease

Many of these conditions (nerve damage, eye disease, heart disease, etc.) are complications of diabetes. In this regard, you can think of diabetes as a repercussion of accelerated aging. This makes sense when I think of my 30-year-old diabetic patients who already have damaged nerves, kidneys, eyes, and other vital organs, afflictions that are more common-place in seniors. Keeping blood sugar and glycohemoglobin levels under control through proper dietary changes not only reduces the threat of diabetic complications, but also slows down aging.

In addition to limiting carb-heavy foods, eating the following foods reduces inflammation and better preserves your telomeres:

Omega-3 fats: oily, coldwater fish such as salmon, sardines, herring, and mackerel are rich sources of omega-3 fats. One study showed that individuals with higher blood levels of omega-3 had longer telomeres.[1]

Monounsaturated fats: add plenty of olive oil, nuts, seeds, and avocados.

Multi-colored vegetables and some fruit: eat copious amounts, especially of berries.

Dark chocolate: consume with a cocoa content of 70 percent or more in moderation.

Green tea: rich in polyphenols that protect against oxidative damage.

Herbs and spices: ginger and turmeric are examples of potent anti-inflammatory herbs and spices.

Alcohol: red wine is healthy when consumed in moderation. Do not start drinking to slow down aging, given alcohol's associated health risks.

2. **Inactivity:** I've touted the benefits of exercise throughout this book. I now want to highlight some genetic proof that physical activity is currently the most effective fountain of youth available. Tim D. Spector, a professor of genetic epidemiology at King's College London, led a study made up of 2,401 twins. Comparing the genetic material of twins who had engaged in disparate exercise habits over their lifetimes allowed investigators to determine the true effects of exercise on cellular aging as represented by telomere length. Study findings indicated that telomere length increased with voluntary physical activity, after controlling for other factors like body mass index, smoking, sex, socioeconomic status, and physical activity at work.[2] As this study demonstrates, genes are not fixed, unchangeable entities. Despite starting off life with the same genetic material, the more active twins actu-

ally transformed their genes by lengthening their telomeres, a process that leads to anti-aging benefits such as a decreased risk for chronic disease (heart disease, cancer, arthritis, etc.), a sharper brain, and fewer wrinkles!

3. **Stress:** In 2004, Nobel prize winning molecular biologist Dr. Elizabeth Blackburn and UCSF scientist Elissa Eppel, sought to find genetic evidence for the link between stress and aging. They compared a group of mothers who cared for children with chronic illness (a high chronic stress group) to a group of mothers with healthy children (a lower stress group). The mothers with sick children were found to have shorter telomeres and less telomerase activity than the mothers with healthy children, thus providing genetic proof of stress-induced accelerated aging.[3] You may have noticed this phenomenon among your own family members or friends who physically appear older after suffering a personal loss or some other major stressor. The good news is that Blackburn and Eppel followed that study up with another that showed that vigorous exercise actually protected individuals undergoing high stress from the otherwise expected damage to telomeres.[4] Exercise not only reduces your feelings of stress, it actually helps shield your genes from their damaging effects.

4. **Low vitamin D:** Mass paranoia over skin cancer and wrinkles has forced more people to seek shelter from the sun by spending too much time indoors and by shielding their skin with layers of sunscreen. The irony is that these behaviors are instead causing rampant vitamin D deficiency, which has far greater effects in promoting aging and chronic disease, than the relatively lower risk of skin cancer from sun exposure. Vitamin D is a hormone involved in nearly every major metabolic process in the body, and vitamin D deficiency is linked to a growing list of conditions. It's no surprise then that vitamin D deficiency also affects telomere length. One study revealed that individuals with higher vitamin D levels not only had longer telomeres, but also had lower levels of CRP (C-reactive

protein), a blood marker for inflammation.[5] We discussed in earlier chapters how inflammation and oxidation are critical processes in promoting cellular damage and chronic diseases such as atherosclerosis. This study suggests that vitamin D is a key player that may tie together the connection between inflammation, telomere health, and the overall aging process.

Let's summarize some of the major factors that accelerate aging:

- Chronically high glucose levels from excess carbohydrates and insulin resistance (as revealed by elevated HbAlC blood tests)

- High stress levels

- Sedentary lifestyle

- Vitamin D deficiency

The majority of South Asians I encounter have all four of these risk factors. Fortunately, simple lifestyle modifications can impact all of these simultaneously. A single outdoor exercise session improves your ability to metabolize glucose and manage stress, and affords a natural dose of vitamin D.

VITAMIN D HEALTH

A growing body of research is now supporting the role of vitamin D in vital metabolic processes that prevent premature aging and chronic disease. A simple vitamin D supplement isn't going to make up for an unhealthy diet and a sedentary, high-stress lifestyle. Vitamin D isn't a magical pill, but a hormone that helps your lifestyle efforts work together more efficiently and effectively so that you can make further gains when you've hit a wall with some of your goals. For example, vitamin D may help lift your HDL a few more points or reduce your blood sugar and blood pressure just enough to get you out of the prediabetes range or help you avoid the need for blood pressure medications. It may help you lose those stubborn remaining pounds that don't want to budge despite your best efforts with nutrition and exercise. I've seen a lot of chronic aches and pains suddenly disappear when vitamin D levels are replenished. Vitamin D may even help prevent cancer by regulating healthy cell division in the body.

Numerous studies confirm that vitamin D helps to lower the very insulin resistant conditions South Asians are most at risk for, such as diabetes, heart disease, abnormal cholesterol, and high blood pressure. I'm not saying replenishing vitamin D is a guaranteed path to success, but there is enough existing evidence to support adequate vitamin D intake as a key part of your health management.

The Science of Vitamin D

When the ultraviolet (UV) rays of sunlight strike the skin's surface, they trigger a series of biochemical reactions that convert cholesterol underneath the skin to vitamin D via the liver and kidneys. The fact that our bodies depend on sunlight to create a hormone as essential as vitamin D should serve as proof that humans were meant to spend more time outdoors, not self-imprisoned in the indoor spaces of work and home. Vitamin D made from sunlight cannot cause toxicity, and lasts longer in your body (typically stored for 30-60 days) than vitamin D taken from a pill.

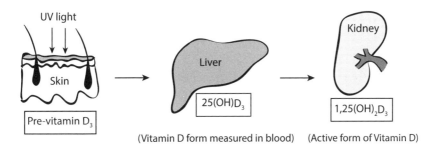

(Vitamin D form measured in blood)   (Active form of Vitamin D)

Why is Vitamin D Low in Most South Asians?

We must go back to our ancestral roots to understand how the color of our skin is an evolutionary adaptation to the region of Earth we originally inhabited. The geographic location of South Asia imparts an abundant amount of sunlight because of its proximity to the equator. The dark skin of South Asians evolved due to an increased level of the pigment melanin, developed as a protective shield from the harsh effects of the sun. There's a tradeoff, however. More melanin means less vitamin D production, since melanin reduces the amount of penetrating UV light. Location compensated for decreased vitamin D synthesis in darker skin, especially since our ancestors spent most of their time outdoors and got plenty of sun exposure. In contrast, those of European ancestry who migrated further from the sunlit equator adapted with lighter skin pigment, which enables more vitamin D production to occur with less sun exposure.

So what happens when you take a darker-skinned South Asian out of the subtropical, sunlit land of his ancestry, and export him to the northern latitudes of Silicon Valley, London, or Toronto, where he spends extended amounts of time indoors in a high-tech workplace? You dramatically lower his exposure to sun-induced vitamin D synthesis. Of course, in today's world, even living in an ancestrally aligned geographic location has little meaning to most South Asians. If you're a software engineer who spends most of your time indoors, it doesn't matter whether you live in Canada, Silicon Valley, or Bangalore. If you spend the majority of your time bathing in screenlight rather than sunlight, you'll suffer from some degree of vitamin D deficiency.

Reduced sunlight exposure in the presence of darker skin is the most significant reason South Asians lack sufficient vitamin D; however, there are two other factors that drive low vitamin D production.

Excess belly (visceral) fat: Vitamin D is fat soluble—when it enters the body it has the tendency to migrate towards and enter into our fat cells for storage. The more fat you have, the greater the likelihood vitamin D is sequestered inside fat cells instead of available to help power essential biochemical reactions in your body. Excess body fat is quite literally a vitamin D trap! As a result, individuals with extra body fat require higher vitamin D doses.

I mentioned earlier that often patients lose extra pounds when vitamin D is replenished. Vitamin D encourages weight loss by boosting metabolism and allowing you to burn rather than store fat. Our primitive ancestors depended on the body's ability to store fat during the winter months when food was scarce. Low vitamin D levels helped to lower metabolism and activate fat storage. Unfortunately, in modern times, our already low vitamin D levels drop even further in the winter, but our year-round feasting continues, leading to fat accumulation around the clock, regardless of season. The combination of persistent vitamin D deficiency and a sedentary lifestyle locks our bodies in a perpetual state of metabolic hibernation.

Abnormal vitamin D metabolism: A study published in the *Journal of Clinical Endocrinology and Metabolism* confirms that South Asians are at a much higher risk of vitamin D deficiency and its associated conditions than Caucasians. The study found that South Asians living in the Southern United States had a decreased ability to metabolize vitamin D compared to Caucasians living in the same region. Compromised vitamin D metabolism may be an additional factor that keeps vitamin D levels low.[6] Researchers specifically studied an enzyme called 25 (OH)D-24-hydroxylase, which normally inactivates the functional form of vitamin D. They found that this enzyme was significantly more active in South Asian subjects. The authors postulated that the increased activity of this vitamin D inactivating enzyme might partially account for lower vitamin D levels in South Asians.

Diagnosing Vitamin D Deficiency
Vitamin D levels in the blood are measured with a test called the "25-vitamin D" or "serum 25(OH)D." Levels are expressed in nanograms per milliliter (ng/ml). Vitamin D expert Dr. Michael Holick, author of *The Vitamin D Solution*, considers less than 20 ng/ml deficient, less than 30 ng/ml insufficient, and between 40 and 60 ng/ml optimal. A recent study of over 400,000 subjects found that a vitamin D range of 20-36 ng/ml was associated with the lowest risk of heart disease, in addition to lower overall rates of death and disease from other causes.[7] While vitamin D advocates suggest slightly higher levels, it's clear that getting your level up to 30 offers protection from serious disease, while a level below 20 can suggest a serious health problem requiring immediate attention.

Vitamin D Production

I recommend a three-pronged strategy consisting of sunlight, diet, and supplementation for replacing vitamin D in deficient individuals.

Sunlight: Sunlight is by far the most abundant source of vitamin D. Unlike supplements, sun-driven vitamin D production carries no toxicity and lasts at least twice as long as dietary vitamin D. How much vitamin D you obtain from sunlight depends on your skin type, the latitude you live in, the season and time of day you expose your skin, and the reflectiveness of the earth's surface around you. You can only manufacture vitamin D during the periods of the year when the sun's rays are powerful enough. This ranges from most of the year in the tropical latitudes, to perhaps two-thirds of the year over most of the contiguous United States, to only a few months per year above the 45th parallel. (The 45th parallel lies halfway between the equator and the poles, near the US/Canadian border, Portland/Seattle, Toronto, upstate New York and the South of France, and in the Southern Hemisphere, New Zealand, and Southern Chile/Argentina.)

Dr. Holick provides exposure time recommendations based on a percentage of how long it takes your skin to develop mild pinkness (slight sunburn), which he refers to as one minimal erythemal dose or 1 MED. If you expose your arms and legs—which make up over half your body's total surface area—to 25-50 percent of 1 MED, 2-3 days a week, then you will obtain sufficient amounts of sunlight to make enough vitamin D. For example, if your skin turns pink after an hour in the sun, then you only need to spend 20-30 minutes in the sun 2-3 times a week.

Key points to remember:

- Spend 25-50 percent of 1 MED 2-3 days a week in the sun.

- Your prime sun exposure interval is between 10 am and 3 pm, when UV rays from sunlight are optimal.

- Apply sunscreen to your face, neck, and hands to avoid sun damage, but do not apply to other exposed surfaces (arms, legs, chest, abdomen, etc) during the sun exposure interval.

- Expose 25-50 percent of your body surface area during sun exposure sessions. In terms of skin surface area, your legs make up 36 percent, arms 18 percent, abdomen and chest 18 percent, and back 18 percent.

- If you stay in the sun longer than your sun exposure interval, be sure to apply a broad-spectrum sunscreen with an SPF of 15 or greater.

Dr. Holick provides "Sensible Sun Tables" based on the above factors in his book *The Vitamin D Solution*. For example, a lighter skinned North Indian living at a mid-latitude location on the globe (such as San Francisco or New York), requires about 30-40 minutes of sun exposure three times a week between 11 am and 3 pm during the months of March to May, and 20-30 minutes three times a week during June to August. A darker skinned South Indian living in the same regions would need 40-60 minutes between March and May, and 25-35 minutes between June and August. If the South Indian spent his summer in his home country (tropical latitude), then the sun exposure time would drop down to 20-30 minutes. There are also smartphone vitamin D apps such as "D Minder" that provide recommended sun exposure times based on the variables discussed.

Diet: While diet provides only a fraction of the vitamin D potential that optimal sun exposure does, it just so happens that many vitamin D-rich foods are extremely healthy. Vitamin D-rich foods include salmon (especially fresh wild caught), herring, mackerel, cod liver oil, sardines, mushrooms, egg yolks, and tuna. Vitamin D-fortified foods—often heavily processed carbohydrate products—offer very minimal levels of an inferior source of vitamin D called D2; these foods are not even worth considering in the vitamin D equation. A typical South Asian diet, especially among vegetarians, is deficient in vitamin D, which makes sun exposure and supplements a necessity for most.

For many, a day without sunshine is a day of metabolic confusion, mild depression, and disrupted sleep.

Supplements: Although sunlight is the preferred source of vitamin D, supplementation may be necessary for individuals with low sun tolerance (which induces symptoms such as headaches, excessive fatigue, etc.), or those who lead sun-challenged lifestyles, such as those who spend the majority of their days indoors or live in regions where sunlight is limited. Even if you think you get adequate sun exposure, it is still advisable to take additional supplements during the periods of the year when vitamin D production from sunlight is hindered or impossible. Depending on your vitamin D level, you may need over-the-counter vitamin D3 supplements at a typical daily dose between 1,000 to 2,000 international units. If you have very low vitamin D levels (under 20 ng/ml), you may need to take a higher prescription dose of 50,000 international units (IUs) once a week for eight weeks, followed by a maintenance dose. In my experience, 2,000 IUs daily is the average maintenance dose for South Asians, with some patients requiring higher doses.

Vitamin D Big Picture

When patients find out they are vitamin D deficient, the first question they ask is "how much vitamin D should I take?" I'd rather have them ask, "how much sunlight should I get?" Sunlight is so much more than just an abundant vitamin D source. Sunshine also reduces stress, enhances mood, reconnects us with nature, and helps regulate our body's internal clock (i.e., circadian rhythm) to help us sleep better at night and keep our hormones in balance. For many, a day without sunshine is a day of metabolic confusion, mild depression, and disrupted sleep. Low vitamin D levels are reflective of typical indoor workaholics or homebound, high-stress individuals who have completely lost their connection to nature and the benefits of intermittent, healthy doses of sunshine.

In addition to expanding your approach to low vitamin D beyond just popping a pill, try to avoid the all or nothing mentality when soaking in some sunrays. If you can't get your recommended half MED dose, then take just a few minutes out of a busy day that has you suffocating inside from work overload.

Practical Ways to Incorporate Sunlight into Your Indoor Days

Below are some practical strategies for bringing some sunshine into your darker days.

Get outside: Replace some of your indoor workouts with outdoor ones, keeping your arms and legs exposed. If you're too modest to show sufficient skin, end your workout with some stretches in the privacy of your backyard where you can peel off some layers or roll up your pant legs and sleeves.

Workday walks: I realize dress codes may not allow adequate skin exposure, but even rolling up your sleeves while you walk provides some essential vitamin D.

Work outdoors: Scan some emails on your smartphone or laptop while basking in the sun...and encourage your kids to take their homework outside as well! Sun glare on screens often prevents individuals from taking their devices outdoors. Try increasing the brightness setting on your screen, purchase/make a "laptop hood," or use an adjustable patio or beach umbrella to provide shade.

Outdoor housework: How about taking mundane chores outdoors? Fold laundry (lay a bed sheet on your lawn and fold away), cut vegetables, or go through mail. Change into shorts and a t-shirt to maximize sun exposure.

TAKING BETTER CARE OF SOUTH ASIAN SENIORS

Most South Asians either live in an extended family with senior members or have elder family visiting for several months at a time. For many South Asians, aging parents who remain in their native country are a source of constant worry and even guilt since it's difficult to provide adequate elder support and care over long distances. Routine preventive care is sorely lacking for South Asian seniors, and the difference in medical practices between the US and South Asian countries leaves South Asians in the dark as to whether their elder family members are receiving appropriate care. A physician from India may have a different approach to blood pressure management or preventive screening tests than a US physician, and the varying protocols can be confusing. For this reason, I've put together a list of the most important health measures to help South Asian seniors prevent chronic diseases and maintain an acceptable quality of life. These are just some guidelines. Be sure to connect seniors to a trusted physician and schedule regular visits.

Vision: Schedule routine eye exams. By the time seniors start to complain about their vision, eye conditions like glaucoma and retinal disease may be in the advanced stages. Cataracts, characterized by progressive clouding of the eye lens, are three times more common in South Asians and occur up to 12 years earlier than they do in other ethnic groups.[8] All the major medical conditions prevalent in South Asians (insulin resistance, high blood pressure, etc.) have a cumulative impact on eye health. Even subtle defects in vision can impair everyday activities like walking and driving, which put seniors at risk for falls and accidents. Be sure to keep up with the following:

- All healthy adults should have a baseline vision exam by age 40—sooner if there is a family history of early eye disease, or if diagnosed with diabetes or high blood pressure. Subsequent intervals will be determined by the eye specialist.

- Diabetics of any age must have a dilated exam once a year to screen for disease of the retina.

- Seniors above age 60 should have a comprehensive eye exam with dilation. Subsequent screening intervals will be confirmed by the eye specialist.

Mobility: As seniors age, they need to move more, not less. Sarcopenia, the gradual wasting of muscle that occurs naturally with chronological aging, becomes more prominent after age 50, when the rate of muscle loss (if not challenged by a well-formulated strength training program and/or enthusiastic participation in sports) averages one to two percent per year. In South Asian culture, seniors often adopt the mindset that life naturally becomes more sedentary as the years go by, and behave according to these perceptions. This accelerates sarcopenia further. Furthermore, when they do experience physical decline, pride often prevents them from walking outdoors with a cane, walker, or other assistive device. The more limited they are with walking, the more they need to do stationary leg exercises such as seated leg extensions, partial squats in a chair, etc. These should be done under close supervision. For motivation, realize that a senior who can't walk or exercise quickly becomes a bed bound, chronically ill senior who requires around-the-clock care.

Immobile South Asian seniors are also at high risk for developing painful and potentially fatal bedsores (aka pressure ulcers). I have had close family members and patients suffer terribly from neglected bedsores that penetrate through the skin, down to the bone. It's important to emphasize the following mobility guidelines in seniors:

- Frequent walking—even if assistive devices are required.

- Regular leg strengthening for balance and stability. See Chapter 7 on exercises that include senior-specific recommendations.

- Adequate vitamin D exposure to reduce the risk of falls.

- Diligent inspection of body surfaces each day for bedsores, especially along the spine, tailbone, buttocks, hips, heels, and other contact points. Any skin changes should be reported immediately to a nurse or physician.

Mind and mood: It is often easy to overlook the mental status of elderly family members, especially because they have been culturally conditioned to internalize emotions like loneliness, low self-worth, pain, and hopelessness. Such persistent emotions are forms of chronic stress that can lead to depression, memory loss, and even physical disease. Encourage your older loved ones to socialize with peers their own age in order to garner mutual support for shared life stage stressors. Schedule a variety of productive activities that enhance self-worth and physical well-being, such as gardening, housework, childcare, community service, etc. Be sure to compliment and acknowledge the service they are providing.

It can also be helpful to screen seniors for depression. Here are three quick diagnostic home tests that measure either physical or mental well-being:

1. **"TUG" (Timed Up and Go) test:** This is one of the best ways to measure walking stability and fall risk in seniors. Use a chair, preferably with arm rests, and mark an area 10 feet from the chair using tape or some other marker. Perform as follows:

    *   Have the person sit in the chair with their arms resting on the armrests

    *   Time how long it takes them to stand up, walk to the marked area, turn around, return to the chair, and sit back down

    *   Give the individual one practice trial before the timed test

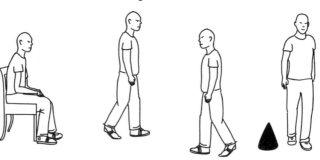

<10 seconds	Freely mobile
<20 seconds	Mostly independent
20-29 seconds	Variable mobility
>30 seconds	Impaired mobility

Geriatric depression screen (GDS): I've included the short four-question version (GDS-4) below, but you can find an intermediate version with 15 questions (GDS-15) or the complete 30-question version (GDS-30) online. I suggest using the GDS-4 as a quick screen and if any questions are positive, following up with the GDS-15 or GDS-30.

To start, answer the following as yes or no:

1. Are you basically satisfied with your life? (No = 1 point)

2. Do you feel that your life is empty? (Yes = 1 point)

3. Are you afraid something bad is going to happen to you? (Yes = 1 point)

4. Do you feel happy most of the time? (No = 1 point)

Scoring:
0 = Unlikely depressed; 1 = Possibly depressed; 2-4 = Depressed

No test is 100-percent accurate, so if you suspect depression despite a score of 0, be sure to consult a physician.

2. **Mini-cog for dementia:** This quick screening test is valid among different ethnic groups. A more comprehensive test is the MMSE (mini mental status exam), which can be found online. For individuals already diagnosed with dementia, the MMSE should be performed and scored by a healthcare professional at periodic intervals. Perform the following three assessments in order:

• **Three-word recall:** Once you have the individual's attention say, "I am going to call out three words that I want you to remember" (choose three unrelated words like "banana, watch, and chair"). Have the person repeat the three words out loud. They will have to recall these words later.

- **Clock drawing test (CDT):** Say, "Please draw a clock. Start by drawing a large circle." When done, instruct them to "put all the numbers in the circle." After they've completed this second step, say, "Now set the hands to show 11:10 (10 past 11)."

- **Three-word recall:** Ask the individual to recall the three words mentioned in the first assessment.

Scoring:
2 points = correctly drawn clock (0 points if incorrectly drawn);
1 point for each word recalled (3 points maximum)

A score of 0-3 means there is some degree of cognitive impairment
A score of 4-5 means there is no significant cognitive impairment

Bones: Osteoporosis is very common in South Asians. A sedentary, indoor lifestyle deficient in bone-building, weight-bearing exercises and vitamin D is a major cause. A lack of age-appropriate screening often means osteoporosis is identified as a hip fracture from a fall rather than caught by early diagnosis from a screening bone density test. Bone density screening age depends on risk factors such as a history of previous bone fracture without injury ("fragility fracture"), history of long-term steroid use, smoking, alcohol, and a family history of fracture. Based on current guidelines, all women 65 and over should screen with a baseline bone density test. If a woman undergoes menopause before age 65 and has one of the aforementioned risk factors, she should get screened for osteoporosis earlier. Men do not routinely need to screen for bone density unless risk factors are present. Below are some recommendations for keeping your bones healthy and strong.

- Weight-bearing activities should be performed upright so that your body works against gravity...even walking is a weight-bearing exercise.

- Vitamin D levels should be checked and replenished if low. It's as easy as spending 10-15 minutes a day in the sun!

- A nutritious diet rich in antioxidants, calcium, and other vitamins and minerals is recommended.

Blood pressure: High blood pressure is often overlooked and undertreated in South Asian seniors. This may be because hypertension is so common and usually doesn't cause symptoms, making it easy to push aside. I recommend seniors with high blood pressure record blood pressures regularly with a portable home monitor and take these readings to doctor visits. This will give physicians a better sense of the average home-measured blood pressure, which is more relevant than occasional office-based results. Please review Chapter 4 for more details on high blood pressure.

Medications: Because insulin resistance triggers multiple conditions, such as high blood pressure, cholesterol, and diabetes, the average South Asian senior is typically prescribed a long list of medications. Often medication doses need to be adjusted or even discontinued since blood pressure levels don't remain constant. Blood pressure may gradually increase over time, or even improve if healthy changes are made. Be sure seniors schedule regular medication checks with their physician and pharmacist to review the following items:

- Do all medications need to be continued?

- Can dosages be adjusted?

- Are there any drug-drug interactions that are of concern? Be sure to bring in a list of all vitamins, supplements, homeopathic, and Ayurvedic medications that can interact with prescription medications.

Many seniors who split their time between the United States and India are taking a mix of medications from both countries. The different drug names can easily confuse physicians. Use an online medication guide like the one found at www.medguideindia.com/show_brand.php to determine the chemical name for each drug so that your doctor knows exactly what you are taking and can account for any negative interactions between prescriptions.

Advanced directives: Sadly, end of life care is a taboo topic among South Asian families. Lack of open discussion often results in family members experiencing confusion and conflict about what their ailing family member truly desires at the end of life. It is important to plan for the inevitable while family members are still healthy and capable enough to make their own decisions. I realize this is a difficult topic to discuss, but avoiding it makes end of life care inherently more stressful than it needs to be. Take the following steps to ensure smoother sailing in a time of crisis:

- Initiate a discussion with family members about end of life care and wishes. Any age is appropriate to start this discussion and outline a plan.

- Complete a living will or advanced directive. An advanced directive is a legal document that directly addresses end of life decisions so that you can provide detailed instructions about your health care wishes to an appointed agent (family member, close friend, etc.) who has power of attorney to make care and treatment decisions on your behalf if you are unable.

- A POLST (physician orders for life-sustaining treatment) is an even more specific document outlining whether the individual wants interventions such as CPR (cardiopulmonary resuscitation), breathing machines, etc. You can discuss this document in detail with your physician.

Once you have completed the forms mentioned above, be sure to give your primary care physician a copy to keep in your chart to ensure that health care wishes are carried out.

Vaccines: Preventive health is often neglected in South Asian patients, especially seniors. Patients neglect routine vaccines and subsequently develop potentially crippling conditions like shingles or life-threatening pneumonia. Be sure to inquire about age-appropriate vaccines at every doctor's visit. I've included four of the most important vaccines to maintain senior health. Keep in mind that vaccine recommendations are subject to change, so discuss with a doctor.

Annual influenza (flu) vaccine: The flu can manifest as a serious infection in seniors. This vaccine should be given yearly.

Zoster (shingles) vaccine: Shingles materializes as a very painful, blistering rash that is a reactivation of a prior herpes zoster infection within the nerves. In seniors, shingles can have a prolonged course and may even lead to chronic pain. The vaccine can reduce your risk of getting shingles by half and can also minimize the severity of symptoms. The vaccine is recommended for seniors ages 60 and above.

Tetanus-Diphtheria-Pertussis (Tdap) vaccine: This combination vaccine protects against tetanus-diphtheria infection and also reduces the risk of pertussis (whooping cough), which is becoming more prevalent in seniors. All adults should get a single dose of Tdap to protect against pertussis, with subsequent boosters of standard Td vaccine given every 10 years.

Pneumococcal vaccine (pneumonia): This is typically a one-time vaccine administered at age 65 to reduce the risk of contracting pneumonia. Although young adults usually recover completely from pneumonia, seniors tend to have weaker immune systems and can die from a bout.

Be sure to discuss appropriate vaccine intervals with your doctor, who will also outline any potential risks or contraindications for each immunization.

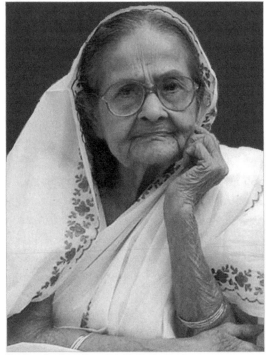

Prativa Sarkar, Age 85 Kolkata, India

MY GRANDMOTHER: OPTIMAL AGING IN ACTION

We often take a reductionist approach to our health, zoning in on specific nutrients and vitamins while neglecting the big picture. When I reflect on my late grandmother's life, I realize how her daily routine in her home in Kolkata, a city in the northern region of India, was a symphony of individual parts—optimal nutrition, physical activity, and sunlight exposure—working together effortlessly to carry her through 86 years of life in incredible physical and mental health. Unlike me, she didn't spend thousands of hours researching these topics. She didn't have a computer to answer common health questions, a pedometer to track her activity, a nutrition counter to monitor what she ate, or a vitamin D table to tell her how much sensible sun exposure to get each day. Instead she used instinct and intuition to make natural lifestyle choices that kept her in great health. I realize the world we live in today is vastly different, but it is still possible to filter through the abundant distractions and reconnect with what's natural. If my grandmother were alive today she'd attribute her longevity and health to the following principles.

Leg strength: In her eighties, my grandmother was able to perform a deep squat while sweeping the floor, making tea and breakfast from a ground level stove, eating from a banana leaf on the floor, performing her temple ceremonies twice daily, and using a squat toilet before the days of the modern toilet. She also had extraordinary hamstring flexibility, which allowed her to do a full hip hinge with straight knees. All of these attributes, which are essential for spinal health, are disturbed by prolonged sitting, which explains the chronic neck and back pain so many of us suffer from. In addition to leg exercises, find ways to incorporate squatting into your day. Squat while brushing your teeth in the morning, squat while reading the paper, tablet, or your favorite device on the floor between your feet, squat while watching TV, while cutting vegetables, etc.

> *"My late grandmother's daily routine in India was a symphony of individual parts—optimal nutrition, physical activity, and sunlight exposure—that worked together effortlessly to carry her through 86 years of life in incredible physical and mental health."*

Sunlight: After bathing, my grandmother would spend a good 15-20 minutes sitting in the sun and letting her hair dry. Often she brought the cutting board out into the sunlit courtyard and chopped vegetables, descaled fish, and grated fresh coconuts. She had no idea about the connection between vitamin D and sunlight. She did it because it felt natural and good to perform her chores while sunbathing.

Prayer: My grandmother engaged in a daily meditation practice of managing her temple affairs and performing worship to deities. These activities helped her manage stress levels. Although she did not suffer from digital overload, she did face the huge responsibility of managing a large household of multiple family members and housekeepers who came with their own sets of emotional stressors, financial hardships, and illnesses. Regardless of whether you are a person of faith, devoting some time during the day for quiet reflection and meditation is a proven technique to manage stress, lower inflammation, and slow down aging of both mind and body.

Food: Most of my grandmother's life predated the onslaught of processed and fast foods. Her diet consisted of an abundant amount and diversity of vegetables, fruits, nuts, fish, chicken, lamb, and goat prepared with traditional fats like ghee and coconut milk. Being of Bengali origin, she consumed plenty of the staple rice, bread, and sweets, but she never faced diabetes or premature heart disease. She was slightly overweight, likely due to these excess carbs, but because she was healthy in all other areas, this excess body fat did not translate into insulin resistance.

I'll never forget my grandmother's visit to the US one summer. Although she was happy to be with us, her mood was dramatically different. She was quiet, withdrawn, and anxious to get back to her life in India. The natural rhythms of her usual life were disrupted. She was mostly cooped up indoors in front of the TV while we were away at school and work. She wasn't a fan of Western food, and she lacked the sense of worth and family connection she had back in India. If she had stayed with us any longer, she may have even become borderline depressed.

I bring this up only to illustrate the importance of recreating at least part of the traditional lifestyle and responsibilities elder family members are used to when they move to the US or stay for extended periods. Seniors often experience depression resulting from isolation and a lack of self-esteem. They do not receive the same degree of respect and attention they did in their native land. No matter how much you care about your elders, you might not catch that they are suffering. Most seniors will not openly express their feelings and frustrations. They have been conditioned to internalize and do not want to seem like a burden. Suppressed negative emotions can lead to depression, dementia, and chronic illness in South Asian seniors. Be proactive and co-create an environment and daily schedule that promotes physical activity, mental stimulation, social communion, and tasks that promote self-worth. Restoring some of the old traditions and natural lifestyle habits discussed in this chapter will not only benefit seniors, but will also improve the health and well-being of the entire family.

Summary

- South Asians are susceptible to accelerated aging due to factors such as inactivity, posture, high-carb diet, stress, and low vitamin D.

- Vitamin D deficiency is extremely common in South Asians and can be screened with a simple blood test.

- Vitamin D deficiency should be remedied with adequate sun exposure over large skin surface areas. Supplementing in the winter months is advised, particularly for people with sun-challenged lifestyles.

- Be vigilant in regularly monitoring health-screening items in seniors, such as vision, mobility, and mental health.

- Encourage leg strength exercises and activities in seniors.

- Create a productive, nurturing environment that promotes optimal mental and physical health.

For Professionals

- Pay attention to signs of accelerated aging in patients.

- Explain to patients that an elevated blood sugar or glycohemoglobin is not just a diabetes risk marker, but also signals advanced aging.

- Screen for vitamin D deficiency in all adults, especially seniors.

- Encourage seniors to self-monitor their blood pressure if there is a history of any abnormal readings.

- Emphasize the importance of preventive screening to South Asian seniors and their family members.

- Reconnect South Asian seniors to old traditions that promote good health, such as increased physical activity, more natural food intake, and plenty of outdoor time.

CHAPTER 12

ACHIEVING YOUR GOALS

YOU HAVE MORE THAN ENOUGH INFORMATION to make significant improvements in your life. Unfortunately, knowledge is often not sufficient to drive behavior change. You may understand fully that the foods you habitually eat have a negative impact on your health, but may still succumb to temptation. You may realize that prolonged sitting is a significant health hazard, but cannot summon the motivation to increase activity levels. The trick isn't to tap into that innate South Asian discipline that defines us as hard-driving, goal-achieving individuals, especially in the areas of academics and professional work. When we apply this type of discipline to lifestyle changes and follow overly regimented, restrictive diets and exercise programs, we inevitably fail over the long run. Lifestyle changes should not be adding stress to an already stressful life. In order to apply your newfound health knowledge, go easy on yourself by setting realistic goals and sustainable life habits.

SETTING GOALS

Many individuals fail to achieve success because they are overambitious with goal setting. Fresh out of medical training, I encouraged this proclivity. After a health check-up, I would often tell a patient to "eat healthier, exercise, stop smoking, and manage your stress," and off I'd send them with a stack of handouts. Overwhelmed, most patients failed to accomplish a single one of these goals. The lesson I learned over the years is to start with a very specific, achievable goal that can be built upon. When it comes to high-risk South Asian patients who have struggled with dietary and lifestyle modifications, I narrow the focus to diet on the first visit. Many patients have already seen another physician or nutritionist who advised them to cut back on fat, cut back on carbs, cut back on salt, etc. This list of no nos goes far beyond one's mental capacity for change. If they are insulin resistant, as most are, I focus specifically on restricting carbohydrate intake. Carbohydrate reduction stimulates rapid and significant changes that the patient can feel (improved energy and reduced hunger and digestive symptoms) and see (weight loss and improved lab results). If the thought of considerably cutting back carbohydrates is overwhelming, start with carb restriction at a single meal—perhaps you forgo that piece of toast at breakfast or the chapati at lunch. You could also start with a single specific food, like eliminating or significantly cutting back on rice.

There is no hard, fast rule for goal setting. You could choose to modify a lifestyle behavior, like tackling activity or stress levels, before embarking on a nutrition goal. If you're a little more motivated, implement one goal from each category. If you embark upon ambitious lifestyle/dietary change and find that it's not going so well, scale back on the number of goals you're striving for, and/or scale back on the quantifiable elements of your goals. For example, if you've reduced your daily carbohydrate intake from 400 grams to 100 grams and this modification is proving too difficult, then approach in a more step-by-step fashion. Reduce carbohydrate intake in 100-gram increments with each passing month. Stay positive at all times, and realize that some change is better than no change.

Sample goals may include a mix of the following:

Nutrition:
- Drop daily net carb intake to less than 150 grams

- Cut out one problem food (sodas, sweets, white rice, etc.)

- Replace wheat chapatis with coconut flour chapatis

- Introduce "carb copycat" vegetable replacements

- Replace grain-based breakfast with an egg-based breakfast or other low-carbohydrate alternative

Activity:
- Initial walking goal of 5,000 or more steps per day

- 20 squats or push-ups daily (adjust to your own goal)

- Increase plank time by one minute

- Sit less, and implement a standing or treadmill desk

Stress/Sleep:
- Meditate for 10 minutes a day

- Do sun salutation every morning

- No screen time for the final hour before bedtime

- Play once a week—pick a hobby or physical activity you truly enjoy

BUILDING YOUR HEALTH TEAM

Even when armed with the right knowledge and specific goals, you may not succeed without the support of others. If you are self-driven and highly motivated, you may be able to achieve your health goals with minimal supervision from a physician. However, most of us need to work with a supportive health team to help keep us on track with our goals and to catch us when we fall.

When I say "health team," I don't just mean doctors and nurses. I mean the people who have the most significant positive impact on your health. Surround yourself with people who share your passion for prioritizing health, and find a way to work with those who may unknowingly be putting you at risk or otherwise having a negative impact on the pursuit of your health goals. A family member who loves you but is consistently putting high-carbohydrate meals on your plate becomes a health risk no matter how good the intentions. I recommend sitting down with that person and having an honest discussion about the impact these foods are having on your health. Hopefully you can agree upon healthier options. Likewise, when it comes to social occasions, don't bend to peer pressure to eat unhealthy, drink, or smoke. If you have a group of friends who are not sympathetic to your efforts and are a barrier to your goals, you may need to rethink your social circle.

Let's categorize the different members of your health team:

- **Home:** anyone who lives with you, visits frequently, or controls the food that comes into your house

- **Work:** your co-workers, your manager, and your onsite health resources (fitness facilities, cafeteria, human resource employees dedicated to wellness)

- **Medical:** your doctor, your nutritionist, your therapist, your naturopath, your chiropractor…anyone with a certified area of expertise that allows them to prescribe drugs, an eating plan or herbals, or perform procedures or interventions (acupuncture, physical therapy, psychotherapy, etc.)

- **Community:** your physical environment, including your social circle, your child's school, your place of worship, or an online community that promotes healthy practices

Home
Take control of your home environment, especially the kitchen. Go through your pantry and clear out all those junk food snacks that tempt you after work or late at night. If you insist on keeping

some, seal them up well and stick them in an inconvenient location, like on a high shelf. Some people even put these snacks in a locked safe and hand the key over to a more disciplined family member. If the shopping and/or cooking falls to another family member who insists on stocking the kitchen with unhealthy snacks and meal items, it's time for a serious discussion. These "talks" are never easy, but the alternative is a family with all members at high risk for insulin resistance.

Work with the cook in your house to stock plenty of low-carb foods (cauliflower rice, low-carb chapatis, shredded vegetable curries) to easily replace white rice and flat breads. Also, be sure your children's caretakers provide nutritious snacks and meals.

To summarize:

- Give your pantry and fridge a complete makeover by replacing unhealthy foods with healthier choices

- Have a frank discussion with family members or anyone who is consistently contributing unhealthy meals and snacks

- Keep close tabs on what your children are eating

Work

Most of us spend more waking hours at work than at home. Work can be a high-stress environment that drives hunger and poor food choices, especially if you have easy access to junk food. It's easy to fall victim to the company cafeteria or a stocked break room located too close to your cubicle, not to mention the mouth-watering catering options offered up at meetings. To optimize your work environment, try the following:

- Pack home-made nutritious meals and snacks whenever possible

- Watch out for the so-called "heart healthy" foods in the cafeteria or vending machine, as they often contain excess carbs

- If catering options are consistently unhealthy and you cannot influence food choices, eat a healthy meal or snack of your own before or after work events

- Identify a handful of restaurants near the office where you can eat low-carbohydrate, high-nutrient value foods

- Start or join a walking group at work; aspire to grand lunch-time efforts of a mile or more, but don't forget that five-minute walks can also contribute to improved health over time

- Reach out to your employer's human resources (HR) team for additional support; I work with the HR teams for over 20 Silicon Valley companies and many employees find me through HR sponsored events

Medical

Your doctor may not be fully onboard with a lifestyle plan focused on reducing excessive carbohydrates rather than saturated fats. Many physicians may actually disagree with this less common approach. Don't give up on your doctor, or the plan! Look for a doctor who is open-minded and supportive of some dietary "self-experimentation" while monitoring your key numbers at appropriate intervals. For example, your doctor should be willing to conduct a repeat cholesterol panel two to three months after you've implemented significant dietary changes. If instead your doctor insists on semi-annual or annual cholesterol checks only, then it may be time to go doctor hunting. In general, check labs when you've lost at least an inch off your waistline or dropped at least six pounds. It's unlikely you'll see significant improvements in your labs until you notice such improvements in your body.

If you like your doctor but he or she remains a stickler for labs at strict intervals, you can order your own tests by visiting websites, such as directlabs.com, that allow you to select tests from a menu (typically at a substantial discount from the rates charged through insurance providers), print out your orders, and then visit a certified lab in or near your zip code. You may also purchase a home device that monitors numbers like blood pressure or blood sugar for additional information and motivation. There are home cholesterol testing kits that can measure triglycerides and HDL, but as of now, their results are not as accurate or as consistent as those of standard blood draws, and test strips can be pricey.

There are other members of your team aside from your doctor who can help you reach your health goals. I've had patients, family members, and friends who were inspired by their personal trainers, mental health therapists, acupuncturists, naturopathic specialists, or spiritual leaders. Anyone who encourages healthy living and helps you manage stress is of great value. You may have to spend a little extra time and money to build your health team, but the returns are priceless when it comes to preventing chronic illness and maintaining optimal health.

Community

One of the greatest temptations South Asians face is the abundance of food-centric social gatherings. Inviting friends over entails elaborate hosting with unhealthy carb-laden appetizers, entrees, and desserts. This type of meal can really turn your efforts upside down, especially in the early stages when you are trying to make significant progress with habit modification. Once you reach your goal body composition, indulging sensibly on occasion shouldn't take you too far off course. My hope is that, as our community becomes more knowledgeable about the health crisis, we can start to form healthier social alliances.

Remember, insulin resistance is essentially carbohydrate intolerance. Perhaps it's best to think of insulin resistance as a "carbohydrate allergy." For some individuals, even small doses lead to profound metabolic problems. If you invite friends to your house and know that one of your guests has a severe peanut allergy, would you serve a bowl of spiced peanuts as an appetizer, thai curry with spicy peanut sauce as an entrée, and top the meal off with a delicious peanut-filled dessert? That would be insensitive and irresponsible, right? Bringing other people on board with your health goals is no less important than alerting them to any food allergies you might have. Sit down with your closest circle of friends, the ones with whom you socialize frequently, and have a heart-to-heart about some of the health issues discussed in this book. Your friends are most likely also grappling with insulin resistance, and uniting as a joint force will make it easier to use innovation and culinary creativity to create healthier social gatherings. Here are some guidelines that you may find useful:

- Schedule some <u>non</u>-food physical activities, like meeting for a hike or a bike ride, or gathering at a local park

- Enjoy non-food entertainment like movie night, karaoke to bollywood hits, or board game night

- Set some "food rules" for social get-togethers; serve up crispy vegetable appetizers with creamy dip and offer low-carb options for you and your guests, like cauliflower rice or coconut flour chapatis

- Serve lower carb fruits such as berries for dessert, learn to bake with coconut flour or almond flour, and try the Indian sweets in the recipe section for special occasions like Diwali

Try setting invitation times between meals or after dinner. Often the work involved with cooking and cleaning up after parties prevents busy families from meeting more regularly. The real entree at social gatherings is not the food, it's the laughter...the connection to culture through shared experiences and the community building... that help break up our fast-paced, stressful lives.

Online Community

If you are unable to build the right health team to support your efforts, realize that there are some wonderful online communities that offer valuable information and support. I personally found that the tremendous online community at marksdailyapple.com sparked my passion for ancestral health practices and inspired me to take a new approach to implementing successful lifestyle changes that challenged many of the common conventions I learned during medical training.

Now that you have a solid understanding of what drives the high-risk health status of South Asians, you can seek out worldwide communities that share your views on health. Finding recipes, exercises, and lifestyle advice aligned with your culture and individual health goals can be a powerful catalyst for success. Today, in an effort to serve a high-risk population that I feel compelled to assist, and to help connect this culturally distinct group online, I publish a blog at southasianhealthsolution.org. This is a great place to start making connections and getting the support you deserve.

SOME FINAL THOUGHTS FROM DR. RON

I greatly appreciate your interest in this book and hope you have enjoyed the material. If you went to the trouble to purchase this book and read it all the way to this point, I consider this a predictor of your success with lifestyle transformation. Yes, modern life is busy and we have assorted real-life priorities and responsibilities that can often get in the way of achieving a basic passing score in healthy living. I am here to suggest that this no longer be acceptable for you. Whether you are a breadwinner with intense career demands and pressures, a multitasking parent trying to make it through the day and looking forward to collapsing into bed, a college student trying to keep your grades respectable, or a single person with plenty of free time and disposable income, it is critical to prioritize your health above everything else in your life.

Yes, I said everything else. When you travel on an airplane, you are reminded that the emergency protocol is to put your oxygen mask on first, so that you can be better equipped to help your child in an emergency situation. Today, the health of the general population, and in particular the South Asian community, is nothing short of a state of emergency.

I can speak emphatically here because I see firsthand the fallout at street view with my medical practice. Day after day, I greet kind, intelligent, hard-working South Asian folks pursuing the American Dream, only to receive the bad news, or very bad news, that I often must dispense. And mind you, most of what I do, most of the data I measure, most of the medication and treatments I deliver, fall into the "needless suffering" category. Only a slight percentage of any doctor or hospital's patients are there for genetic abnormalities or fateful, random illness. The vast majority of my work includes battling against cultural forces that create diet- and lifestyle-related health conditions and disease. This battle was my inspiration for this book—to try and promote a cultural transformation not through the medication, hospitalization, surgery, or death that frames my daily reality, but through easy-to-read, innovative, and inspiring medical truths.

Alas, it is not the information that is lacking today as much as the motivation. If you paid even moderate attention to the words you've read, if you walk away remembering only the simplest insights—like restrict carbohydrate intake to moderate insulin production; or move your body more throughout the day to counter the negatives of sedentary patterns; or mellow out your evenings by restricting the use of bright lights and digital screens and getting to bed earlier—then you have all the information you need to achieve remarkable improvements in your health, energy levels, mood, and body composition in just a short time.

It's not a big deal to implement baby steps along these lines, and your actions can create a ripple effect among family members, friends, co-workers, neighbors...anyone with whom you interact! As a parent of pre-teenagers, it's interesting to observe that even youngsters are pretty darn good at absorbing the behavior and lifestyle examples they are exposed to...what they learn now has a lasting impact on future habits. What we do as parents delivers vastly more influence than what we say. In the workplace, which is a competitive environment by design, people pay attention to excellence, to positive energy, and to dramatic changes in usual patterns. When one person achieves a breakthrough with weight loss, fitness, or any form of personal growth, the effect on others is tremendous. The positive steps you take now will literally have a transformative effect on everyone around you, which makes your personal goals and motivations larger than you. I wish you the best of success!

SAMINA'S STORY

Samina is a 25-year old Asian Indian woman who recently moved from England to California and was referred to me for a South Asian consult regarding her polycystic ovarian syndrome (PCOS).

I HAVE SUFFERED FROM polycystic ovarian syndrome (PCOS) since my teenage years. I've battled acne, obesity, and irregular periods, but it wasn't until I discovered that years of unchecked PCOS threatened my ability to conceive that I became an active participant in change. A one-hour consultation with Dr. Sinha changed my life, and not only was I able to manage PCOS with the combination of a low-carb diet, exercise, and medication, but I was also able to have a child.

I experienced the first signs of PCOS during my teenage years: acne, irregular periods, excess facial hair, and fluctuating weight. My poor mother, concerned with my spots and my increasingly irregular periods, dragged me to countless doctors, but the advice was always the same—it was only a matter of time before my hormones settled and the symptoms faded…but they never did. I faced many family gatherings where the topic of my acne and weight were hot topics—everyone had a different remedy that would "fix" me.

It wasn't until I was 17 that I was officially diagnosed with PCOS. The list of future health-related problems was unnerving, but I was ready for college and too excited to take these concerns seriously. I continued to eat a Bangladeshi diet (rice and curry) at home, and enjoyed the British cuisine of potatoes and all things fried.

During my college years, I put a whole stone (14 lbs) on my 112 lb frame. My periods got worse as my activity levels declined and my weight increased. By graduation I was 133 lbs, and my BMI officially stated I was overweight.

The most dramatic changes to my body and my life occurred after college when I married and entered grad school all in the same year. As the pounds packed on I remained in denial and refused to weigh myself, but I'd venture to guess I weighed about 160 lbs—a weight gain of 30 pounds in a single year! The rapid weight gain affected me on an emotional level—I regularly got asked if I was pregnant—and also had a tremendous impact on my cycle. I started missing periods…sometimes for three months or more. And when they came, the periods were heavy and extremely painful, and I had to take sick days off work.

It was obvious I couldn't ignore my weight any longer. I followed the standard advice: exercise three to five times a week and eat a balanced meal. I stuck to a 1200-calorie per day diet and cut out all the obvious offenders—sugary sweets, fats, cheeses—and switched to "good" carbs—brown rice, brown bread, fruits, porridge, oats, and vegetables. Despite my diligence, I couldn't seem to drop below 153 lbs, far from my ideal weight.

At the same time, I started feeling a little broody. Although we weren't quite ready to have a baby, I decided to speak to a doctor about getting pregnant and address any underlying issues. It became evident that my PCOS was going to make it difficult to conceive. The doctor put me on metformin, a diabetes pill used to treat insulin resistance, and told me to lose more weight. If symptoms didn't improve, my next stop would be the infertility clinic. My carelessness with my health in my teens and early twenties was manifesting as the most devastating of consequences.

I worked hard for the next year and continued to follow the standard diet and exercise protocol. My periods responded favourably by showing up every six to eight weeks, but still with no regularity. Despite eating less and exercising, I plateaued at about 145 lbs and was unable to lose any more weight.

At 25, things changed for me. I moved from England to California where I actively pursued getting pregnant. When I was first referred to Dr. Sinha, I was extremely skeptical. I was certain he'd be another doctor piling on the same diet and exercise philosophy that wasn't helping me lose weight. On the contrary, Dr. Sinha explained the link between insulin resistance, PCOS, and the effects of carbohydrates on the body. A light bulb went off and I could see how his guidance applied to my health history.

I made changes to my diet over the next few months. I swapped high-carb foods with low-carb/high-protein alternatives. A typical breakfast that used to consist of oats and porridge was now replaced by eggs; my lunch sandwiches were traded in for soups; and my rice and curry dinners for vegetables and proteins. I was able to keep my net carbs to 80 grams a day and used the MyFitnessPal app to make tracking carbs easy. Within a few weeks I lost a few pounds, and within months my periods became regular. Best of all…I became pregnant!

To say I was shocked would be an understatement. We had planned for a difficult conception and were already looking at infertility treatments! I firmly believe the low-carb diet Dr. Sinha recommended led to my weight loss, my regular periods, and my successful pregnancy. It's no coincidence that I saw Dr. Sinha in April and by September of that year I fell pregnant. And even though I never reached the ideal BMI (128 lbs according to standard BMI tables), dropping to 132 lbs improved my fertility.

Post-pregnancy found me back at the beginning, with several pounds of baby weight to lose. The difference this time is that I have the right tools and knowledge to reach my weight and health goals. I will certainly stick to a low-carb diet and continue managing insulin resistance, PCOS, and my overall weight, while enjoying motherhood. I only have Dr. Sinha to thank for this!

HARISH'S STORY

Harish is a 34-year-old Asian Indian male I met at a health and fitness seminar in Lake Tahoe called Primalcon, who later came to see me in my office for a consultation.

IF YOU HAD TOLD ME six months ago that I'd be a featured success story in a health book written by Dr. Ronesh Sinha and published by health and fitness expert Mark Sisson, I would have laughed in disbelief! Partly because at that time my health goals seemed extraordinarily daunting…but mostly because I owe my remarkable transformation in body and health to these two men. Having grown up as the fat kid, and never having had success with weight loss goals as an adult, the 71 lbs I dropped following a low-carb diet, along with the better health and improved energy levels I now enjoy, should serve as inspiration to all South Asians struggling with diet, weight, and less-than-optimal health.

Growing up in Bangalore, India, I was fueled on a vegetarian diet consisting primarily of white rice, lentils, legumes, potatoes, vegetables (which I must admit I wasn't very fond of), dairy, fried snacks, and sweets, along with Indian breads such as chapati, paratha, puri, and nan. This diet primed me for obesity, but it wasn't until the teenage years that I started to feel self-conscious about my weight. I internalized my feelings, but was incredibly frustrated, and my self-esteem suffered. Rather than tackling my weight, I indulged in spicy, greasy restaurant foods. By the time I was 21, I weighed 220 lbs, quite a lot for a 5'11" guy.

My health took a turn from bad to worse when I moved to the United States to pursue higher education. Western food took its toll, and my grain-based vegetarian diet gave way to conventionally raised chicken tainted with antibiotics and hormones. There was no time for exercise, and I immersed myself in work.

Upon moving to San Francisco in May 2013 and hitting rock bottom with my weight and health, I decided to take some time off work and focus exclusively on my health, fitness, and well-being.

Ready to make changes but unsure where to start I began searching online for Primal/Paleo restaurants (the Primal diet had always intrigued me and was an approach I could easily follow). I found plenty of unhealthy Indian restaurants nearby, but didn't find many eateries that would support my new eating plan. I decided instead to start with a narrow selection of healthier foods. My new daily diet consisted of eggs, low-fat dairy, cheese, avocados, grilled chicken, hummus, nuts, and the occasional vegetable. Eventually, I became more Primal-aligned and replaced low-fat dairy with raw, full-fat dairy, store-bought eggs with organic pastured eggs, and added grass-fed butter and more vegetables.

My biggest challenge in terms of fitness was finding an exercise program that was sustainable. I had rarely exercised before and knew very little about fitness. I was looking for a personal trainer when I stumbled upon a training facility in the Bay Area by the name of FNS360. While they did offer training services, they also offered several group classes that focused on functional fitness (similar in some ways to CrossFit). These classes were a game changer as far as my fitness was concerned and I have seen steady improvements in my strength, speed, agility, endurance, balance, and flexibility. I also started playing tennis regularly and have incorporated hiking and walking into my lifestyle.

I met Dr. Ronesh Sinha for the first time in Lake Tahoe at Mark Sisson's PrimalCon event in September 2013. My interest was immediately sparked, since Dr. Sinha is an MD of Indian origin who has incorporated Primal/Paleo principles to successfully treat high-risk South Asian vegetarian and non-vegetarian patients.

I immediately scheduled a consultation with Dr. Sinha. We did some baseline blood work and I was amazed that all of my blood markers had improved, and many of them significantly! Thanks to this new lifestyle I now…

- Feel better about myself…the way I look and feel

- Am happier

- Have more energy

- Am fitter, stronger, and faster

- Enjoy physical activity and try activities I previously shied away from

- Have a healthier relationship with food

- Enjoy improved body composition

- Have disposed of all my old "fat" clothes

- Am in better control of my health

- Have improved health markers (blood pressure, LDL-C, HDL-C, LDL-C density, triglycerides, hemoglobin A1c, C-reactive protein) and a reduced risk of heart disease and diabetes

I didn't take control of my health until I was 34 years old. It is never too late to change habits and change your life, and Dr. Sinha offers a foolproof method of success in this book!

Harish's Labs	June 2012	October 2013
Triglyceride	153 mg/dL	65 mg/dL
HDL	33 mg/dL	39 mg/dL
LDL	116 mg/dL	88 mg/dL
LDL Pattern	B	A
hsCRP	5.0 mg/dL	2.8 mg/dL
Triglyceride/HDL	4.6	1.7
HbA1C	6.1 %	5.4 %

Dr. Sinha's Comments:

Notice how Harish's labs initially showed an abnormal triglyceride/HDL ratio with the expected pattern B LDL (small, deadly boats), elevated inflammation evidenced by his high hsCRP, and prediabetes with an elevated HbA1C level. Through his lifestyle changes, all of which are aligned with the principles in this book, he dropped his ratio to target levels, reduced inflammation, reversed prediabetes, and dropped over 70 pounds!

RAJESH'S STORY

Rajesh is a 41-year-old Asian Indian engineer who was referred to me for metabolic syndrome and fatigue.

AFTER YEARS OF STRUGGLING with flagging energy levels, obesity, and looming health disasters, I finally got my weight and health under control...and I owe my success to Dr. Sinha's sound lifestyle and nutrition recommendations. My wakeup call came on the heels of my yearly checkup at Palo Alto Medical Foundation in January 2013. I can't say I was surprised by the lab results, but seeing the numbers in front of me did make an impact. My weight was 210 lbs, my blood glucose measured 107 and my triglycerides were elevated at 217. At the time, I could barely walk I was feeling so exhausted. My primary care physician referred me to Dr. Ronesh Sinha.

During my first consult, Dr. Sinha outlined an eating plan that cut my carbohydrate consumption and replaced the rice, fried foods, and bread I was so fond of with more nutritive food items. I diligently incorporated the plan, filling up on salads and dense protein sources like chicken. I also got moving, and make it a daily practice to walk one hour every morning on the treadmill, a routine I've been able to stick to since February 14th, 2013.

Just one month of healthy lifestyle and nutrition changes was all it took to turn my lab results around…or should I say down! Blood glucose decreased to 91 and triglycerides to 141. After three months, my weight had dropped to 190 lbs and my blood glucose to less than 80! Seeing the quantitative proof fortified my resolve to continue with Dr. Sinha's suggestions. My weight is now around 180 lbs and my energy levels in the green zone! I can walk and play cricket and tennis without any issues. I recently visited India, and was thrilled by the stunned reactions of my friends and relatives. My transformation was so inspiring, that many of my loved ones are also implementing Dr. Sinha's recommendations—eating fewer carbohydrates, more fruits and vegetables, and moving their bodies! Thank you Dr. Sinha, for changing not only my life, but the lives of my family and friends as well!

Rajesh's Labs	February 2013	April 2013
Fasting Glucose	107 mg/dL	80 mg/dL
Triglyceride	217 mg/dL	91 mg/dL
HDL	42 mg/dL	50 mg/dL
LDL	76 mg/dL	78 mg/dL
Triglyceride/HDL Ratio	5.2	1.8

Dr. Sinha's Comments:

Notice how Rajesh significantly improved his triglyceride/HDL ratio and blood glucose in just two months simply by reducing extra carbohydrates and increasing activity levels. Well done!

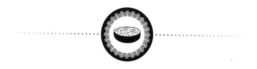

INDIAN RECIPES REINVENTED

IF THERE'S ONE THING I don't need to teach most Indians, it's how to cook. Low-carb strategies, however, may be less familiar, so I've included some key recommendations for preparing low carb substitutes for starch staples like rice, noodles, and bread. Rice, noodles, and bread don't make meals delicious. It's the spices and sauces we add to them! I will leave it to your imagination to spice these up in your own unique way, and by all means, if you concoct recipes worth sharing, send them to southasianhealthsolution.org where I can post them.

BREADS

The staples below use coconut flour and almond flour to make quick and easy bread substitutes that have low NCs and plenty of protein. You can create all types of "BLSs" (Bread-Like Substances), from muffins and cookies to cakes and pies. These are the basics, but if you search online, you will find many more creative options. Say goodbye to bread and hello to higher protein, lower carbohydrate substitutes.

Ma's Coconut Flour Chapatis (makes 10 chapatis)

Be patient. It may take a few attempts since they can be fragile and crumble. Err on the side of overcooking before flipping. It's very tough to burn coconut flour chapatis, but very easy to flip early and break apart.

Ingredients:
  1 cup coconut flour
  4 eggs
  3 cups water (add to desired consistency)
  Half of a finely chopped onion
  1 chopped green chili (optional)
  3 tsp salt (salt to taste)
  3 tsp whole cumin seeds

1. Add all ingredients to mixing bowl.

2. Use a hand mixer to blend ingredients to a fairly thin consistency. You may need to add more or less water to achieve desired thickness.

3. Spoon batter onto non-stick pan. Works great on an electric non-stick griddle.

4. Don't flip chapatis too early. Wait 10-12 minutes with griddle on 300° F. The top of the chapati should be dry and almost fully cooked before flipping.

Some of my patients create a paratha by adding vegetables, like peas and carrots, and even meat, like ground lamb, to the batter. It's nutritious enough to eat as a standalone meal. Try different fillings to add variety.

Five-Minute Loaf of Guilt-Free Microwave Bread

This may seem too good to be true, but yes it is possible to make five-minute, high-protein flourless bread in your microwave. I store leftovers in the fridge and eat them as a quick breakfast or a meal accompaniment. On "spaghetti night," I toast a five-minute loaf, dip it in an olive oil/balsamic mixture, and top with Parmesan cheese. Very versatile!

Ingredients:
   1 cup almond meal or flax meal (I prefer almond meal)
   2 tsp baking powder
   4 large eggs
   4 tsp butter
   1 ripe banana

1. Mix almond or flax meal, eggs, baking powder, and melted butter in a bowl until you reach a smooth consistency.

2. Pour into a pyrex loaf dish (9 in x 5 in) and microwave to four minutes. Cooking times vary depending on microwave power, but once the bread rises give it another minute or so.

3. Refrigerate until firm.

4. Toast it (often needs to be double toasted until dark brown and crispy) and spread on almond butter, sunflower seed butter, cream cheese, etc.

You don't have to add the banana, but it does make the bread moister. Add blueberries (or mix in dark cacao powder for chocolate cake) to make sweeter, or opt for savory with jalapeno peppers and cheddar cheese.

Cauliflower Pizza

Pizza is probably the most universally loved food. I was in disbelief about the ability to make pizza crust out of vegetables, eggs, and cheese, but it is possible and it actually tastes great. Like the coconut flour chapatis, this takes a little practice, but even when the crust breaks apart it's still delicious!

Ingredients:
    1 medium head cauliflower
    ½ cup soft cheese (mozzarella, goat, etc.)
    1 large egg
    Tomato sauce (homemade is best)
    Shredded cheese and your favorite toppings (traditional or
        Indian-paneer, chicken tikka, etc.)
    1 tsp dried basil
    1 tsp dried oregano
    ½ tsp garlic powder
    1 tbsp olive oil
    1 tbsp coconut flour or 2 tbsp almond meal

Additional items:
    Food processor or grater for cauliflower
    Parchment paper
    Thin towel or cheese cloth for squeezing moisture out of cauliflower

1. Preheat oven to 450 degrees.

2. "Rice" one head of cauliflower by adding florets to a food processor or using a hand grater. Blend until cauliflower is a rice-like consistency. Set aside any extra for the cauliflower rice recipe below...that way you only have to clean up once!

3. Transfer cauliflower rice into a covered microwave safe bowl and microwave for five minutes.

4. Pour onto a thin dishtowel or cheesecloth and let cool for one to two minutes.

5. Wrap cauliflower tight with dishtowel and squeeze hard to remove as much moisture as possible. It's helpful to separate into two bundles to maximize moisture removal.

6. Add cauliflower to bowl with cheese, oil, coconut flour (or almond meal), herbs, garlic powder, and eggs. Hand mix to achieve dough-like consistency.

7. Spray non-stick spray onto parchment paper and place on pizza stone or baking pan.

8. Roll cauliflower dough into a ball and plop on pan. Shape into pizza rectangle or circle, with a half-inch crust. Don't make crust too thin or it will break.

9. Put crust in oven for 8-10 minutes until golden brown.

10. Remove pizza crust and add pizza sauce, cheese, and favorite toppings.

11. Place pizza back in oven for 5 minutes.

Indian pizza is becoming a popular spinoff of the traditional Italian dish. Make your own version by adding toppings like paneer or chicken tikka. You don't have to stick with cauliflower crust; carve some eggplant or portobello mushroom into large, flat slices of pizza crust. Just roast and top with pizza sauce, your favorite toppings, and cheese.

RICE SUBSTITUTES

The following rice substitutes replace an extremely high NC starch with no nutritional value with very low NC, highly nutritious vegetables. Use any of your favorite chopped or shredded vegetables as your base.

Indian Coconut Cauliflower Rice

Ingredients:
2 cups cauliflower
½ red onion
4 garlic cloves minced
¼ cup sliced almonds
¼ cup coconut flakes
½ tsp turmeric
1 tsp cumin
¼ cup chopped cilantro
Coconut oil or ghee
Salt and pepper to taste

1. "Rice" the cauliflower (use a food processor to chop cauliflower into rice-sized pieces).

2. Heat coconut oil in a pot and then add whole cumin seeds. When the seeds crackle, add onion until light brown, followed by cauliflower, chili (optional), cumin powder, salt, and turmeric.

3. Cook over low heat for 10 minutes and add chopped cilantro at end.

4. A great dish to cook in bulk, coconut cauliflower rice is even more filling and high protein when you add fish, meat, eggs, nuts, and vegetables, transforming it into a biryani or fried rice dish.

5. You can also substitute broccoli for cauliflower. Yes, you'll have green-colored rice, but given the incredible nutritional value of broccoli, the extra color is worth it. Or get the best of both worlds with broccoflower, a brocolli/cauliflower hybrid.

Shredded Cabbage Sabji

I've included a very simple version of this South Asian staple, so feel free to jazz it up with your own culinary creativity. Shredded Cabbage Sabji, however, isn't the usual South Asian side dish, but a substitute for rice that will fill your plate and your stomach. Pour curries over your cabbage sabji. I often request cabbage sabji at restaurants and then enjoy a side of meat or paneer curry and raita (yogurt).

Ingredients:
2-3 cups shredded cabbage (buy pre-packaged or shred it yourself)
Coconut oil or ghee
Handful of shredded coconut
Handful of peas
6 curry leaves
1 tsp cumin seeds
1 tsp mustard seeds
1 tsp coriander powder
½ tsp turmeric powder
1 onion chopped
4-5 cloves garlic

1. Heat oil or ghee in a pan and add cumin, mustard seeds, curry leaves, and garlic until color just changes.

2. Add chopped onion and stir until soft.

3. Add turmeric powder, coriander powder, and garam malasa, and stir until even color.

4. Add cabbage and shredded coconut. Stir until soft or desired consistency (I like it a little crisp).

5. Add salt to taste.

You can follow this same formula for nearly any vegetable, so add a variety to your daily plate.

NOODLES

Replace your high-carb, fat-storage-promoting noodles (and pasta) with low-carb, nutrient-packed vegetables or versatile shirataki noodles.

Spaghetti Squash

Ingredients:
1 whole spaghetti squash
Extra virgin olive oil or butter
Fresh parmesan
Chili flakes
Your favorite spaghetti sauce (meat or vegetarian)

1. Poke 10-15 holes into whole spaghetti squash to prevent squash from exploding in the microwave.

2. Stick spaghetti squash in the microwave for 8-10 minutes (time varies based on your microwave power). If it's soft enough to be easily pierced with a fork, it's done.

3. Let spaghetti squash cool for 8-10 minutes and then slice open lengthwise.

4. Scoop out seeds.

5. Use fork to remove spaghetti squash strands, pulling the strands from the skin to the center.

6. Plop onto a baking dish and mix in some extra virgin olive oil, salt and pepper, and your favorite meat or vegetarian spaghetti sauce.

7. Top with fresh parmesan and chili flakes.

Shirataki noodles

Shirataki noodles are thin, shiny, low-carb noodles made from the Japanese konjac yam. Traditional shirataki noodles have zero carbs, while the tofu-based ones have very few carbohydrates. Commonly sold wet in a plastic package, shirataki noodles can be found in most grocery stores in the soy section or in Asian markets. Don't be turned off by the unpleasant odor when you open the package.

1. Rinse noodles well, drain, and cut into smaller pieces.

2. Pan fry noodles on high heat with no oil ("dry fry") for about 5-8 minutes, stirring continually until you hear "squeaking."

3. Use these versatile noodles for soup, curries, salads, or pasta substitutes.

4. Use a flavorful sauce or base to subdue the flavor of the noodles. Be generous with your use of garlic, herbs, spices, chili, etc.

5. Mix in vegetables, meat, fish, egg, nuts, and/or seeds to enhance antioxidants, protein, and healthy fats.

6. If you still notice an undesirable flavor (some people are very sensitive to the taste), try boiling noodles in water for five minutes after draining (step 1) and then dry fry.

Other Vegetable Noodle Options

Use a julienne slicer or spiralizer device to carve vegetables into noodles. Green or yellow zucchinis, carrots, parsnips, and sweet potatoes work well. Many grocery stores also sell shredded vegetables like broccoli slaw, which can work as a quick noodle substitute.

WRAPS AND BOWLS

Get familiar with the wraps and bowls approach to eating at home and in restaurants. This is a great way to enjoy delicious foods without the abundant fat-storing carbohydrates found in rice, noodles, and bread.

Wraps: Use leaves in place of breads to wrap all types of tasty fillings, from lettuce-wrap tacos and burgers to Asian chicken salad. Use romaine lettuce or butter lettuce for softer wraps, and iceberg lettuce for crispy wraps. Even if a restaurant doesn't offer lettuce wraps on the menu, chefs will often make them on request since nearly every restaurant kitchen stocks lettuce.

Bowls: Most Mexican restaurants, Asian restaurants, and even some Indian restaurants are starting to offer "bowl" meals like burrito bowls, stir-fry bowls, and tandoori bowls. These bowls are typically full of meat, paneer, vegetables, flavorful sauces, and spices, and can be easily whipped up at home. Top burrito bowls off with shredded cheese, sour cream, and guacamole. Like wraps, many food places can make low carb bowls upon request.

INDIAN SWEETS

Interestingly, many of the ingredients in Indian sweets that are commonly considered unhealthy (coconut and ghee) are actually highly nutritious and don't stimulate insulin production. The key is to replace sugar with smaller amounts of more nutritious sweeteners like organic honey and coconut sugar, which are still highly insulin generating, so you want to use the smallest amount possible. I've included two recipes that are acceptable for special occasions.

Gajar Halwa (Indian Carrot Pudding)

Ingredients:
  2 cups grated carrots (handgrate or use food processor)
  1 can coconut milk
  1 tsp cinnamon
  1 tsp nutmeg
  1 tsp cardamom (elaichi) powder
  2 tbsp ghee or coconut oil
  1 handful dried shredded coconut
  1 handful sliced almonds
  1 handful raisins

1. Heat 2 tbsp ghee in non-stick pan.

2. Add grated carrots and cook gently for 3-4 minutes.

3. Add coconut milk, stir well, and cook for another 15 minutes while covered.

4. Add cardamom powder, cinnamon, and nutmeg to carrots.

5. Simmer on medium heat for another 30 minutes.

6. Garnish with almonds, raisins, and shredded coconut.

Simmering longer ensures a thicker consistency. Coconut milk is ideal, but you can substitute with almond milk or organic whole milk if you wish. Carrot has its own natural sweetness for those with an extra sweet tooth. You can also mix in organic honey when you add the cinnamon and nutmeg, or add a small spoonful to your serving bowl.

Coconut Ladoo (Coconut Balls)

This recipe takes advantage of the incredible multipurpose nature of coconut. You can use four different forms of coconut for this recipe: coconut oil, dried coconut, coconut milk, and coconut sugar.

Ingredients:
- 1 cup grated coconut (use fresh, ripe, or dried)
- 1 can coconut milk
- ¼ cup coconut sugar or organic honey
- 2 tbsp ghee or coconut oil
- ¼ tsp cardamom powder

1. Heat ghee or coconut oil in a frying pan.

2. Add coconut and stir-fry for 1-2 minutes.

3. Pour in coconut milk and stir frequently on medium-low, making sure not to burn the milk.

4. When all the milk is absorbed, add the sugar (or honey) and cardamom powder.

5. Cook until mixture is nice and sticky, so you can form round balls.

6. Let coconut cool for 10-15 minutes.

7. Grease your hands with ghee and make round balls out of coconut mixture.

8. Coat the ladoos by dipping into dried coconut

APPENDIX B

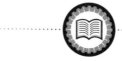

REFERENCE NUMBERS AND RESOURCES

BIOMETRICS:

World Health Organization (WHO) Waist-to-Hip Ratio (WHR) cutoffs

<u>MALES</u>: > 0.90 is abnormal   <u>FEMALES</u>: > 0.85 is abnormal

http://whqlibdoc.who.int/publications/2011/9789241501491_eng.pdf

International Diabetes Federation (IDF) Ethnic Values for Waist Circumference (WC):

Ethnic Group	Men	Women
Europid	≥ 94 cm (37.0 in)	≥ 80 cm (31.5 in)
South Asian	≥ 90 cm (35.4 in)	≥ 80cm (31.5 in)
Chinese	≥ 90cm (35.4 in)	≥ 80cm (31.5 in)
Japanese	≥ 90cm (35.4 in)	≥ 80cm (31.5 in)

Until further data is compiled, the IDF recommends using South Asian cutoffs for South and Central Americans, and European cutoffs for Sub-Saharan Africans, Eastern Mediterranean, and Middle East (Arab) populations. These are general cutoffs that require individual customization. For example, a highly insulin resistant South Asian male may need to achieve a WC closer to 33 inches or below. Aim for a WC that helps you achieve your Metabolic 6-pack.

www.idf.org/webdata/docs/MetS_def_update2006.pdf

Lipid Numbers

A standard lipid panel gives you most of the information you need, especially when you track ratios. Advanced lipid tests that assess particle numbers and size may be indicated in select cases only. Advanced tests may not be covered by insurance and it is not normally necessary to check them repeatedly. Reference values may vary depending on the specific test.

Test	Goal	Comments
Triglyceride/HDL ratio	< 3.0	Marker for insulin resistance
Total cholesterol/ HDL ratio	< 3.5	
Triglycerides	< 100 mg/dL (1.3 mmol/L)	
HDL	Male: > 40 mg/dl (1 mmol/L) Female: > 50 mg/dl (1.3 mmol/L)	
hsCRP	< 1.0 mg/dl	Marker for inflammation
LDL-P (particle number)[1]	< 1,000 nmol/L	Direct measurement of LDL particle numbers
Apo B[2]	< 60 mg/dL	Surrogate marker for LDL particle number (LDL-P)
LDL size (A,A/B,B)[3]	Predominant pattern A	
Lp (a)[4]	< 10 mg/dl (based on VAP test)	Measured if early family history of heart disease.

[1]LDL-P: The most accurate way to measure particle number is using nuclear magnetic resonance (NMR) technology. The *NMR Lipoprofile* test uses this technology.

[2]Apo B: Apo B is a protein present on each LDL particle, so Apo B measurements serve as markers for LDL-P. *BHL (Berkeley Heart Lab), HDL (Health Diagnostic Laboratory), and VAP (Vertical Auto Profile)* are some of the tests that offer Apo B measurements. *VAP's* Apo B measurement does not use the gold standard technique.

[3] LDL size: Assessed by various tests, including *VAP, BHL, HDL,* and *NMR Lipoprofile.* LDL size is not as effective at assessing heart disease risk as LDL-P or Apo B measurements.

[4]Lp (a): Reference range varies depending on lab.

Blood Pressure Table:

Blood Pressure	Systolic (upper number)		Diastolic (lower number)
Normal	less than 120	and	less than 80
Prehypertension	120-139	or	80-89
High blood pressure (Stage 1)	140-159	or	90-99
High blood pressure (Stage 2)	160 or higher	or	100 or higher

Blood Glucose Ranges:

Test	Normal	Prediabetes	Diabetes
Fasting blood glucose	< 100 mg/dL	100 to < 125 mg/dL	≥ 126 mg/dL
A1C test	< 5.7%	5.7-6.4%	≥ 6.5%
OGTT*	< 140 mg/dL	140 to < 200 mg/dL	≥ 200 mg/dL

*OGTT is the Oral Glucose Tolerance Test, which is a two-hour test that checks blood glucose levels before and two hours after you drink a special sweet drink. This test is most commonly used to screen pregnant women for gestational diabetes (diabetes during pregnancy) and is sometimes given when standard tests (fasting blood glucose, A1C) offer conflicting results.

RECOMMENDED SMARTPHONE APPS

Nutrition Apps

- MyFitnessPal

- LoseIt

- SparkPeople

Exercise Apps

- Body weight exercises: squats, push-ups, and pull-ups by Runtastic (accelerometer-based motion tracking during exercises)

- Pedometer by Runtastic (accelerometer-based step tracking)

- Interval training: Tabata app (four-minute high-intensity exercise timer)

- Yoga: Yoga Studio by Modern Lotus

Stress Management

- Apps by Azumio: Stress Doctor, Stress Check (based on heart rate variability)

- Pranayama app by Saagara (sound-cued breath control)

Sleep Apps

- Justgetflux.com (reduces sleep-disrupting blue light from screens)

- Sleep cycle (motion-sensitive app allowing you to wake in light phase sleep)

- Sleep pillow (white noise app to prevent noise-induced awakenings)

ONLINE RESOURCE LIST

1. www.southasianhealthsolution.org: My personal blog where I share cutting edge, culturally tailored information.

2. www.marksdailyapple.com: Incredibly prolific resource on health, nutrition, and exercise. A "must-subscribe."

3. www.pamf.org/southasian: Comprehensive online resource on South Asian health. Not all dietary recommendations may be compatible with the material in this book.

4. www.nomnompaleo.com: Fantastic online resource for low-carb, high-flavor ethnically diverse recipes with beautifully illustrated step-by-step instructions.

5. aapiusa.org/uploads/files/docs/APPI_Guide_To_Health_And_Nutrition__2nd_Edition.pdf: Not all dietary recommendations compatible with this book, but an extensive resource on the Asian Indian diet broken down by geographical region.

6. www.mysahana.org: Excellent website on South Asian mental health.

NOTES

Inflammation and Insulin: The Real Culprits

1. JV Neel, "Diabetes mellitus: A Thrifty Genotype Rendered Detrimental by Progress," *The American Journal of Human Genetics*, (December 1962): 14(4): 353–362.
2. Jonathan CK Wells, "Commentary: Why are South Asians susceptible to central obesity? — The El Niño hypothesis," *International Journal of Epidemiology*, Volume 36, Issue 1, Pp. 226-227.
3. Raj S Bhopal, Snorri B Rafnsson, "Could mitochondrial efficiency explain the susceptibility to adiposity, metabolic syndrome, diabetes and cardiovascular diseases in South Asian populations?" *International Journal of Epidemiology*, Volume 38, Issue 4, Pp. 1072-1081.
4. Wells JCK, "Ethnic variability in adiposity and cardiovascular risk: the variable disease selection hypothesis," *International Journal ofEpidemiology*, 2009;38:63-71.
5. Dorner TE, Schwarz F, et al., "Body mass index and the risk of infections in institutionalized geriatric patients," *British Journal of Nutrition*, 103(12) (June 2010):1830-5.
6. Yajnik CS, Lubree HG, Rege SS, et al. "Adiposity and hyperinsulinaemia in Indians are present at birth," *The Journal of Clinical Endocrinology & Metabolism*, 2002;87:5575-80.
7. Shirley N. Bryan, Mark S. Tremblay, et al., "Physical Activity and Ethnicity Evidence from the Canadian Community Health Survey," *Revue Canadienne de Sante Publique*, Vol 97, No.4:271-6.
8. Fischbacher CM, Hunt S, Alexander L., "How physically active are South Asians in the United Kingdom? A literature review," *Journal of Public Health*, 2004;26:250-58.
9. Patra SK, Nasrat H, Goswami B, Jain A, "Vitamin D as a predictor of insulin resistance in polycystic ovarian syndrome," *Diabetes and Metabolic Syndrome*, 2012 Jul-Sep; 6(3):146-9.
10. A. K. Bhalla, E. P. Amento, B. Serog, and L. H. Glimcher, "1,25-dihydroxyvitamin D3 inhibits antigen-induced T cell activation," *Journal of Immunology*, vol. 133, no. 4, 1984: 1748–1754.
11. P.R. von Hurst, W.Stonehouse, J.Coad, "Vitamin D supplementation reduces insulin resistance in South Asian women living in New Zealand who are insulin resistant and vitamin D deficient– a randomised, placebo-controlled trial," *British Journal of Nutrition*, Vol. 103, Issue 04 (February 2010): pp 549-555.
12. Abate N, Chandalia M. Ethnicity, "Type 2 diabetes & migrant Asian Indians,"*Indian Journal of Medical Research*, 2007;125:251-8.

Cholesterol and Heart Disease

1. A. Sachdeva, C.P. Cannon, et al., "Lipid levels in patients hospitalized with coronary artery disease: An analysis of 136,905 hospitalizations in Get With The Guidelines,"*American Heart Journal*, Volume 157, Issue 1 (January 2009): 111-117.e2.

2. Siri-Tarino PW, Sun Q, Hu FB, Krauss RM, "Meta-analysis of prospective cohort studies evaluating the association of saturated fat with cardiovascular disease," *The American Journal of Clinical Nutrition*, 2010;91:535-46.

3. Howard B, Manson J, Stefanick M, et al., "Low-fat dietary pattern and weight change over 7 years: the Women's Health Initiative Dietary Modification Trial," *JAMA*. 2006;295:39-49.

4. Hu F, Stampfer M, Manson J, et al., "Dietary fat intake and the risk of coronary heart disease in women," *The New England Journal of Medicine*, 1997;337:1491-9.

5. Ascherio A, Rimm E, Giovannucci E, Spiegelman D, Stampfer M, Willett W. "Dietary fat and risk of coronary heart disease in men: cohort follow up study in the United States," *BMJ.com,* 1996;313:84-90.

6. Kirkham R. Hamilton, "Heart Disease Risk: Cholesterol and Lipids in 2011,What Do We Really Know? An Interview with William Castelli, M.D.," (February 18, 2011), http://www.prescription2000.com/Interview-Transcripts/2011-02-18-william-castelli-heart-disease-lipids-transcript.html.

7. Enas EA, Chacko V, Senthilkumar A, Puthumana N, Mohan V., "Elevated lipoprotein(a)–a genetic risk factor for premature vascular disease in people with and without standard risk factors: a review," *Disease-A-Month,* Jan 2006;52(1):5-50.

8. T. Vepsäläinen, M. Soinio, et al., "Physical Activity, High-Sensitivity C-Reactive Protein, and Total and Cardiovascular Disease Mortality in Type 2 Diabetes," *Diabetes Care*, 2011 July; 34(7): 1492–1496.

9. Steven W. Cole, et al., "Meditation Reduces Proinflammatory Gene Expression," *Brain, Behavior, and Immunity Journal*, Published online July 20, 2012.

10. Ahmad Esmaillzadeh, Masoud Kimiagar, et al., "Fruit and vegetable intake, C-reactive protein, and the metabolic syndrome," *The American Journal of Clinical Nutrition,* (December 2006) vol. 84, no. 6: 1489-1497.

11. Radhika G, Ganesan A, et al., Sathya RM, "Dietary carbohydrates, glycemic load and serum high-density lipoprotein cholesterol concentrations among South Indian adults," *The European Journal of Clinical Nutrition*, (Nov 7 2007):413-420.

Your Body: Width over Weight

1. J.P. Reis, C.M. Loria, et al., "Association Between Duration of Overall and Abdominal Obesity Beginning in Young Adulthood and Coronary Artery Calcification in Middle Age," *The Journal of the American Medical Association,* 2013;310(3):280-288, doi:10.1001/jama.2013.7833.

2. Lesley M. L. Hall, Colin N. Moran, et al., "Fat Oxidation, Fitness and Skeletal Muscle Expression of Oxidative/Lipid Metabolism Genes in South Asians: Implications for Insulin Resistance?" http://www.plosone.org/article/info:doi/10.1371/journal.pone.0014197.

3. Carnethon MR, De Chavez PJ, et al., "Association of weight status with mortality in adults with incident diabetes," *The Journal of the American Medical Association,* (Aug 8, 2012), 308(6):581-90.

4. WHO expert consultation, "Appropriate body-mass index for Asian populations and its implications for policy and intervention strategies," *The Lancet* (Jan 10 2004), 363(9403):157-63.

5. Yusuf S, et al., *The Lancet* (2005), 366:1640-1649.

Blood Pressure: The Pressure Is Killing Me

1. Yang Q, Liu T, et al., *Archives of Internal Medicine*, "Sodium and potassium intake and mortality among US adults: prospective data from the Third National Health and Nutrition Examination Survey," (Jul 11, 2011), 171(13):1183-1191.

2. Ferrara, et al., "Olive Oil and Reduced Need for Antihypertensive Medications," *Archives of Internal Medicine,* 2000;160(6):837-842.

3. Morris MC, Sacks F, Rosner B., "Does fish oil lower blood pressure? A meta-analysis of controlled trials," *Circulation*, 1993 Aug;88(2):523-33.

4. Davis, D.R., Epp, M.D., Riordan, H.D., "Changes in USDA Food Composition Data for 43 Garden Crops, 1950 to 1999," *The Journal of the American College of Nutrition,* (Dec 2004), vol. 23 no. 6 669-682.

5. John P. Forman, Jamil B. Scott, et al., "Effect of Vitamin D Supplementation on Blood Pressure in Blacks," *Hypertension*, 2013; 61: 779-785.

Why South Asians Struggle with Fat Loss and Weight Loss

1. Emily A Hu, An Pan, et al., "White rice consumption and risk of type 2 diabetes: meta-analysis and systematic review," *BMJ.com*, 2012;344:e1454.

2. D.Mozaffrian, MB Katan, et al., "Trans Fatty Acids and Cardiovascular Disease," *New England Journal of Medicine* (April 13, 2006), 354 (15): 1601–1613.

CARBS Approach to Burning Fat

1. Emily A Hu, An Pan, et al., "White rice consumption and risk of type 2 diabetes: meta-analysis and systematic review," *BMJ.com*, 2012;344:e1454.

2. Christopher N. Blesson, Catherine J. Andersen, et al., "Whole egg consumption improves lipoprotein profiles and insulin sensitivity to a greater extent than yolk-free egg substitute in individuals with metabolic syndrome," *Metabolism-Clinical and Experimental,* Volume 62, Issue 3 (March 2013), pp.400-410.

Exercise

1. Misra, Alappan, et.al, "Resistance Exercise in Asian Indians with T2DM," *Diabetes Care*, May 5, 2008.

2. Jason M.R. Gill, PHD, Raj Bhopal, et al., "Sitting Time and Waist Circumference Are Associated With Glycemia in U.K. South Asians," *Diabetes Care*, (2011 May), 34(5): 1214–1218.

3. S. Gupta, A. Rohatgi, et al., "Cardiorespiratory Fitness and Classification of Risk of Cardiovascular Disease Mortality," *Circulation*, 2011; 123: 1377-1383.

4. Cooney MT, Vartiainen E, et al., "Elevated resting heart rate is an independent risk factor for cardiovascular disease in healthy men and women," *American Heart Journal* (2010 Apr), 159(4):612-619.

Fatigue and Stress

1. Hisako Tsuji, MD, Martin G. Larson, ScD, et al., "Impact of Reduced Heart Rate Variability on Risk for Cardiac Events, The Framingham Heart Study," *Circulation* 1996; 94: 2850-2855.

2. D.S. Black, S.W. Cole, et al., "Yogic meditation reverses NF-κB and IRF-related transcriptome dynamics in leukocytes of family dementia caregivers in a randomized controlled trial," *Psychneuroendocrinology*, Vol. 38, Issue 3 (March 2013): 348–355.

3. Van Cauter E, Holmback U, et al., "Impact of sleep and sleep loss on neuroendocrine and metabolic function," *Hormone Research*, 2007;67Suppl 1:2-9. Epub 2007 Feb 15.

4. Center for Science In the Public Interest (CSPI) website, "Caffeine Content of Food and Drugs," http://www.cspinet.org/new/cafchart.htm.

5. Women's Health

6. Rodin DA, Bano G, et al., "Polycystic ovaries and associated metabolic abnormalities in Indian subcontinent Asian women," *Clinical Endocrinology*, (Oxf) 1998 Jul;49(1):91-9.

7. Wijeyaratne CN, Balen AH, et al., "Clinical manifestations and insulin resistance (IR) in polycystic ovary syndrome (PCOS) among South Asians and Caucasians: is there a difference?" *Clinical Endocrinology*, 2002;57:343–350.

8. Palaniappan L, Wang Y, Fortmann SP, "Coronary heart disease mortality for six ethnic groups in California, 1990-2000," *Annals of Epidemiology*, 2004 Aug;14(7):499-506.

9. James F. Clapp III, MD, "Long-term outcome after exercising throughout pregnancy: fitness and cardiovascular risk," *American Journal of Obstetrics & Gynecology*, **Nov 2008;** Vol. 199, Issue 5, pp 489.e1-489.e6.

10. Muthayya S, Kurpad AV, et al., "Low maternal vitamin B12 status is associated with intrauterine growth retardation in urban South Indians," *European Journal of Clinical Nutrition*, 2006 Jun;60(6):791-801,Epub 2006 Jan 11.

11. Gernand AD, Simhan HN, et al., "Maternal serum 25-hydroxyvitamin D and measures of newborn and placental weight in a U.S. multicenter cohort study," *The Journal of Clinical Endocrinology & Metabolism*, 2013 Jan;98(1):398-404.

12. B. A. Haider, ScD candidate, I. Olofin, et al., "Anaemia, prenatal iron use, and risk of adverse pregnancy outcomes: systematic review and meta-analysis," *BMJ.com*, 2013;346:f3443.

Children's Health

1. Healthy Weight Journal May/June 1999 Vol. 13 #3.
2. FJ Elgar, W Craig, SJ Trites, "Family dinners, communication, and mental health in Canadian adolescents," *J Adolesc Health.* 2013 Apr;52(4):433-8.
3. M.Joshi, "Young Indian children obtain less sleep than their Caucasian counterparts," *Top News,* (June 12, 2008), http://www.topnews.in/health/young-indian-children-obtain-less-sleep-their-caucasian-counterparts-23000.
4. Council on Communications and Media, "Media Use by Children Younger Than 2 Years," *Pediatrics,* Published online on Oct 17, 2011, http://pediatrics.aappublications.org/content/early/2011/10/12/peds.2011-1753.full.pdf.
5. Dimitri A. Christakis, Frederick J. Zimmerman, et al., "Early Television Exposure and Subsequent Attentional Problems in Children," *Pediatrics,* Vol. 113 No. 4 April 1, 2004 pp. 708 -713.
6. Gurvinder Aujla, "South Asian children 'less active' than peers," *BBC News Health,* (Nov 3, 2011), http://www.clarendonmedicalcentre.com/2011/12/03/south-asian-children-less-active-than-peers/.
7. Eyre EL, Fisher JP, et al., "Ethnicity and long-term heart rate variability in children," *Archives of Disease in Childhood,* 2013 Apr;98(4):292-8.
8. J. M. Tanner, H. Goldstein, R. H. Whitehouse, "Standards for Children's Height at Ages 2-9 Years Allowing for Height of Parents," *Archives of Disease in Childhood,* 1970;45:755-762.
9. C.V. Harinarayan, Ramalakshmi T., et al., "High prevalence of low dietary calcium, high phytate consumption, and vitamin D deficiency in healthy south Indians," *The American Journal of Clinical Nutrition,* April 2007,vol. 85 no. 4,1062-1067.
10. Tikotzky L, DE Marcas G., et al., "Sleep and physical growth in infants during the first 6 months," *Journal of Sleep Research,* (2010 Mar);19(1 Pt 1):103-10.
11. Jennifer M. Walsh, Mark Kilbane, Fionnuala M. McAuliffe, et al., "Pregnancy in dark winters: implications for fetal bone growth?" *Fertility and Sterility,* (January 2013), Vol. 99, Issue 1, 206-211.
12. R. Kremer, P.P. Campbell, et al., "Vitamin D Status and Its Relationship to Body Fat, Final Height, and Peak Bone Mass in Young Women," *The Journal of Clinical Endocrinology & Metabolism,* Vol. 94 no.1 (January 1, 2009), 67-73.
13. Villamor E, Marin C, et al., "Vitamin D deficiency and age at menarche: a prospective study," *The American Journal of Clinical Nutrition,* 2011 Oct; 94(4):1020-5.
14. Biro FM, Galvez MP, Greenspan LC, et al., "Pubertal assessment method and baseline characteristics in a mixed longitudinal study of girls," *Pediatrics,* 2010 Sep;126(3):e58.
15. Elizabeth Weil, "Puberty Before Age 10: A New Normal," *New York Times Magazine,* March 30, 2012, http://www.nytimes.com/2012/04/01/magazine/puberty-before-age-10-a-new-normal.html?pagewanted.

16. Paavonen EJ, Räikkönen K, et al., "Sleep quality and cognitive perfor-mance in 8-year-old children," *Sleep Medical,* 2010 Apr;11(4):386-92.

17. Gillen-O'Neel, C., Huynh, V. W. and Fuligni, A. J. (2013), "To Study or to Sleep? The Academic Costs of Extra Studying at the Expense of Sleep," *Child Development,* 84: 133–142.

18. Dan Schreiber, "Meditation program mends troubled Visitacion Valley Middle School," *SF Gate* (Jun 15, 2013), http://blog.sfgate.com/cityin-sider/2013/05/06/barry-zito-russell-brand-david-lynch-meditate-at-sf-school/.

19. Yajnik CS, Fall CH, et al., "Neonatal anthropometry: the thin-fat Indian baby. The Pune Maternal Nutrition Study," *International Journal of Obesity,* 2003 Feb; 27(2): 173-80.

Aging

1. Farzaneh-Far R, Lin J, et al., "Association of marine omega-3 fatty acid lev-els with telomeric aging in patients with coronary heart disease," *The Jour-nal of the American Medical Association,* (2010 Jan 20);303(3):250-7.

2. Cherkas LF, Hunkin JL, et al., "The association between physical activity in leisure time and leukocyte telomere length," *Archives of Internal Medicine,* (2008 Jan 28);168(2):154-8.

3. E.S. Epel, E. Blackburn, et al., "Accelerated telomere shortening in response to life stress," *Proceedings of the National Academy of Sciences,* (Sep 28, 2004), Vol. 101 no. 49, 17312–17315.

4. Puterman E, Lin J, Blackburn E, O'Donovan A, Adler N, et al., (2010), "The Power of Exercise: Buffering the Effect of Chronic Stress on Telomere Length," *PLOS ONE,* 5(5): e10837. doi:10.1371/journal.pone.0010837.

5. J.B. Richards, A.M. Valdes, et al., "Higher serum vitamin D concentra-tions are associated with longer leukocyte telomere length in women," *The American Journal of Clinical Nutrition,* (November 2007), Vol. 86 no. 5 1420-1425.

6. Emmanuel M. K. Awumey, Devashis A. Mitra, et al., "Vitamin D Metabo-lism Is Altered in Asian Indians in the Southern United States: A Clinical Research Center Study," *The Journal of Clinical Endocrinology & Metabo-lism,* (January 1, 1998) Vol. 83 no. 1169-173.

7. Y. Dror, S. Giveon, et al., "Vitamin D Levels for Preventing Acute Coro-nary Syndrome and Mortality: Evidence of a Non-Linear Association," *The Journal of Clinical Endocrinology & Metabolism,* March 26, 2013 jc.2013-1185.

8. Nathan G Congdon, "Prevention strategies for age related cataract: pres-ent limitations and future possibilities," *British Journal of Ophthalmology,* 2001;85:516-520.

INDEX

diet. *See* low-fat diet; low-insulin lifestyle; vegetarian diet

dietary fats, 105–107
  cholesterol fallacy, 30–31, 34–35, 52
  healthy, 66–67, 117, 134–136, 243–245
  unhealthy, 34, 107, 118, 242

dieting. *See* weight loss

doctors. *See* health professionals

E

energy management. *See also* fatigue
  advice for professionals, 224
  journaling, 204–205, 218, 224
  peak performance, 218–219
  traffic light analogy, 192–193, 224

Eppel, Elissa, 307

exercise
  avoiding, 151–154
  beginning steps, 154–156, 188
  benefits, 156–157, 160–161, 307
  bone health and, 234, 320
  children's, 283–285, 291–292
  family activities, 219, 280, 284–285, 335–336
  habits, forming, 181–183, 187
  pregnancy and, 249–250
  for seniors, 317, 320, 327
  tracking progress, 184–188
  tree analogy, 160–173
  walking, 176–177, 285, 292, 317–318, 320
  working workouts, 178–179

exercise equipment, 161, 183–184

exercises
  burpees, 175
  lunges, 165–170
  planks, 170–173
  squats, 162–165
  sun salutation, 174
  timesaving workouts, 178–181

F

family activities, 219, 280, 284–285, 335–336

family history, risk factors, 32

fast carbs, 102

fasting, intermittent, 141–142, 144–147, 150

fat storage
  car analogy, 97–101, 203–204
  factors, 112–113
  and insulin resistance, 109–111

fat-burning. *See* low-insulin lifestyle

fatigue. *See also* energy management
  Manish's story, 190
  medical conditions, 220–224
  Rajesh's story, 344–345
  reducing, 224
  S-factors, 193–217, 224
  understanding, 103, 190–191
  VikramVikram's story, 219

fat/muscle ratio, 78–81, 94

fats. *See* dietary fats

fatty liver. *See* non-alcoholic steatohepatitis

fish, 243–245

Freakonomics (Levitt), 157

fructose, reducing, 131–133

fruits, net carbs, 131–133

G

genetic factors of obesity, 16–18

gestational diabetes, 18, 239–241, 253

Goldstein, Harold, 273

Goyal, Deepak, 250

grains, 65

Greenspan, Louise, 288

growth charts, interpreting, 258–266

H

health goals, 104–105, 329–338

health professionals. *See also* advice for
professionals
building your team, 331–332, 335
working with, 43–44, 334–335
heart disease. *See also* atherosclerosis;
cholesterol
causal factors, 2, 25, 26, 52, 94
cholesterol role, 31
Vinod's story, 27
women and, 229
heart rate measures, 22, 185–187,
197–198
HFCS, 131
high blood pressure. *See* hypertension
high fructose corn syrup, 131
Holick, Michael, 19, 311–313
hydrogenated fats, 34, 107
hypertension. *See also* blood pressure
advice for professionals, 74
factors, 12, 55, 74
lack of symptoms, 56, 74, 189
lowering, 63–74
Nirmala's story, 56

I

IF (intermittent fasting), 141–142,
144–147, 150
infertility and PCOS, 227–228,
339–340
inflammation
age acceleration, 304–306
causal factors, 22–24, 26
and chronic disease, 2, 26, 52
Ravi's story, 3, 297–299
reducing, 23, 47–50, 52, 94, 305–306
sprained artery analogy, 4–6
insulin resistance. *See also*
CARBS approach; diabetes;
low-insulin lifestyle
advice for professionals, 150
age acceleration, 304–306

and carbohydrates, 103–104, 203–204
chronic disease factor, 2, 11–13
detecting, 13–16
fatigue factor, 187, 224
hypertension, 60, 74
obesity link, 13
Ravi's story, 3, 297–299
reducing, 25, 47–50
train station analogy, 9–10
weight loss inhibitor, 109–111
intermittent fasting (IF), 141–142,
144–147, 150

J

journal, energy ratings, 204–205, 218,
224

K

Kabat-Zinn, Jon, 201
Keys, Ancel, 30

L

LBW, 18, 60, 235–239, 253
legumes. *See* beans and lentils
Levitt, Steven D., 157
low birth weight, 18, 60, 235–239, 253
low-fat diet, 51–52, 136, 150
apparent success of, 113–114
commercial products for, 116
evidence against, 30
myths, 97
stress of, 95
low-insulin lifestyle. *See also*
6-S strategy; CARBS approach;
S-factors of fatigue
adopting, 329–338
fat-burning, 104–105, 109–111, 118,
135
increased energy and, 204–205
Metabolic 6-pack and, 13–15
as "new norm," 2, 113–117

Y